The Rehabilitation Handbook

Edited by **Cynthia Wison**

FOSTER
ACADEMICS
New Jersey

Published by Foster Academics,
61 Van Reypen Street,
Jersey City, NJ 07306, USA
www.fosteracademics.com

The Rehabilitation Handbook
Edited by Cynthia Wison

International Standard Book Number: 978-1-63242-392-4 (Hardback)

Printed in China.

Contents

Preface

The simplest definition of rehabilitation would be the restoration of someone or something to its rightful place or state. As the modern age progresses, our health is slowly coming into focus. Medical science is advancing speedily and new cures for diseases and disorders are discovered on a regular basis. There are many instances though, which cannot only rely on medicine but also needs extra effort to restore back to a previous state of being.

Rehabilitation is understood by most people to be related to a medical term, and for most parts it is true. There are many different types of rehabs and they can be extremely varied. Rehabilitation for drug addiction, gambling, alcohol, physical trauma, restoration of mobility and even land and wildlife rehabilitation are many of the different paths that rehab can take. Each has their own methodology towards achieving recovery. Rehabilitation has gained recognition as a viable and medically approved choice for so many struggling to find and gain a foothold in society and get healthy after some event or the other. In a way rehabilitation, especially medical and addiction related rehab, needs a lot of outside support as well. A support system to fall back is always hoped for with any person undergoing rehabilitation. Motivation and encouragement are also big factors in helping people succeed in rehab.

This book is a collation of data that presents researches on rehabilitation studies all over the world. I am thankful to those whose hard work resulted in these researches as well as my family for their support.

Editor

Injured Workers Perspectives on Recovery following Non-Life-Threatening Acute Orthopaedic Trauma: A Descriptive Study

Fiona J. Clay,[1] Swati Shourie,[1] Priscilla Robinson,[2] Donna McKenzie,[3] and Emily Kerr[1]

[1] *Injury Outcomes Research Unit, Monash Injury Research Institute, Monash University, Building 70, Level 1, Clayton Campus, Melbourne, VIC 3800, Australia*
[2] *School of Public Health, Faculty of Health Sciences, La Trobe University, Bundoora, Melbourne, VIC 3086, Australia*
[3] *Institute for Safety Compensation and Recovery Research, Monash University, Melbourne, VIC 3004, Australia*

Correspondence should be addressed to Fiona J. Clay; fionajclay@gmail.com

Academic Editors: M.-R. Lin and F.-Z. Shaw

Background. Little is known about the recovery process following non-life-threatening acute orthopaedic trauma from the viewpoint of the injured person. A better understanding could facilitate optimal rehabilitative planning. *Objective.* To explore patients' views on factors important to them in recovery following non-life threatening acute orthopaedic trauma. *Methods.* Descriptive study utilizing content analysis and chi-square analysis. To better understand recovery expectations, 168 adults who had sustained non-life threatening acute orthopaedic trauma were surveyed at 2, 12, and 26 weeks after injury and invited to respond to the following question "what are the most important things necessary for you to best recover?" *Results.* According to participant's responses, major themes on recovery involved a return to health and a return to health but with an ongoing plan, and for a minority (12%) recovery involved a focus on their current status. The study found that some recovery expectations changed over time. *Conclusion.* The journey to recovery is complex, often prolonged, and highly individual. Responses suggest that some injured persons need more assistance for a successful recovery than others. Those who appeared "caught in the moment" of the injury may benefit from clinical and rehabilitative management focusing on long-term recovery and acceptance of the injury event.

1. Introduction

Acute traumatic injury is a major contributor to the global burden of injury [1]. Fortunately, with the continued evolution of advanced trauma systems, an increasing number of people are surviving traumatic injuries. Despite this, the dimensions of recovery from the viewpoint of the injured person are not well understood. Recovery is often measured in terms of return to work (RTW), pain levels, and activities of daily living using standardized patient report instruments [2–6]. However, it is clear that these instruments only account for certain aspects of the recovery process as research indicates they do not align well with the injured person's experience of recovery.

Positive recovery expectations predict better outcomes for a variety of health conditions including recovery from whiplash-associated disorders and lower back pain [7]. Quantitative studies have measured the association of recovery expectations with time lost from work, pain, and functional status as well as factors associated with recovery expectations [7, 8]. However, quantitative studies have limited ability to explore individual experiences and identify the finer intricacies of recovery from the point of view of the injured worker.

Qualitative research has explored recovery from the perspective of the injured person following physical trauma, lower back pain, hand injuries, and upper limb musculoskeletal disorders [9–12]. Various themes have emerged from these studies including the "importance of the injury event" and "moving on from the trauma" as well as the role of family and work support. Other studies have described recovery in terms of symptom attenuation, improved capacity to perform, and quality of life. Overall though, it is clear that the actual process of recovery for an injured person is a complex issue and if patient care, prognosis, and rehabilitation are to be improved then further research to address the intricacies of recovery from the viewpoint of the injured person is needed.

Injured persons' views on recovery following non-life-threatening acute orthopaedic injuries have rarely been addressed. However, research findings indicate that the journey to recovery and independence even among those with minor traumatic injuries can be slow and vary considerably. The few studies undertaken in this area suggest that some people recover well following acute orthopaedic injuries but others have prolonged periods of poor health experiencing persistent pain, poor mental health, and extended inability to perform duties at work. With an increasing emphasis being placed on self-management of health, exploring the participant's viewpoint of recovery will be vital to empowering the patient to participate in the management of their injury.

The current analysis forms part of a prospective cohort follow-up study that examined biopsychosocial factors associated with work disability and persistent pain following non-life-threatening acute orthopaedic trauma. The aim of the current study is to explore injured workers' views on what would aid their recovery following non-life-threatening acute orthopaedic trauma. The study was designed to establish if there were commonalities of responses provided by study participants at each particular time point, whether these responses changed with time following the injury, and the potential impact of these responses. The study is grounded in a theoretically biopsychosocial framework approach [13], that postulates that factors related to the person's own experience and understanding of their psychosocial functioning and their environment are as important as physical factors relating to the injury in determining recovery. In this paper, we present the recovery expectations of a cohort of patients with range of non-life-threatening orthopaedic injuries over time.

2. Method

2.1. Study Design and Setting. Full details of the study design, setting, and participants have been published elsewhere [3, 6]; however we provide a synopsis of our methods here. The Determinants of Outcome in Orthopaedic Trauma is a multicentre prospective follow-up cohort study conducted in the state of Victoria, Australia. In 2005 the year the study commenced, the population of the state of Victoria was listed as 5.02 million.

This study utilizes data collected as part of the Determinants of Outcome in Orthopaedic Trauma study. The primary focus of the main DOOT cohort study was to establish the predictive determinants of work disability and persistent pain following non-life-threatening acute orthopaedic trauma. The focus of the current analysis is to explore patient's views on important factors that would enable recovery following non-life-threatening acute orthopaedic trauma.

2.2. Participants and Procedures. Patients presenting to one of four hospitals in Victoria as a result of sustaining a non-life-threatening acute orthopaedic trauma were recruited to the study. The Victorian Admitted Episodes Dataset (VAED) is a dataset of acute patient hospital admissions representing 100% coverage of hospital admissions to public hospitals in Victoria [14]. The VAED was used to select study hospitals in different geographical regions in order to achieve a representative sample of Victorian working age population admitted to its public hospitals annually as a consequence of sustaining acute unintentional trauma. The hospitals selected for the study broadly reflected a range of socioeconomic status in patients admitted to hospitals. The choice of hospitals was also based on their trauma status under the Victorian State trauma system in order to facilitate the recruitment of patients with a range of orthopaedic injuries. Four hospitals took part, one regional hospital, two metropolitan hospitals, and one level 1 major trauma hospital. The level 1 trauma hospital receives more serious injuries or concerning presentations.

For the purpose of this study, an unintentional injury was defined as what could be coded as an accident using the International Statistical Classification of Disease-Australian Modification (ICD10-AM) codes "V01–V99" [15]. Injury was further defined according to the ICD10–AM codes "S00-T98" [15]. These codes do not include psychological injury.

Injury factors were retrieved from the patient's medical record in order to allow for the coding of the injury according to the Abbreviated Injury Severity (AIS) Scale [16] and the subsequent calculation of the Injury Severity Score (ISS) [17]. Patients were classed as having a minor injury if they had an ISS of 1–8, moderate injury ISS 9–15, and a major injury ISS > 15.

The inclusion criteria were people aged 18 to 64 in paid employment during the 4 weeks prior to the injury, with sufficient English language skills to allow completion of questionnaires. Patients were excluded if they had sustained an intentional injury, were not employed, or if medical staff considered them to be medically unfit to provide informed consent. Patients with a significant traumatic brain injury associated with prolonged loss of consciousness were excluded because of the documented cognitive sequelae that are not comparable to other types of injury.

Patients were recruited following presentation to the hospital emergency department. After obtaining informed consent, demographic and occupation data was collected and a retrospective assessment of preinjury health was conducted at recruitment. In addition, patients were further surveyed by phone or in person if they were still in hospital, 2 weeks, 12 weeks, and 26 weeks following their injury. Follow-up time-points were chosen based on the different phases of disability (acute, subacute, and chronic) following injury. All participants for this study were recruited and followed up between March 2005 and October 2006.

2.3. Injury Compensation in the State of Victoria. In the Australian state of Victoria, all employers are required to have workers' compensation insurance. Employers maintain this insurance either through the Victorian WorkCover Authority (VWA) unless they are entitled to self-insure or obtain insurance through *Comcare,* the national workers' compensation scheme. The majority of Victorian workers (85%) are insured by the VWA. A claim may be lodged once the employee has been off work for 10 days or if a medical excess threshold has been exceeded. Any driver, passenger, pedestrian, motorcyclist, or cyclist that is injured on a designated Victorian road and/or in a designated vehicle is covered by the Transport Accident Commission. The injured person must meet the initial costs of medical treatment ($564.00) and the first week of sick leave.

Injuries with no entitlement to state-based compensation include those sustained at home, most sporting injuries, and transport accidents that occur on a nondesignated road. Self-employed workers are not entitled to coverage by VWA or Comcare.

2.4. Study Factors and Measures. At each post-injury time-point, participants were asked if they had returned to work. Those who answered in the affirmative were asked when they returned and if they had had any periods of sick leave since their return to work.

At recruitment, participants were asked whether they had experienced any difficulties with pain prior to the injury. Pain intensity was measured at the first followup using the short-form McGill Pain Questionnaire [18], a validated dedicated pain measurement tool [19]. Participants were asked to rate their overall pain since the injury using a 6-item adjectival scale. The scale is scored: 1 = no pain, 2 = mild, 3 = discomforting, 4 = distressing, 5 = horrible, and 6 = excruciating. Responses were dichotomised into the following groups (high: distressing/horrible/excruciating and mild: no pain/mild/ discomforting).

Participants reporting negative emotional states of depression, anxiety, and stress were assessed using the DASS21 a generic measure comprising three self-report scales [20]. The scales were scored and categorized according to recommended cut-offs (normal, mild, moderate, severe, and extremely severe) [21]. The DASS21 was collected prospectively at two weeks followup. The reported symptoms do not infer a clinical diagnosis [21].

Recovery expectations were measured at each post-injury follow-up time-point by asking participants to rate on a numerical 0–10 rating scale if they believed they would recover enough to return to their usual preinjury activities. The recovery expectations question was derived from work by Cole et al. [22]. High scores represented strong recovery beliefs.

Compensable status was measured by asking participants if they were receiving injury compensation medical treatment or wage from state-based compensation authorities responsible for work injury and/or transport related injury.

Comorbid health conditions were obtained from the medical records pertaining to the current injury. Age was assessed as a continuous variable. Dichotomous categories defined for some factors were educational status completed university degree versus completed less than university degree, ISS scores (ISS < 9 versus ISS ≥ 9) based on the common groupings for minor, moderate, and major trauma and comorbid health conditions (none versus one or more).

Participants were asked to indicate their occupation. In some cases the response provided was not their occupation but the industry in which they were employed.

2.5. Questionnaire Data Collection and Synthesis. At each postinjury time-point, participants were invited to respond to the question: "What are the most important things necessary for you to best recover?" This was an open ended question. Participants were invited to voice the primary concerns and no coaching of responses or suggested answers were provided. A qualitative approach was taken to the analysis of these data. Responses were transcribed verbatim.

The coding process involved two stages. The open text responses were first analysed for common themes using qualitative content analysis themes by FC, EK, and SS separately [23, 24]. As participant responses can illustrate themes, each response was at first grouped into broad emerging themes based on the common words used in their actual response. For example, the category time and rest included responses like person A who indicated "I need *time* to get over my injury." The category "following instructions" broadly classified responses such as those from person B who stated "*doing what I am told* by the physio." After this initial step, FC and SS met several times to discuss the emerging themes. Following discussions, the common themes seem to fall under eleven preliminary themes, which were then reorganised into themes that reflected a core thought process of the participant. The themes allow the researchers to bring together the different views and perspectives about recovery expectations in a structured manner and assist in exploring the journey from injury to recovery [23, 24].

Recovery has been described as a journey where the "event of the injury" has been used as a demarcating line categorising a patient's life into "before the trauma" and "after the trauma" [10]. In addition, taking the "event of the injury" as a starting point of recovery, the same study categorised the journey to recovery as "event" where the "event becomes a defining moment"; "fall-out" where the individuals become increasingly aware of the effect of injury, and "moving on" which involves overcoming dependence. The "event," "fall-out," and "moving-on" appear to describe the recovery process as a continuum. In our content analysis, we wanted to assess "where the attention or focus" of the participant was at each time point and how this changes over time. So in the current analysis, we examined the "focus" of the participants' responses.

2.6. Quantitative Data Analysis. Frequencies were used to report the broad themes. Chi square χ^2 analysis (3 × 2) was used to determine significant differences in the frequency of common responses. The SPSS 19.0 program (SPSS Release 19.0, Chicago, USA) was used for all data analysis. Descriptive data are presented as means (standard deviations) or number of subjects (percentages). The baseline characteristics of patients with complete data at six months were compared

TABLE 1: Characteristics of the study participants. Recovery expectations measured according to the question: "Do you believe you will recover enough to return to your pre-injury activities?" measured on a 0–10 Likert scale. High scores represent stronger expectations.

Age last birthday	37.7 years (18–62) (mean/range)	
	N	(%)
Gender		
Male	126	(75.0)
Female	42	(25.0)
Injury severity score		
Minor: 1–8	88	(52.4)
Moderate and major: >9	80	(47.6)
Education		
Less than university	136	(81.0)
University	32	(19.0)
Receipt of compensation for injury*		
No	91	(55.8)
Yes	72	(44.2)
Returned to work after 26 weeks after injury*		
Yes	104	(68.4)
No	48	(31.6)
Pain intensity at 2 weeks after injury		
Low pain intensity	104	(61.9)
High pain intensity	64	(38.1)
Presence of pain at 26 weeks after injury		
Yes	81	(54.0)
No	69	(46.0)
	Mean	SD
Recovery expectations#		
Week 2 (n = 161)	8.60	1.90
Week 12 (n = 148)	8.49	1.92
Week 26 (n = 108)	7.77	2.07

*Missing responses. #Significant difference $P < 0.05$: week 2 versus week 26 and week 12 versus week 26.

with participants with incomplete followup using chi-square tests or t-tests. A probability (P) value of <0.05 was considered significant.

2.7. Ethics. The research was conducted in accordance with the Declaration of Helsinki [25]. The study and all interviews were conducted with the understanding and consent of all study participants. Ethics approval was obtained from the Standing Committee on Ethics in Research Involving Humans of Monash University and the corresponding Ethics Committees at all participating hospitals.

3. Results

3.1. Demographics and Injury Characteristics. Baseline surveys were completed by 168 Victorian workers who had sustained nonlife-threatening acute orthopaedic trauma leading to hospitalization and were recruited to the study. Over the course of the study, 18 persons were lost to followup (89% followup). A comparison of those lost to followup with those that remained in the study revealed no significant differences with respect to age, gender, education, compensable status, injury severity, and hospital of admission (data not shown). In addition, there was no difference in terms of hospital location with regards to those who declined to take part in the study and those who took part. The median time to followup was 17 days (2-week followup), 82 days (12-week followup), and 181 days (six-month followup).

3.2. Participants. All participants were in salaried employment at the time of their injury. The mean age of the sample was 37.7 years and the cohort consisted primarily of men (75%). Descriptive characteristics of the study cohort are presented in Table 1. One-third of the cohort presented with one or more comorbid conditions at study entry and 91 participants (56%) sustained an injury that provided entitlement to injury compensation. Using the ISS to classify injuries, 88 patients sustained minor injuries (ISS 1–8), 69 moderate injuries (ISS 9–15), and 11 major injuries (ISS > 15).

3.3. Outcome Measures. Return to work and pain outcomes for participants were the main outcomes in this cohort study and have been described in detail elsewhere. However, to provide context to this substudy, key findings are summarised

Table 2: Grouped response to question according to follow-up time-point: What are the most important things necessary for you to best recover? Chi square analysis for differences in the frequency of the most common responses according to the three postinjury time-points.

	Week 2		Week 12		Week 26		Chi square	df	*P*
	N	%	*N*	%	*N*	%			
Time and rest	82	35.2	**29**	**15.5**	10	8.5	39.9	2	0.000
Positive attitude looking after myself	19	8.1	**29**	**15.5**	23	19.5	10.2	2	0.006
Doing the therapy or exercises that have been prescribed	37	15.8	**39**	**20.9**	29	24.5	4.13	2	0.127
Following instructions	24	10.3	**4**	**2.1**	1	0.85	19.6	2	0.000
Further repair of the injury (including further treatment)	23	9.8	**25**	**13.4**	8	6.7	3.57	2	0.168
Family support	9	3.8	**3**	**1.6**	12	10.1			
Returning to work	4	1.7	**5**	**2.6**	5	4.2			
Support from workplace including income support	5	2.15	**7**	**3.7**	3	2.5			
Quality care	4	1.7	**6**	**3.2**	3	2.5			
Get back into a normal routine	9	3.8	**6**	**3.2**	0				
I have recovered			**5**	**2.6**	7	5.9			
Nothing as it will not change			**9**	**4.8**	1	0.84			
Total number of responses	233		**186**		118				
Number and proportion of participants who provided responses	161	(86.6%)	**148**	**(79.6%)**	108	(50.1%)			
Mean number of responses/responding participant	1.4		**1.3**		1.1				

Responses were separated for doing the therapy and exercise and following instructions. Following instructions involved no mention of therapy or exercises. The chi square analysis (3 × 2) compared each response for the three time-points. Numerator is the response under consideration e.g., time and rest, denominator all other responses, df: degrees of freedom, *P*: probability. The bold numbers refer to the number of responses and proportions for the responses provided at 12 weeks post injury.

here. Follow-up data on return to work was available for 152 participants as 18 participants were lost to followup. Sixty-eight percent of participants ($n = 104$) returned to work within 6 months [6]. The prevalence of pain was common with nearly a half (54%) of participants reporting the presence of persistent pain at 6 months, and over two-thirds (87%) reporting that their pain interfered with their normal work activities [3].

At the first followup, moderate, severe, or extremely severe symptoms of depression, anxiety, and stress were reported by 32 participants (depression 19.8%), 40 participants (anxiety 24.8%), and 26 participants (stress 16.1%). The levels of symptoms reported by participants as measured by the DASS21 at the first follow-up time-point are outlined in Table 5.

3.4. Recovery Expectations. Participant views on recovery, including their expectations, were measured at each follow-up time-point using a Likert scale from 0 to 10 on "whether they believed they would recover?" (Table 1). The mean score at each time-point indicated a statistically significant reduction in recovery expectations between two weeks and six months after injury ($P < 0.05$).

3.5. Question on Recovery-Quantitative Analysis. The open ended question revealed personal circumstances, including an insight into the feelings of patients and their views on recovery. Responses are summarised according to the time-point at which they were provided: 2, 12, and 26 weeks post-injury (Table 2).

At week 2 after injury, the most common response to the question "important things that will help you best recover" was "time and rest" (35.2%) followed by "doing the therapy" and exercises prescribed to them as aiding their recovery (15.5%). Time and rest as a response was less important 12 weeks after injury. At that time-point, "doing the therapy and exercises" was the most common response (23.4%) followed by "maintaining a positive outlook." At 26 weeks after injury these responses were again the most common with "doing therapy and exercise" scoring 28.5% of the responses and "having a positive attitude" 22.5%.

Chi square analysis was used to determine if there was a statistically significant change for the most common responses over the three follow-up time-points. In this analysis, the numerator comprised the particular response, for example, "time and rest" and the denominator included the total number of all other responses provided at that time-point. The chi-square analysis indicated a statistically significant difference in the frequency of the grouped responses over the three follow-up time-points for: (1) time and rest; (2) maintaining a positive outlook; and (3) doing what health providers told them to do. There was a nonsignificant difference in the frequency of responses for the grouped responses: (1) therapy and exercises and (2) further repair of the injury.

3.6. Open Ended Question Exploring Participants' Views on Recovery. In order to explore patients' views about what would aid their recovery following non-life-threatening acute orthopaedic trauma, content analysis was carried out on the brief open text responses provided by participants to the question "what are the most important things that will help you best recover?" Responses were broadly categorized into

TABLE 3: Characteristics of study participants provided to add context to outlined open ended responses according to return to work status at 6 months.

Participant code	Age	Gender	Compensable injury	Occupation/industry	DASS21 Symptoms 2 weeks*	Returned to work by 6 months	Pain intensity 2 weeks	Presence of pain at 12 weeks	Recovery beliefs at 2 weeks
RTW1	18	Male	no	Bus driver	No	Yes	Low	No	4
RTW2	18	Female	no	Horticulture	Yes	Yes	Low	No	9
RTW3	61	Female	No	Bakery assistant	No	Yes	Low	Yes	10
RTW4	47	Female	Yes	Assembler worker	No	Yes	Low	No	10
RTW5	58	Female	No	Psychologist	No	Yes	Low	Yes	10
RTW6	18	Female	Yes	Cattery	Yes	Yes	Low	No	6
RTW7	51	Female	Yes	Library officer	Yes	Yes	High	Yes	10
RTW8	54	Male	No	Courier	Yes	Yes	Low	No	10
RTW9	62	Male	No	Air conditioning technician	No	Yes	Low	Yes	9
RTW10	44	Male	No	Manufacturing	No	Yes	Low	Yes	5
RTW11	34	Male	No	Construction	Yes	Yes	Low	Yes	6
RTW12	48	Male	No	Carpenter	No	Yes	Low	Yes	9
RTW13	35	Male	No	Electrical inspector	No	Yes	Low	No	10
RTW14	41	Male	No	Information technology	No	Yes	Low	Yes	10
RTW15	34	Female	No	Healthcare	No	Yes	Low	Yes	10
RTW16	31	Male	Yes	Information technology	Yes	Yes	Low	Yes	7
NO1	27	Male	no	Car industry	Yes	No	Low	No	6
NO2	25	Male	Yes	Radiographer	No	No	High	Yes	10
NO3	47	Female	No	Factory worker	No	No	Low	No	5
NO4	30	Male	Yes	Labourer	No	No	Low	Yes	10
NO5	56	Male	Yes	Construction	No	No	Low	No	9
NO6	58	Female	Yes	Nurse	Yes	No	Low	Yes	8
NO7	49	Male	Yes	Education	No	No	high	Yes	10
NO8	26	Male	Yes	Groundsman	Yes	No	High	No	10
NO9	62	Male	Yes	Construction	Yes	No	High	Yes	—
NO10	39	Male	Yes	Plasterer	No	No	High	Yes	9
NO11	51	Male	Yes	Truck driver	Yes	No	Low	Yes	7

*Participant reported symptoms of anxiety, depression, and/or stress (one or more).

three primary themes and the expression of these themes based on the participant's main focus.

3.7. Open Ended Responses on Recovery: Descriptors. While open ended responses were received from most participants, Table 3 provides the range of descriptors for those participants whose open ended response is reported in this paper. The descriptors are provided to add context and depth to responses. The choice of descriptors was based on the data collected, the biopsychosocial focus of the overall study, and the literature on factors associated with recovery.

Three key themes emerged, the first recovery focused on a return to health with an ongoing plan, the second Ideal recovery involves a focus on return to health, and the third recovery involves a focus on current status. Brief illustrative responses of the different ways of expressing the same theme are provided in Table 4. Around half of the participants seemed to focus on their immediate situation, namely, a "return to health." A small number of participants (12%) were focused on their current status with the remainder being those participants who had an ongoing plan for after their return to health. Individual participant comments are included in both the tables and the text and include reference to the participant code. For example, (RTW2) refers to the second participant who returned to work and (NO5) refers to the 5th participant who did not return to work as listed in Table 4.

3.8. Recovery Themes

3.8.1. Recovery Focused on a Return to Health with an Ongoing Plan. The first theme included those participants who

TABLE 4: Recovery themes, subthemes, and illustrative quotes.

Themes	Subthemes	Illustrative quotes
Recovery involves a focus on return to health	Focused on a return to physical functioning	"Turn my head more as I have a restricted range of movement" (RTW2)
		"First rest, then learning how to walk on two legs again" (NO3)
	Focused on complete or partial symptom resolution	"Leg healing, once that is right, I am happy" (NO8)
		"Pins to come out of (leg) and for it (the bone) to knit" (RTW4)
		"Hand therapy for my little finger on right hand so that I can recover movement and feeling" (NO6)
	Focused on following instructions and/or advice of their health providers	"That I follow the therapist's instructions as closely as possible" (NO12)
		"Listening to advice of medical/physio people and adhering to their advice" (RTW1)
		"Rest and keeping my leg elevated, don't overdo it" (RTW3)
	Focused on healthcare, providers, and resources	"Better sling for my arm, one that doesn't cut the circulation off at my neck" (RTW16)
		"Get strength back in my leg, different doctors all the time doesn't help me recover" (RTW14)
	Focused on others: unsure of their role	"Up to the doctors and physios- I don't want to start doing things without seeing the doctor" (NO11)
		"Keep going back to Dr for tests and x-rays" (RTW11)
	Focused on their own mental health	"Good healthy outlook, I need to believe that I am going to recover" (RTW9)
		"Keep my mind active, feel as if I am contributing" (RTW7)
	Focused on quality of life	"Keep up the social activities with family and friends" (RTW15)
		"Family support, enjoy life and my hobbies" (NO2)
Recovery involves an ongoing plan after they had returned to health	Focused on recovery with an emphasis on financial or employer support	"Having my job held open for me, not working till I am well enough " (RTW12)
		"Not having the financial burden of not working" (RTW13)
		"Confidence of my employer to look after me" (RTW8)
		"Flexibility in working hours, understanding from my employer re mobility restrictions" (RTW5)
		"Consideration at work for my temporary limitations, I will need assistance with parking" (RTW5)
	Focused on a return to physical functioning without expressed concern about their work or employer	"Different tasks at work, no heavy lifting" (RTW6)
		"Strengthen my heel so that I get full movement back in my foot and can return to work" (RTW10)
		"Being able to work again normally, get back to where I was" (NO5)
Recovery involves a focus on current status	Focused on the injury and the impact of the event	"So your injury never occurred, to turn back time" (NO9)
		"Nothing will help, doctors say I won't improve" (NO7)
		"Being told the truth by my doctors to allow me to heal myself" (NO4)
		"My thumb needs to be perfect for me to do my job properly and I can't see that happening" (NO1)

articulated a plan for return to health and had given some thought towards an ongoing plan (i.e., plans after recovery). "Consideration at work for my temporary limitations, I will need assistance with parking" (RTW5). Two different aspects emerged. In the first subtheme, the ongoing plan primarily focused around a return to physical functioning without expressed concern about their work situation or their employer. "Being able to work again normally, get back to where I was" (NO5). The desire to get back to work and for normality was characteristic of responses provided by many others. While participants did not articulate concerns about their employer in their ongoing plan, a second subtheme

Table 5: Participants reported symptoms of depression, anxiety and stress as measured by the DASS21 at each follow-up.

Symptoms	2 weeks (n = 161)	
	N	%
Depression		
Normal	114	60.8
Mild	15	22.9
Moderate	20	8.6
Severe	7	5.5
Extremely severe	5	1.8
Anxiety		
Normal	99	61.4
Mild	22	13.6
Moderate	21	13.0
Severe	10	6.2
Extremely severe	9	5.6
Stress		
Normal	98	70.8
Mild	37	9.3
Moderate	14	12.4
Severe	9	4.3
Extremely severe	3	3.1

was also apparent, namely, those whose recovery involved an ongoing plan after a return to health but which emphasised financial and employer support. Such responses included "Having my job held open for me, not working till I am well enough" (RTW12), "Different tasks at work, no heavy lifting" (RTW6), and "Not having the financial burden of not working" (RTW13). Employer support was primarily in relation to workplace accommodations and understanding from their employer, possibly because the nature of their occupation and the injuries sustained would need to be supported by workplace accommodations if a successful return to work was going to be achieved. Injured workers wanted confidence that their employer would do the right thing by them whether it was holding open their job till they were better or providing workplace accommodations like parking or having different duties.

3.8.2. Ideal Recovery Involves a Focus on Return to Health. The second theme covered the majority of open ended responses received by the study participants and strongly focused on factors that would aid their recovery. For this theme, there was no mention of an ongoing plan after a RTH (i.e., plans after recovery). Even though all the participants in this study were in employment, only a proportion of the participants spoke about their employment, financial status, or what support they would need when they get back to work after recovery. Different ways of expressing this theme emerged depending on the importance/focus of factors to the injured participant. These included a return to physical functioning, symptom resolution, mental health, following instructions, and quality of life. Responses were generally positive with an emphasis on themselves and with clear ideas on how they would return to health. Overall planning involved goal setting and intended actions in order to regain a reasonable or preinjury level of physical functioning. While the majority of responses in this theme reflected active engagement by the injured participant in their recovery, a minority (n = 20) of the responses seemed unsure of their role in recovery, instead focusing on the actions of others.

Around a quarter of the participants identified complete and partial symptom resolution or a resolution of complications stemming from the injury as important aspects of their return to health plan. "Pins to come out of (leg) and for it (the bone) to knit" (RTW4) "Leg healing, once that is right, I am happy" (NO8). A similar proportion of participants regarding their "return to health plan" mentioned following instructions and/or therapy of their health care providers, "That I follow the therapist's instructions as closely as possible" (NO12). However this participant did not speak of an ongoing plan for after recovery.

For others, the most important thing necessary for their recovery related to healthcare issues. This included access to additional resources "Better sling for my arm, one that doesn't cut the circulation off at my neck" (RTW16) and for others it was communication with their healthcare providers.

Few participants (<5%) had a RTH plan that involved consultation with their healthcare providers "Keep going back to Dr for tests and X-rays" (RTW11). Some seemed unsure of their role in their own recovery.

Some injured workers, while making positive statements, had no clear RTH plan. These participants all reported symptoms of depression, anxiety, or stress as measured by the DASS21 two weeks following their injury. When talking about recovery, they were strongly focused on their injury, they did not mention physiotherapy or following the therapists' instructions but appeared more focused on their own mental health such as "being positive during their recovery period" with no mention of plans for "after they have recovered".

3.8.3. Recovery Involves a Focus on Current Status. While many participants indicated the need for rest and time, a minority (12%) provided comments that suggested they may be "stuck in the moment of the injury and its impact." Regret and generally pessimistic statements served as reminders about the traumatic nature of their injury had restrained their lives "My thumb needs to be perfect for me to do my job properly and I can't see that happening" (NO1), "I need to be allowed to be angry about what has happened" (NO8). For this group of participants, it seemed they were still struggling with the notion that "life would not be the same." Their comments reflected a sense of being "unable to move on" and they appeared in need of psychological assistance. What was noticeable in this theme was the high percentage (90%) of responses provided by workers who did not RTW during the six month follow-up period. These responses seem similar to the "fall out" phase mentioned in other study described as "an ever increasing awareness of the effect of the injury on their lives."

4. Discussion

Patients' views on recovery following non-life-threatening acute traumatic injuries have received little research attention to date. The aim of the current analysis was to explore patients' views on what would aid their recovery, establish whether there were commonalities in the responses, and determine any change in responses with time following the injury. Participants were asked for a brief response to the following question: "What are the most important things necessary for you to best recover" and what they thought at the time. Responses were received from 168 employed persons who had sustained a range of non-life-threatening acute orthopaedic injuries leading to hospitalization. Analysis of responses revealed common themes regarding participant's perceptions of what they considered "key" to their recovery. The themes derived from the data provide insight into the ways injured people negotiate the recovery process and include having a clear plan for returning to health, a plan for returning to employment, and maintaining recovery strategies including social interaction. Overall the study findings suggest that the most important aspect of recovery for the injured workers was a return to what they perceived as their life before the accident. The attitude of the participant regarding their own recovery seems to influence their immediate decisions regarding return to health and return to work. In particular, returning to "prior to accident" physical functioning, advice from health care specialists, environment provided by the employer, financial situation, and social interactions dominated their responses.

Clay et al. examined the biopsychosocial predictors of RTW using the same dataset as the current study [3]. In that study, participants with strong recovery expectations had 16.7 greater odds of returning to work by 12 weeks than participants with weak recovery expectations. In contrast a Swedish study that examined the association between self-perceived recovery and the SF36 following minor traffic related musculoskeletal injuries found that physical aspects of functional health status were more strongly associated with recovery than emotional or social aspects [26].

The biomedical model of health considers recovery as universal in which all injured persons have a predictable recovery trajectory and "patients" need to follow the instructions of their health care providers to achieve optimal results, sometimes referred to as "structural functionalism" [27]. However our findings and other research studies indicate that while this may be true for a percentage of injured people, recovery overall following injury can be both complex and subjective and may not always follow a predictable trajectory. We would like to emphasise that the use of quotations marks around the responses should not be inferred as representing the injured workers unchanging world view on recovery [28] because as we see in this study, recovery is both individually experienced and a dynamic state.

The recovery process as a continuum influenced the identification of emerging themes that reflected the core thought process of the participant and the different views and perspectives about recovery expectations. For example, we grouped the responses, time and rest because that's how most people think of rehabilitation. Recovery takes time and often it's by resting from the context in which the injury occurred (i.e., work/driving/sport). Had other questions been asked—a limitation of the current study—it is feasible that the grouping of responses may have slightly differed.

This study, while small in nature and exploratory provides evidence to support a relationship between participant responses and time after injury. For example, at the first postinjury time-point (around 2 weeks postinjury), time and rest was the most common response. At this stage many participants remained in the acute/subacute post-injury phase with more than 25% still in hospital. However, as time passed, a decrease in the frequency of this response was observed. This is perhaps not unexpected in the early post-injury stages given the injury required hospitalisation. That, "time and rest" was offered as a response at later time-points may suggest barriers to ideal recovery for some participants such as depression or chronic pain.

Our findings are similar to another study on the psychological aspects of people with hand injuries under treatment and rehabilitation, which asked its participants the question "What is the single most important thing that will enable the best recovery for you? [29]." Responses in that study included time, caution, attitude to the follow the instructions of the doctor or therapist, and to do the prescribed therapy or exercises for the hand. The study found that caution was considered more important than time in the initial stages. In the current analysis, time and rest was a common and important response. In agreement with our findings, the study by Haese found that responses changed according to the phase of treatment [29]. This is not unusual as recovery is a dynamic process.

Hush et al. (2009) explored patient's perceptions of recovery from low back pain, finding that symptom resolution, and an improved capacity to perform a broad scope of self-defined functional activities were considered important aspects of recovery by the participants [11]. This is in keeping with our findings of the importance of getting back to health and activities following a return to health. In previous studies, psychological health has been identified by participants as a marker of recovery, with particular mention of "having a more positive outlook" and the "importance of not getting depressed". Our study found similar attitudes among participants, for example, "Good healthy outlook, I need to believe I am going to recover." In both studies, psychological health was identified by participants as a marker of recovery, particularly in terms of having a more positive outlook and the importance of not getting depressed.

The focus of the current study was on Victorian workers who were all in salaried employment at the time of their injury. Nearly half were entitled to injury compensation which may have included wage replacement. This may be one reason why the majority of participants were focused on "returning to health" and did not have a "return to work" plan if financial needs could be met via wage replacement. Our study did not specifically ask whether their injury affected their employment; which is a limitation of the study. Work is a central aspect of adult life and provides a sense of social identity [30]. For most, working is a financial necessity so recovery [3] and RTW from an unexpected injury are important to workers and their families if only for financial reasons. Murgatroyd et al. (2010) considered the effect of compensation on recovery following severe motor vehicle crash injuries and suggested that recovery was particularly stressful for those claiming compensation [9]. In the current study, around half of the participants were in receipt of injury compensation. Compensable injury status does not appear to have had an impact on participants' views on recovery. While one participant (data not shown) did provide the response of "income support, home support, work support, financial support", few participants responded similarly and no participant made any direct reference to any compensation system.

The current analysis utilized responses from participants to the question—What are the most important things necessary for you to best recover?. The advantage of opened ended responses is that it *permits one to understand the world as seen by the respondents. This enables the researcher to capture the points of view of other people without pre-determining those points of view."* [31]. As not all participants provided a response to the open ended question on recovery at each follow-up time-point (see Table 2), the study findings reflect a baseline of concerns. While this needs to be acknowledged as a potential limitation of the study, this baseline of concerns could form the basis of outcome measurements or be explored more rigorously in further studies using in depth interviews that explore in more depth the intricacies associated with recovery. The consistency of some responses for example on workplace and employer accommodations suggests that these issues need further exploration. While government policies and organisations like the Transport Accident Commission encourage communication between employers and employees following injury, our thematic analysis suggests that depending upon the person and the injury, some participants needed more assistance from employers for a successful recovery and RTW than others. This may be due to the nature of their injury or alternately it could be that some people need more assistance than others during the recovery process. This is highlighted by responses such as "Confidence of my employer to look after me" or "Flexibility in working hours, understanding from my employer re mobility restrictions" which reflects their concerns about the circumstances at work. It was not possible to explore these psychological aspects in order to make any inferences with regard to this factor.

The inclusion of pain intensity [6] and participant-reported symptoms of depression, anxiety and stress as measured at 2 weeks post-injury reflect the contributions of these factors measured in the early post injury stages as strong predictors of long term recovery [2, 4, 5]. We found participants who reported symptoms of depression, anxiety or stress tended to focus more on their recovery and in their responses did not appear to think about RTW or what they would do after their recovery. This group of participants did not mention what they would do after they recover they seemed to have "no going plan" but were concentrating on their injury status. In addition, our study found that even participants who did not report any symptoms of depression, anxiety or stress as measured by the DASS21 may need some encouragement or guidance to think about an ongoing plan (i.e., plan following recovery or a RTW plan), for example, "Up to the doctors and physios—I don't want to start doing things without seeing the doctor". Bodenheimer et al. (2002) has argued that people with health-related conditions who self-manage their health have an improved chance for a rewarding lifestyle because they take part in their own care [32]. Health behaviour is a product of an individual's feelings, beliefs, and cultural practices. For the injured workers in the current study, moving on and planning were not straightforward. While some within weeks of the injury offered comments on recovery that indicated they were planning beyond the injury, others were focused on a return to health, and a minority overall appeared unable to move from the moment of the injury and its impact.

Research suggests that a single recovery question may be a useful for conducting an overview or overall assessments of recovery following injury [33]. A better understanding of injured workers views on recovery is critical to how recovery is measured in clinical and rehabilitative practice the findings of this study further contribute towards the current debate on how recovery following acute nonlife-threatening traumatic injuries is influenced by more than just physical factors and how recovery could be better measured if the spectrum of factors patients consider key for their recovery are addressed.

4.1. Strengths and Limitations. Statistics derived from quantitative health surveys offer little insight into the human motivation behind certain preferences and behaviours which led us to conclude that a combination of quantitative and qualitative research, would offer a greater breadth of perspectives on the impact of how patients view recovery than just a survey. Participant's perspective on their recovery is one of the strengths of this study as is the use of different methods approach for data collection. Such an approach has provided for greater rigour by reducing the likelihood of "gaps" in the information collected. Other key strengths include its prospective longitudinal design and high follow-up rate and the measurement of recovery expectations at three post-injury time-points.

Limitations that need to be considered include the need for multiple stages of data collection and the potential loss of flexibility and depth due to quantizing the open text comments [33]. We acknowledge the potential for collinearity in the quantized data. Selection bias may have affected the frequency and type of responses provided at the six month time-point. There was a significant amount of missing data (35%) at this time point due to participants who felt they had recovered declining to provide a response. We cannot rule out the influence of the healthcare provider on the participant's responses. If a healthcare provider strongly reinforced the message of having to do the therapy or exercise, it is feasible that the participant's responses may not be an unbiased reflection of their own views. Finally, the subjective nature of the recovery comments raises concern of recall bias. While this cannot be ruled out, research has established a high degree of accuracy in recall for important single events including pregnancy and later recall about delivery [34]. We assume that injury that results in hospitalization would be an important event and therefore less subject to recall bias.

5. Conclusions

In conclusion, the findings of this study indicate that the journey to recovery following non-life-threatening acute orthopaedic trauma is complex, often prolonged, and highly individual. The path can vary considerably between persons who have sustained similar injuries and are influenced by individual perceptions of their own recovery and by family and work situations. These findings need to be confirmed with more homogenous injury populations. They highlight the importance of exploring the patient's views on recovery and provide additional evidence that postinjury recovery cannot easily be explained within a biomedical model that focuses only on factors related to the physical injury. While acknowledging potential methodological limitations, this study has identified some key aspects that injured persons consider will assist their recovery. Some of these aspects are central to the injured person and others to family, treating providers, and the workplace. Further exploration of these aspects and how they affect clinical, rehabilitative, and social outcomes are warranted.

Abbreviations

RTW: Return to work
RTH: Return to health
NO: No return to work
ISS: Injury Severity Score
VAED: Victorian Admitted Episodes Dataset
VWA: Victorian WorkCover Authority.

Conflict of Interests

The authors declare that there is no conflict of interests regarding the publication of this paper.

Acknowledgments

The Transport Accident Commission and the Monash University Accident Research Centre Postgraduate Students Fund funded the data collection phase of this study. The funding bodies played no role in the design, conduct, analysis or interpretation of the data or in the writing of this paper. Fiona J. Clay was the recipient of an NHMRC Public Health scholarship and VIC-Health scholarship and a participant in the CIHR strategic training program in Work Disability Prevention Program at the time of data collection.

References

[1] D. M. Urquhart, O. D. Williamson, B. J. Gabbe et al., "Outcomes of patients with orthopaedic trauma admitted to level 1 trauma centres," *ANZ Journal of Surgery*, vol. 76, no. 7, pp. 600–606, 2006.

[2] D. Zatzick, G. J. Jurkovich, F. P. Rivara et al., "A national US study of posttraumatic stress disorder, depression, and work and functional outcomes after hospitalization for traumatic injury," *Annals of Surgery*, vol. 248, no. 3, pp. 429–435, 2008.

[3] F. J. Clay, S. V. Newstead, W. L. Watson, J. Ozanne-Smith, J. Guy, and R. J. McClure, "Bio-psychosocial determinants of persistent pain 6 months after non-life-threatening acute orthopaedic trauma," *Journal of Pain*, vol. 11, no. 5, pp. 420–430, 2010.

[4] E. J. MacKenzie, M. J. Bosse, J. F. Kellam et al., "Early predictors of long-term work disability after major limb trauma," *Journal of Trauma*, vol. 61, no. 3, pp. 688–694, 2006.

[5] M. Fitzharris, D. Bowman, and K. Ludlow, "Factors associated with return-to-work and health outcomes among survivors of road crashes in Victoria," *Australian & New Zealand Journal of Public Health*, vol. 34, no. 2, pp. 153–160, 2010.

[6] F. J. Clay, S. V. Newstead, W. L. Watson, and R. J. McClure, "Determinants of return to work following non-life-threatening acute orthopaedic trauma: a prospective cohort study," *Journal of Rehabilitation Medicine*, vol. 42, no. 2, pp. 162–169, 2010.

[7] M. V. Mondloch, D. C. Cole, and J. W. Frank, "Does how you do depend on how you think you'll do? A systematic review of the evidence for a relation between patients' recovery expectations and health outcomes," *Canadian Medical Association Journal*, vol. 165, no. 2, pp. 174–179, 2001.

[8] D. Ozegovic, L. J. Carroll, and J. David Cassidy, "Does expecting mean achieving? the association between expecting to return to work and recovery in whiplash associated disorders: a population-based prospective cohort study," *European Spine Journal*, vol. 18, no. 6, pp. 893–899, 2009.

[9] D. F. Murgatroyd, I. D. Cameron, and I. A. Harris, "Understanding the effect of compensation on recovery from severe motor vehicle crash injuries: a qualitative study," *Injury Prevention*, vol. 17, no. 4, pp. 222–227, 2011.

[10] T. S. Richmond, H. J. Thompson, J. A. Deatrick, and D. R. Kauder, "Journey towards recovery following physical trauma," *Journal of Advanced Nursing*, vol. 32, no. 6, pp. 1341–1347, 2000.

[11] J. M. Hush, K. Refshauge, G. Sullivan, L. De Souza, C. G. Maher, and J. H. McAuley, "Recovery: what does this mean to patients with low back pain?" *Arthritis Care and Research*, vol. 61, no. 1, pp. 124–131, 2009.

[12] D. E. Beaton, V. Tarasuk, J. N. Katz, J. G. Wright, and C. Bombardier, ""Are you better?" A qualitative study of the meaning of recovery," *Arthritis Care and Research*, vol. 45, no. 3, pp. 270–279, 2001.

[13] G. L. Engel, "The need for a new medical model: a challenge for biomedicine," *Science*, vol. 196, no. 4286, pp. 129–136, 1977.

[14] Department Human Services, *The Victorian Admitted Episode Database: An Overview*, Acute Health Division, Department of Human Services, Melbourne, Australia, 14th edition, 2004.

[15] National Centre for Classification in Health, *The International Statistical Classification of Disease and Related Health Problems-Australian Modification (ICD-10-AM)*, Tenth Revision Sydney: National Centre for Classification in Health, 6th edition.

[16] Association for the Advancement of Automotive Medicine, *The Abbreviated Injury Scale 1990*, Barrington, Ill, USA, 1998.

[17] S. P. Baker, B. O'Neill, W. Haddon Jr., and W. B. Long, "The injury severity score: a method for describing patients with multiple injuries and evaluating emergency care," *Journal of Trauma*, vol. 14, no. 3, pp. 187–196, 1974.

[18] R. Melzack, "The short-form McGill pain questionnaire," *Pain*, vol. 30, no. 2, pp. 191–197, 1987.

[19] M. P. Jensen, P. Karoly, and S. Braver, "The measurement of clinical pain intensity: a comparison of six methods," *Pain*, vol. 27, no. 1, pp. 117–126, 1986.

[20] P. F. Lovibond and S. H. Lovibond, "The structure of negative emotional states: comparison of the depression anxiety stress scales (DASS) with the Beck Depression and Anxiety Inventories," *Behaviour Research and Therapy*, vol. 33, no. 3, pp. 335–343, 1995.

[21] S. Lovibond and P. Lovibond, *Manual for the Depression Anxiety Stress Scale*, The Psychology Foundation Monograph, Sydney, Australia, 2nd edition, 1995.

[22] D. C. Cole, M. V. Mondloch, and S. Hogg-Johnson, "Listening to injured workers: how recovery expectations predict outcomes—a prospective study," *CMAJ*, vol. 166, no. 6, pp. 749–754, 2002.

[23] A. G. Tuckett, "Applying thematic analysis theory to practice: a researcher's experience," *Contemporary Nurse*, vol. 19, no. 1-2, pp. 75–87, 2005.

[24] J. W. Cresswell, *Qualitative Inquiry and Research Design: Choosing among Five Approaches*, Sage, Thousand Oaks, Calif, USA, 2nd ed edition, 2007.

[25] World Medical Organization, "Declaration of Helsinki," *British Medical Journal*, vol. 313, no. 7070, pp. 1448–1449, 1996.

[26] C. Ottosson, H. Pettersson, S.-E. Johansson, O. Nyrén, and S. Ponzer, "Recovered? Association between self-perceived recovery and the SF-36 after minor musculoskeletal injuries," *Quality of Life Research*, vol. 16, no. 2, pp. 217–226, 2007.

[27] T. Parsons, "Social structure and dynamic process: the case of modern medical practice," in *The Social System*, chapter 10, Routledge, London, USA.

[28] S. Taylor, "One participant said ...: the implications of quotations from biographical talk," *Qualitative Research*, vol. 12, pp. 388–401, 2012.

[29] J. B. Haese, "Psychological aspects of hand injuries their treatment and rehabilitation," *Journal of Hand Surgery*, vol. 10, no. 3, pp. 283–287, 1985.

[30] M. Corkum, "Mental health: together we do better: marketing meets mental health promotion and work," in *Australian Network for Promotion Prevention and Early Intervention for Mental Health. Mental Health and Work: Issues and Perspectives*, E. Willis, L. Morrow, and I. Verins, Eds., pp. 165–178, Auseinet, Bedford Park, UK, 2002.

[31] M. Q. Patton, *Qualitative Evaluation and Research Methods*, Sage, Newbury Park, Calif, USA, 2nd edition, 1990.

[32] T. Bodenheimer, K. Lorig, H. Holman, and K. Grumbach, "Patient self-management of chronic disease in primary care," *Journal of the American Medical Association*, vol. 288, no. 19, pp. 2469–2475, 2002.

[33] C. W. Roberts, "A conceptual framework for quantitative text analysis: on joining probabilities and substantive inferences about texts," *Quality and Quantity*, vol. 34, no. 3, pp. 259–274, 2000.

[34] M. A. Quigley, C. Hockley, and L. L. Davidson, "Agreement between hospital records and maternal recall of mode of delivery: evidence from 12 391 deliveries in the UK Millennium cohort study," *BJOG*, vol. 114, no. 2, pp. 195–200, 2007.

2

Spine Curve Measures Taken in Individuals with Osteoporosis and Osteopenia Using the IONmed Mobile Phone Application Are Highly Consistent with Digital Inclinometer Measures

Norma J. MacIntyre,[1] Chris P. Recknor,[2] and Julie C. Recknor[2]

[1] *School of Rehabilitation Science, McMaster University, IAHS 403, 1400 Main Street West, Hamilton, ON, Canada L8S 1C7*
[2] *United Osteoporosis Centres, 2350 Limestone Parkway, N.E., Gainesville, GA 30501, USA*

Correspondence should be addressed to Norma J. MacIntyre; macint@mcmaster.ca

Academic Editors: Y.-W. Hsieh, C.-L. Kao, and A. Ozcan Edeer

Introduction. This study determined the agreement between measures of standing posture in individuals at risk of osteoporotic fracture obtained using the IONmed mobile phone application and a digital inclinometer. *Methods.* One experienced rater assessed 20 adults, aged 55–88 years, attending an outpatient osteoporosis clinic. A standardized protocol was duplicated to acquire a single measure of spine curvature (lumbosacral angle, lordosis, kyphosis) using the IONmed mobile phone application and a digital inclinometer. Interdevice agreement was determined using the intraclass correlation coefficient (ICC) with 95% confidence intervals (CI) and standard error of the measurement (SEM) with 95% CI and Bland-Altman plots. *Results.* ICC (95% CI) for lumbosacral angle, lordosis, and kyphosis is 0.97 (0.92, 0.99), 0.97 (0.92, 0.99), and 0.99 (0.98, 1.0), respectively. SEM (95% CI) for lumbosacral angle, lordosis, and kyphosis is 0.99° (0.75, 1.44), 1.33° (1.01, 1.94), and 1.23° (0.94, 1.80), respectively. Measurement bias is small. *Conclusions.* In our sample, the IONmed mobile phone application provides measures highly consistent with the digital inclinometer measures of standing posture. This method offers clinicians a quick, convenient way of identifying alterations in spine alignment which require followup and remediation.

1. Introduction

Thoracic kyphosis increases with age such that kyphotic angle progresses by 3° per decade in men and women over the age of 50 years [1]. Exact prevalence of excessive kyphosis (hyperkyphosis) is difficult to determine due to the lack of a gold standard for diagnosis. Regardless of how it is measured, hyperkyphosis is common in older adults and of particular concern for people with osteoporosis [2]. In a prospective study of 1624 postmenopausal women with osteoporosis followed for three years, Roux and colleagues [3] found that the women in the highest tertile for measures of thoracic kyphosis at baseline were most likely to have suffered a vertebral compression fracture at followup even after adjusting for known risk factors. These findings confirm that hyperkyphosis is an independent risk factor for osteoporotic fractures of the spine. Bruno and colleagues [4] have investigated the compression loading on individual vertebral bodies (T6 to L5) resulting from body weight and muscle loading acting in the axial direction at incremental angles of thoracic hyperkyphosis (50° to 75°) and considered two postural compensation strategies people use to maintain a stable centre of mass and horizontal eye gaze (one of which balances the thoracic and lumbar curvatures). The largest increases in vertebral body compression loading were observed in the thoracolumbar and lumbar regions, particularly in conditions where the spine curvatures were not balanced [4]. Recently, we reported that kyphotic angle is associated with self-reported activities of daily living (ADLs) and performance on a balance test in 36 patients attending an osteoporosis clinic. In our sample of high functioning older adults, 50% were hyperkyphotic according to normative values for digital inclinometer measures whereas only three participants had morphometric vertebral fractures [5]. These findings confirm previous observations that age-related hyperkyphosis develops due to a variety of reasons, only one of which is osteoporotic vertebral fracture. Back extensor muscle weakness is a common cause that is modifiable [6, 7]. Postural training including exercises to improve back extensor muscle endurance or strength have improved kyphosis and physical performance [7] and reduced the incidence of vertebral compression fracture [8]. Therefore, it is important to measure standing posture in order to identify hyperkyphosis and associated compensations in the pelvis and lumbar spine indicative of the need for followup to address the associated impairments and activity limitations in older adults.

Several noninvasive methods have been developed for measuring sagittal plane spine curvatures in standing. Previously, the first author's group assessed the reliability of the flexicurve ruler and the digital inclinometer measures of spine curvatures taken by the same rater and determined that minimal gains in reliability are achieved when performing more than one trial using the digital inclinometer versus a minimum of three measures using the flexicurve ruler [9]. Moreover, test-retest reliability of a single measure of lumbosacral angle, lumbothoracic angle, and thoracocervical angle taken by an experienced rater using the digital inclinometer was very high in older adults attending a rheumatology clinic specializing in osteoporosis care [5]. The factory-calibrated digital inclinometer is relatively inexpensive ($500 USD) and it only takes a few minutes to acquire and manually record the measurements. Therefore, this method was recommended to identify hyperkyphosis and monitor the effectiveness of targeted exercises and education to improve or maintain standing posture [5]. Since the time when that study was conducted, Dr. C. P. Recknor (internist and second author) developed the IONmed mobile phone application for standing posture assessment in order to facilitate the inclusion of this measurement in the clinical setting. This application utilizes the same measurement protocol as that used for the digital inclinometer in combination with an internal calibrated accelerometer system in the mobile phone. The software, which can be downloaded onto a mobile phone that uses either an Android or an Apple operating system, guides the user through the steps to acquire measures of standing posture which are displayed on the device and automatically recorded to a database file. It is expected that the measured spine curvature angles are consistent with those acquired using the digital inclinometer. Therefore, the purpose of this study was to determine the agreement between measures of standing posture obtained using the IONmed mobile phone application designed to assess sagittal spine curvatures in individuals at risk of osteoporotic fracture and a digital inclinometer, previously shown to have excellent test-retest reliability in this population [5].

2. Methods

2.1. Design. Testing was completed during a single visit at an outpatient osteoporosis clinic. All measures were collected by the same rater with seven years of experience using a digital inclinometer to assess standing posture in patients attending the clinic. A single measure of the lumbosacral angle (S), standing lumbar posture (L), and standing thoracic posture (T) was taken using the mobile phone application and duplicated immediately using the digital inclinometer following the same standardized procedure. The measurement protocol described in the Saunder's Digital Inclinometer User's Guide was followed. After removing their shoes and any bulky clothing, participants were instructed to stand erect and maintain their best posture throughout the procedure. The following three landmarks were palpated and the angle was measured: (1) at the sacral midpoint; (2) at the T12-L1 interspace; and (3) at the C7-T1 interspace. The sacral midpoint and the T12-L1 interspace were accessed through light clothing whereas the C7-T1 interspace was exposed. The study protocol was approved by the Northeast Georgia Health System Institutional Review Board. All participants provided written informed consent prior to participating.

2.2. Participants. Patients attending the outpatient osteoporosis clinic between March 2013 and May 2013 were invited to volunteer during their visit in response to a study advertisement posted in the waiting room.

2.3. Spine Curvature Measurements

2.3.1. Mobile Phone Application. The IONmed mobile phone application was downloaded onto an iPhone 5 from https://itunes.apple.com/us/app/spinecurve/id633986164?ls=1&mt=8. (Note that this application also is available for download to mobile phones using the Android operating system at: https://www.ionmed.us/ionmed/android.html.) The application was opened and the onscreen directions were followed. First, the flat surface of the top of the phone was placed against a flat vertical surface as indicated by an arrow on the mobile phone screen. The rater pressed the onscreen prompt to set the pitch to zero degrees. The rater placed the point of the arrow displayed on the mobile phone screen at the sacral midpoint and pressed the labelled bar to automatically record S and reset that angle to zero degrees. The point of the arrow displayed on the mobile phone screen was then placed at the T12-L1 interspace and the labelled bar was pressed to automatically record L and reset that angle to zero degrees. Finally, the point of the arrow displayed on the mobile phone screen was placed at the C7-T1 interspace and the labelled bar was pressed to automatically record T.

2.3.2. Digital Inclinometer. The digital inclinometer (Saunder's digital inclinometer, Empi Therapy Solutions) was placed against a flat vertical surface and the angle output was set to zero degrees. The inclinometer was initially placed at the sacral midpoint and the angle displayed on the digital screen was recorded as S. After recording the angle, the rater pressed the reset button to set that angle to zero degrees. The inclinometer was then positioned at the T12-L1 interspace. The rater recorded the angle displayed on the digital screen as L and pressed the reset button to zero the inclinometer at this

Table 1: Mean (SD) spine curvature angles measured, in degrees, using 2 different devices in 20 older adults standing with their best posture.

	IONmed mobile phone application	Digital inclinometer
Lumbosacral angle	16.2° (5.2)	16.6° (6.2)
Lumbar	32.3° (7.2)	32.8° (7.7)
Thoracic	53.3° (12.9)	53.2° (12.9)

angle. Finally, the rater positioned the inclinometer at the C7-T1 interspace and recorded the angle displayed on the digital screen as T.

2.4. Statistical Analysis. All statistical analyses were performed using SPSS release 20.0 software (SPSS Inc., Chicago, IL). We tested interdevice reliability of measures of S, L, and T with type 2,1 intraclass correlation coefficients (ICCs) [10], and the standard error of the measurement (SEM) which was calculated as the square root of the error variance [11]. Acceptable reliability was determined on the basis of a high ICC in combination with a low SEM. We also used Bland-Altman plots as this is the recommended statistical method for assessing the agreement between any two test methods that purport to measure the same property [12].

3. Results

The participants ($n = 20$, 18 women) were all Caucasian with an average age (SD) of 72.1 (9.8) years. One participant had osteopenia and 19 were diagnosed with osteoporosis, 11 of whom had a history of osteoporotic fracture. Table 1 summarizes the spine curve measures for this sample acquired using each of the two devices.

Interdevice reliability is high for all spine curve measures. ICC (95% CI) for S, L, and T is 0.97 (0.92, 0.99), 0.97 (0.92, 0.99), and 0.99 (0.98, 1.0), respectively. The SEM (95% CI) for S, L, and T is 0.99° (0.75, 1.44), 1.33° (1.01, 1.94), and 1.23° (0.94, 1.80), respectively.

The Bland-Altman plots shown in Figures 1(a)–1(c) illustrate the small measurement bias (varying from 0.1° for T to −0.55° for L). The largest limits of agreement are observed for L (−4.3°, 3.2°). Figure 1 confirms that no systematic differences in the spine angles measured using the two devices are observed as a function of the mean values.

4. Discussion

The purpose of this study was to determine the agreement between measures of standing posture obtained with a user-friendly mobile phone application designed to assess spine curvatures in people with low bone mass and a digital inclinometer, previously shown to have excellent test-retest reliability [5]. For our sample, excellent agreement between the measures of spine curvatures in standing was demonstrated by the high ICCs (≥0.97 with lower 95% confidence bound ≥ 0.92) and the low SEM. For example, we are 95% confident that the "true" value for T is somewhere between 0.94° lower and 1.8° higher than the single measured value obtained using either device. Bland-Altman plots confirm this with biases well within 1° and limits of agreement ≤ 7.5°. There are no apparent systematic errors in the measures obtained using the two devices. This work confirms that the dedicated mobile phone application offers an alternative method for measuring standing posture in older individuals with osteoporosis that is quick and convenient for those healthcare providers who already use information technology to facilitate their clinical practice.

According to the Saunder's Digital Inclinometer User's Guide, normal thoracic standing posture (kyphosis) is between 30° and 40°. Figure 1(c) confirms that only three participants in the current study had a "normal" kyphotic standing posture. There is no gold standard for diagnosing hyperkyphosis; however, 40° is also used as the threshold for classification based on the modified Cobb angle measured on standing lateral spine X-rays [13]. In this method, a goniometer is used to measure the angle at the intersection of lines drawn perpendicular to a line parallel to the superior border of T3 (or the most superior vertebral body border that can be observed) and a line drawn parallel to the inferior border of T12 identified on the radiograph [13]. In the Rancho Bernardo Study cohort of 553 men and 854 women 50 years of age or older recruited from the defined Southern California community, the majority of those over the age of 60 years had kyphotic angles (measured using the modified Cobb angle method) above 40° and mean values increased with age, particularly among those with osteoporotic vertebral fractures [14]. For the group of women 70 to 79 years, the mean kyphotic angle was 51° [14] which is comparable to the average value of 53° for our study sample having an average age of 72 years. The reliability and validity of measures of kyphosis obtained using two common nonradiologic methods, the flexicurve ruler and the Debrunner kyphometer, have been established through comparison with the modified Cobb angle [15]. Previously, generalizability theory was applied to show that single measures obtained using the digital inclinometer are highly reliable in postmenopausal women with one or more osteoporotic vertebral fractures [9]. Subsequently, MacIntyre et al. confirmed that test-retest reliability of single digital inclinometer measures of spine curvatures was high (ICC(SEM) = 0.91(2.5°), 0.90(2.9°), and 0.91(3.5°) for S, L, and T, resp.) [5]. Furthermore, measures of the lumbar lordosis and lumbosacral angle are obtained using this method thus providing important information about postural compensations employed by a person with hyperkyphosis to maintain a stable centre of mass and horizontal eye gaze shown to impact spine loads and fracture risk [4]. Thus, measures of kyphotic angle alone (Debrunner kyphometer) or kyphotic and lordotic indices only (flexicurve ruler) are likely to be inadequate in determining functional restrictions and fracture risk. It can be seen that the level of agreement between the measures obtained using two different devices in the current study is less than the error associated with duplicate measures taken using the digital inclinometer approximately nine days apart

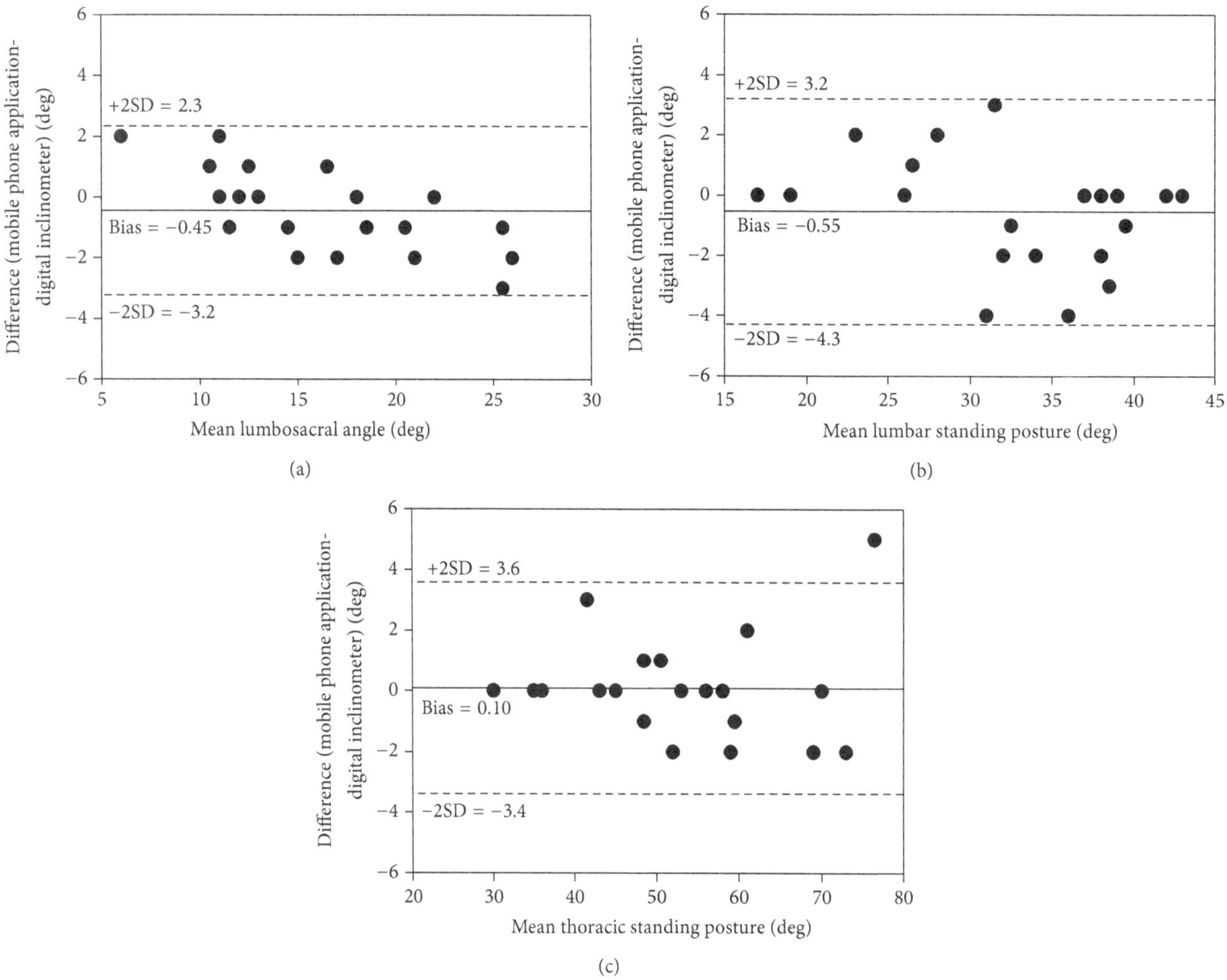

FIGURE 1: Difference in measures acquired using the IONmed mobile phone application and the digital inclinometer plotted as a function of the mean value for each of the 20 volunteers for (a) lumbosacral angle, (b) lumbar standing posture, and (c) thoracic standing posture. Dotted lines represent the 95% limits of agreement and solid lines represent the mean difference in measures (bias).

[5]. Therefore, either device provides quick and reliable values characterizing sagittal plane spine curvatures in standing.

In rehabilitation practice, it is important to have a time-efficient method for measuring standing posture in older adults in order to identify hyperkyphosis and associated compensations in the pelvis and lumbar spine indicative of the need for further assessment or to determine the effect of interventions directed at remediating associated impairments and activity limitations. If impairments that contribute to hyperkyphosis cannot be remediated, as in the case of a prevalent vertebral compression fracture, the effect of appropriate multimodel interventions (e.g., medications, body mechanics and posture reeducation, and modification of tasks) can be monitored by tracking stability of the hyperkyphosis. Other causes of age-related hyperkyphosis are modifiable with appropriate interventions. Postural training for hyperkyphotic women using exercises and education has been shown to reduce kyphosis [7, 16] and improve balance [7, 17, 18] and back extensor muscle strength [7, 16]. These outcomes are particularly important for people at risk of fall-related and vertebral osteoporotic fractures. Improvements in these physical function domains as well as less restrictions in ADLs were reported in a trial of 108 hyperkyphotic women with a recent osteoporotic spine fracture randomized to an experimental group who wore a type of biofeedback-based Spinomed orthosis two hours per day for at least six months compared to the wait list control group [19]. Of note, the postural training intervention must be active since passive treatment (taping versus sham taping or no taping) immediately reduced thoracic kyphosis in a group of women with osteoporotic vertebral fractures but did not improve balance or trunk muscle activation [20]. Based on the available evidence, it is recommended that rehabilitation management of people with osteoporosis include postural reeducation and back extensor strengthening [21, 22]. To evaluate the need for and response to these interventions in the clinical setting, it is critical to have a method that can provide estimates of spine curvatures that are quick and reliable.

We found a very high level of agreement in the estimates of S, L, and T obtained using the IONmed mobile phone application and the digital inclinometer in people attending an osteoporosis outpatient clinic. Although this method could be used to measure spine curvatures in people regardless of their bone health, it must be remembered that these results are context specific and different results may be obtained in a different patient group. Also, the assessor in this study had seven years of clinical experience using the digital inclinometer to measure standing posture in people at risk of osteoporotic fracture. The same protocol is used for the IONmed mobile phone application method. Different results may be obtained by assessors who have more or less experience using the digital inclinometer to measure spine curvatures. Therefore, others should establish the reliability of the values obtained in their particular clinical setting. We used the IONmed mobile phone application to take the first set of measures in all participants. Balancing the order in which the devices were used would have accounted for potential order effects such as fatigue or learning. However, the Bland-Altman plots confirm that the bias characterizing the difference between the measures obtained with these two devices was small and no systematic error was introduced as a result of this design.

5. Conclusions

In our study sample, we found that the IONmed mobile phone application produced estimates for thoracic standing posture, lumbar standing posture, and lumbosacral angle that closely agree with the estimates obtained using the digital inclinometer. The user-friendly application allows the clinician to complete the measurement protocol efficiently with prompts for next steps and automatic recording of measured values. For the growing number of healthcare providers using information technology to facilitate their clinical practice, this mobile phone application offers a quick, convenient method for routine assessment of sagittal spine curvatures.

Conflict of Interests

Chris P. Recknor invented the IONmed mobile phone application for measuring standing posture (patent pending).

Acknowledgments

The authors thank the participants who volunteered for this study and Kavin Sutton for collecting these data.

References

[1] T. Kobayashi, Y. Atsuta, T. Matsuno, and N. Takeda, "A longitudinal study of congruent sagittal spinal alignment in an adult cohort," *Spine*, vol. 29, no. 6, pp. 671–676, 2004.

[2] A. M. Briggs, J. H. Van Dieën, T. V. Wrigley et al., "Thoracic kyphosis affects spinal loads and trunk muscle force," *Physical Therapy*, vol. 87, no. 5, pp. 595–607, 2007.

[3] C. Roux, J. Fechtenbaum, S. Kolta, R. Said-Nahal, K. Briot, and C.-L. Benhamou, "Prospective assessment of thoracic kyphosis in postmenopausal women with osteoporosis," *Journal of Bone and Mineral Research*, vol. 25, no. 2, pp. 362–368, 2010.

[4] A. G. Bruno, D. E. Anderson, J. D'Agostino, and M. L. Bouxsein, "The effect of thoracic kyphosis and sagittal plane alignment on vertebral compressive loading," *Journal of Bone and Mineral Research*, vol. 27, pp. 2144–2151, 2012.

[5] N. J. MacIntyre, A. L. Lorbergs, and J. D. Adachi, "Inclinometer-based measures of standing posture in older adults with low bone mass are reliable and associated with self-reported, but not performance-based, physical function," *Osteoporosis International*, vol. 25, pp. 721–728, 2014.

[6] M. Sinaki, E. Itoi, J. W. Rogers, E. J. Bergstralh, and H. W. Wahner, "Correlation of back extensor strength with thoracic kyphosis and lumbar lordosis in estrogen-deficient women," *American Journal of Physical Medicine and Rehabilitation*, vol. 75, no. 5, pp. 370–374, 1996.

[7] W. B. Katzman, D. E. Sellmeyer, A. L. Stewart, L. Wanek, and K. A. Hamel, "Changes in flexed posture, musculoskeletal impairments, and physical performance after group exercise in community-dwelling older women," *Archives of Physical Medicine and Rehabilitation*, vol. 88, no. 2, pp. 192–199, 2007.

[8] M. Sinaki, E. Itoi, H. W. Wahner et al., "Stronger back muscles reduce the incidence of vertebral fractures: a prospective 10 year follow-up of postmenopausal women," *Bone*, vol. 30, no. 6, pp. 836–841, 2002.

[9] N. J. MacIntyre, L. Bennett, A. M. Bonnyman, and P. W. Stratford, "Optimizing reliability of digital inclinometer and flexicurve ruler measures of spine curvatures in postmenopausal women with osteoporosis of the spine: an illustration of the use of generalizability theory," *ISRN Rheumatology*, vol. 2011, Article ID 571698, 8 pages, 2011.

[10] P. E. Shrout and J. L. Fleiss, "Intraclass correlations: uses in assessing rater reliability," *Psychological Bulletin*, vol. 86, no. 2, pp. 420–428, 1979.

[11] P. W. Stratford, "Getting more from the literature: estimating the standard error of measurement for reliability studies," *Physiotherapy Canada*, vol. 56, pp. 27–30, 2004.

[12] J. M. Bland and D. G. Altman, "Statistical methods for assessing agreement between two methods of clinical measurement," *The Lancet*, vol. 1, no. 8476, pp. 307–310, 1986.

[13] G. J. Fon, M. J. Pitt, and A. C. Thies Jr., "Thoracic kyphosis: range in normal subjects," *American Journal of Roentgenology*, vol. 134, no. 5, pp. 979–983, 1980.

[14] D. L. Schneider, D. G. Von Mühlen, E. Barrett-Connor, and D. J. Sartoris, "Kyphosis does not equal vertebral fractures: the rancho bernardo study," *Journal of Rheumatology*, vol. 31, no. 4, pp. 747–752, 2004.

[15] G. A. Greendale, N. S. Nili, M.-H. Huang, L. Seeger, and A. S. Karlamangla, "The reliability and validity of three non-radiological measures of thoracic kyphosis and their relations to the standing radiological Cobb angle," *Osteoporosis International*, vol. 22, no. 6, pp. 1897–1905, 2011.

[16] E. Itoi and M. Sinaki, "Effect of back-strengthening exercise on posture in healthy women 49 to 65 years of age," *Mayo Clinic Proceedings*, vol. 69, no. 11, pp. 1054–1059, 1994.

[17] C. Cook, "The relationship between posture and balance disturbances in women with osteoporosis," *Physical and Occupational Therapy in Geriatrics*, vol. 20, no. 3-4, pp. 37–49, 2002.

[18] P. Suri, D. K. Kiely, S. G. Leveille, W. R. Frontera, and J. F. Bean, "Increased trunk extension endurance is associated

with meaningful improvement in balance among older adults with mobility problems," *Archives of Physical Medicine and Rehabilitation*, vol. 92, no. 7, pp. 1038–1043, 2011.

[19] M. Pfeifer, L. Kohlwey, B. Begerow, and H. W. Minne, "Effects of two newly developed spinal orthoses on trunk muscle strength, posture, and quality-of-life in women with postmenopausal osteoporosis: a randomized trial," *American Journal of Physical Medicine and Rehabilitation*, vol. 90, no. 10, pp. 805–815, 2011.

[20] A. M. Greig, K. L. Bennell, A. M. Briggs, and P. W. Hodges, "Postural taping decreases thoracic kyphosis but does not influence trunk muscle electromyographic activity or balance in women with osteoporosis," *Manual Therapy*, vol. 13, no. 3, pp. 249–257, 2008.

[21] F. J. Bonner Jr., M. Sinaki, M. Grabois et al., "Health professional's guide to rehabilitation of the patient with osteoporosis," *Osteoporosis International*, vol. 14, supplement 2, pp. S1–S22, 2003.

[22] L. M. Giangregorio, N. J. MacIntyre, L. Thabane, C. J. Skidmore, and A. Papaioannou, "Exercise for improving outcomes after osteoporotic vertebral fracture," *Cochrane Database of Systematic Reviews*, no. 7, Article ID CD008618, 2012.

3

Effect of Box Taping as an Adjunct to Stretching-Strengthening Exercise Program in Correction of Scapular Alignment in People with Forward Shoulder Posture: A Randomised Trial

Neha Dewan,[1] Kavitha Raja,[2] Ganesh Balthillaya Miyaru,[3] and Joy C. MacDermid[1,4]

[1] *School of Rehabilitation Sciences, McMaster University 1400, Main Street West, Hamilton, ON, Canada L8S 1C7*
[2] *JSS College of Physiotherapy, JSS Hospital Campus, Mysore, Karnataka 570004, India*
[3] *Department of Physiotherapy, Manipal College of Allied Health Sciences, Manipal University, Manipal, Karnataka 576104, India*
[4] *Hand and Upper Limb Centre, St. Joseph's Health Centre, London, ON, Canada N6A 4L6*

Correspondence should be addressed to Neha Dewan; dewann@mcmaster.ca

Academic Editors: B. Kuran and K. Masani

Objective. The objective of this study was to provide preliminary estimates of effects of box taping as an adjunct to stretching-strengthening exercise program on scapular alignment in healthy subjects with forward shoulder posture (FSP). *Methods.* Sixty subjects were screened and 38 asymptomatic subjects with FSP were allocated into box taping and standard treatment group using block randomization. Both groups received a supervised stretching-strengthening exercise program and postural advice for 15 sessions over 3 weeks. In addition, box taping was applied to the intervention group. Static and dynamic scapular alignment was recorded at baseline, 7th and 15th sessions. Differences over time and between the treatment groups were determined using repeated measures of analysis of variance (ANOVA). *Results.* Twenty subjects completed the study. Both interventions were well tolerated and resulted in improvements in static and dynamic postural indicators over time in both groups ($P < 0.05$) except for dynamic scapular alignment by the 15th session. We were under powered to detect differences between the groups ($P < 0.05$). *Conclusions.* This study suggests postural exercises improve scapular alignment; but a large RCT is required to determine whether the addition of box taping is indicated, and whether this preventative approach reduces the incidence of upper quarter musculoskeletal disorders. This trial is registered with CTRI/2013/10/004095.

1. Introduction

Patients referred to physical therapy with impaired upper extremity function, often exhibit postural alterations [1]. Forward shoulders is a common maladaptive posture which occurs in up to 73% of the group of healthy subjects between the ages of 20 and 50 years [2, 3]. Kendall et al. described forward shoulders as abduction and elevation of the scapula and a forward position of the shoulders, giving an appearance of a hollow chest [4, 5]. Forward Shoulder Posture (FSP) is characterized by a protracted, downwardly rotated, and anteriorly tipped scapula position with increased cervical lordosis and upper thoracic kyphosis [6]. This pattern may be associated with tightness of serratus anterior, pectoralis minor, pectoralis major and upper trapezius muscle, and weakness of middle and lower trapezius [3]. The imbalance in muscle function is believed to result in reduction of amplitude in posterior tilting and lateral rotation of the scapula during arm elevation [7–9]. The literature has shown that altered scapular kinematics and associated muscle imbalance in FSP places the anterior acromion in close proximity to rotator cuff tendon and increase the potential for subacromial impingement [3, 8, 10–12].

FSP and associated muscle imbalance is one of the factors contributing to episodes of head, neck, and shoulder pain [3, 13, 14] and multiple upper quarter dysfunctions such as bicipital tendinitis [15], thoracic outlet syndrome [16], painful trigger areas [17], and neuropathies [18]. Since few prospective studies have included patients prior to development of these disorders, cause-and-effect has not been clearly established [3]. However, there is an assumption that this association does indicate that FSP is a maladaptive posture that warrants correction.

Many shoulder rehabilitation programs emphasize scapular muscle control [19–21] which indicates that despite limitations in evidence on causal relationship, there is clinical application of the association between scapular malalignment and shoulder pathology [19–25]. Additionally, there are few studies supporting the evidence that changing posture influences impairment [26–28]. Previous researchers have described exercise programs focused on stretching and strengthening exercises to correct the altered posture [13, 29–35]. Few of these studies specifically deal with subjects having shoulder pathology [27] or swimmers [13, 34]. There is a dearth of the literature concerning correction of FSP as a preventive measure against upper quarter dysfunction. Preliminary studies demonstrated that strengthening of the posterior scapular stabilizers combined with stretching of the pectoral muscles given over a period of six weeks can result in improved muscle strength, produce a more erect upper trunk posture, increase scapular stability, and alter scapulohumeral rhythm in healthy subjects [32, 33]. These studies indicated that there was significant change in dynamic position of scapula, but no change in resting position of scapula. A recent scoping review has well recognized the effectiveness of stretching and strengthening of scapular abductors and adductors, respectively, or a combination of both on the resting position of scapula in people with forward shoulder posture [30]. The authors make definite conclusions about relationship between scapular muscle strength and resting position of scapula due to weaknesses in study design. In particular, the review noted that the techniques used to determine the resting position of scapula had questionable validity.

Taping is believed to affect the resting position of the scapula and assist in maintaining the proximal shoulder-girdle stability necessary to perform elevation of the arm [35]. With the tape holding the scapula in a more proper alignment, the patient can then use the shoulder without further reduction of the space between the acromion and humeral head [36]. Additionally, the tape provides a feedback mechanism allowing the patient to feel normal alignment and positioning of the shoulder complex. The two most frequently proposed mechanisms of taping are proprioceptive and mechanical [37]. The benefits of taping are still under contention. However, it is still widely accepted in clinical practice that taping is a useful treatment modality [38–40]. The clinical application of scapular taping has been supported in one case reports [36], one cross over study [41] done with a wash-out period of one hour, one double blinded randomised controlled trial [42], and a recent pilot randomised control trial [39] in which taping was one component of treatment provided to patients with shoulder pain. Over the past decade, taping has been proven to be an effective adjunct in reducing pain, improving proprioception and muscle recruitment pattern, and assists in motor control and function in special populations such as swimmers and violinists with FSP [43, 44]. Although taping is used for the correction of postural abnormalities and many studies are available regarding beneficial effects of taping in symptomatic and specific group of population, nevertheless, there is lack of evidence for its use in clinical practice for upper quarter postural correction in healthy subjects who are at risk of musculoskeletal disorders due to altered posture.

Box Taping is one of the scapular taping techniques explained to correct the scapular position [45]. To our knowledge, this is the first study done to determine additive effects of scapular taping in correction of both static and dynamic scapular alignment over a period of 3 weeks. The objective of this study is to provide preliminary estimates of effects of box taping as an adjunct to stretching-strengthening exercise program on scapular alignment in healthy subjects with forward shoulder posture.

2. Material and Methods

2.1. Prestudy to Establish Cut Offs for Normalized Scapular Abduction Ratio. Normalised scapular abduction ratio (NSA ratio) is considered as one of the reliable measures for scapular position [46] and can be used to discriminate between normal and abnormal scapular mechanics. However, there is no existing data for NSA ratio in Indian population who were the target audience for this study. Data for NSA ratio were collected from participants who had bilateral FSP on visual estimation ($n = 10$). This was to determine an objective cut off point for NSA ratio to include participants in our study.

FSP on visual estimation is decided if any one of the following findings were present [4, 5]:

(i) medial borders of scapula were not parallel to each other;

(ii) anterior shoulder point was anterior to sternal notch/hollowing of the chest present.

The mean NSA ratio in this group was 1.60 which was in close approximation with the mean NSA ratio seen in population from the United States [47, 48]. The group inclusion cut point values for our study were then set at ≥ mean NSA ratio of pilot sample.

2.2. Study Design and Participants. A randomised control trial (RCT) design was used in this study. A NSA ratio on measurement set at ≥1.60 was used as a criterion to define FSP. A convenient sample of 60 healthy participants was screened for FSP among graduate and postgraduate students from various departments of Manipal University. Thirty-eight healthy volunteers with FSP, aged between 18–35 years were included. Participants were excluded if they were symptomatic, had any neurological deficit in upper extremity, or any surgical intervention affecting the thorax and scapula.

All participants who fulfilled screening and eligibility criteria were informed about the study and written informed consent was taken before starting the procedure. The study was approved by institutional research committee of Manipal college of Allied Health Sciences.

2.3. Outcome Measures. Recording of static and dynamic scapular alignment measures was performed bilaterally by

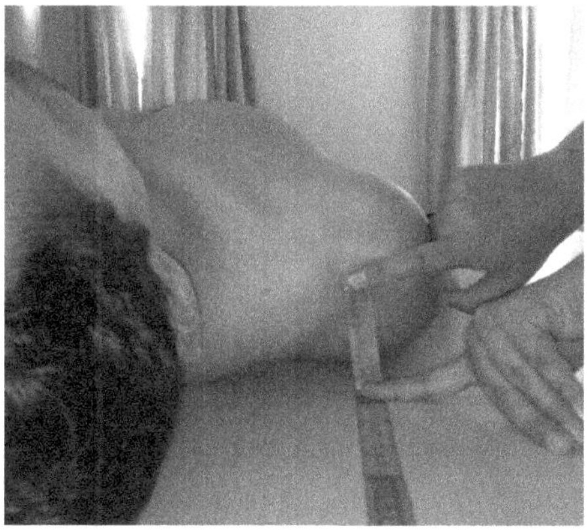

FIGURE 1: Acromial distance: distance between the posterior border of acromion and table surface.

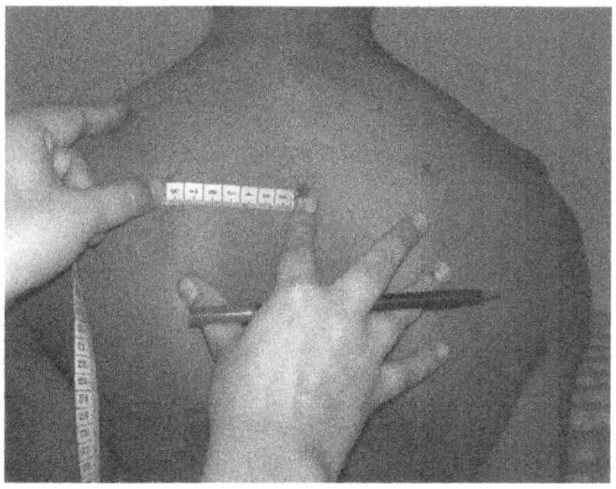

FIGURE 2: T 3 distance: horizontal distance from the third thoracic spinous process to the corresponding point on medial border of the scapula.

the primary investigator. All measurements were taken with measuring tape in centimetres.

For static scapular alignment, three tests were used [49] as follows.

(1) Acromial distance [49–53]: with the participants in supine lying, the distance between the posterior border of acromion and table was measured (Figure 1).

(2) T 3 distance [3, 49, 54]: this test was performed in standing position with the participant instructed to stay relaxed. The measurement of horizontal distance from the third thoracic spinous process to the corresponding point on medial border of the scapula was measured (Figure 2).

(3) Normalised scapular abduction ratio (NSA ratio) [46, 47]: NSA ratio was calculated by dividing the total scapular distance by length of scapula. Total scapular distance is the linear distance from the third thoracic vertebra to inferior angle of acromion. Length of scapula is distance from inferior angle of acromion to root of spine of scapula. The participants stood in relaxed position. Both total scapular distance and length of scapula was measured and NSA ratio was calculated (Figure 3).

For Dynamic scapular alignment: lateral scapular slide test (LSST) was done [46, 51, 53]. The participant stood in relaxed position and measurements were taken from inferior angle of scapula to 7th thoracic spinous process with the participant's arm in 3 different positions at 0 degree (arms relaxed on the sides), 45 degree (hands supported on hip and web space on iliac crest), and 90 degrees (with glenohumeral internal rotation) of abduction (Figure 4).

2.4. Randomisation and Group Allocation. The potential participants were contacted telephonically and were offered an appointment for a baseline assessment. After baseline measurements, participants were randomly assigned by the primary investigator to either of the box taping (n = 20) or standard treatment group (n = 18) using block allocation of 1 : 1. Each block consisted of 4 participants. The primary investigator, a trained physiotherapist who is the primary

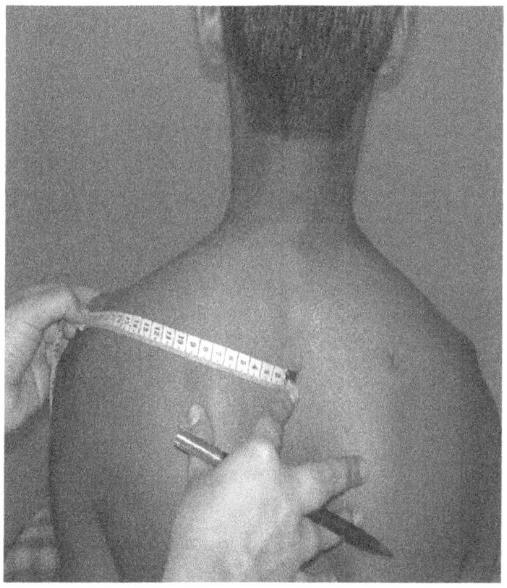

(a)

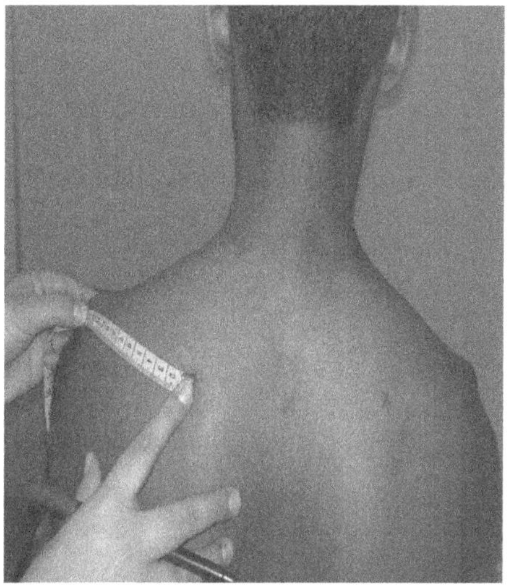

(b)

FIGURE 3: NSA ratio: distance from posterolateral angle of acromion to thoracic spine process, (T 3): distance from posterolateral angle of acromion to root of spine of scapula.

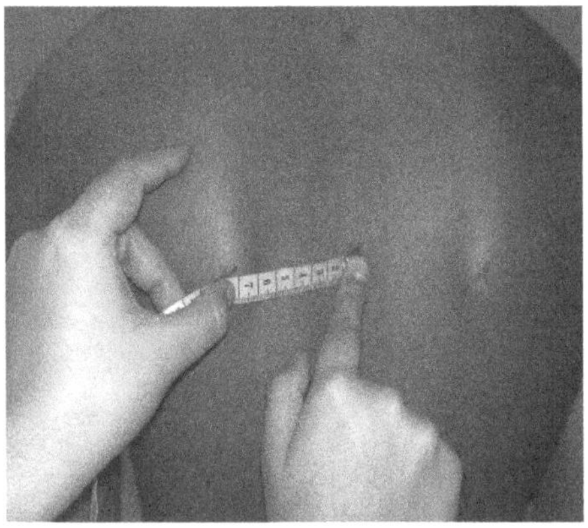

Figure 4: Lateral scapular slide test (LSST): distance from inferior angle of scapula to 7th thoracic spinous process.

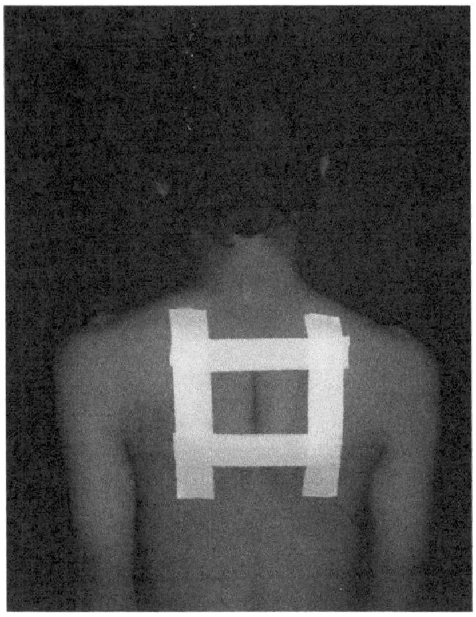

Figure 5: Box taping technique.

author of this paper provided all treatment to both the groups and was not blinded to group allocation.

2.5. Intervention. The standard treatment program consisted of stretching-strengthening exercises and mobilization to counteract the muscle imbalances and joint restrictions that may be associated with FSP. The supervised stretching-strengthening exercise program (Box 1) consisted of passive stretching of tight anterior shoulder girdle muscles (pectoralis minor, pectoralis major, and upper trapezius), strengthening exercises using theraband for posterior scapular muscles (rhomboids, middle, and lower trapezius), and glenohumeral external rotators (infraspinatus and teres minor), thoracic spine mobilization exercise, and strengthening of upper back musculature to maintain proper head position and erect spinal curvature (as forward shoulder posture is found to be associated with forward head posture and thoracic kyphosis [6]). The exercise treatment of approximately 20 minute duration and postural advice to maintain correct shoulder posture were given to both groups. One of the two treatment groups received box taping as an additional intervention to maintain normal scapular alignment. Taping was applied as per guidelines given by Morrissey [55]. Both groups received treatment for 15 sessions over a period of 3 weeks. Subjects were instructed to maintain the tape for about 4 hours/session. Outcome measures for scapular alignment were taken pretreatment and repeated after the 7th and 15th treatment sessions.

At the first session of the exercise program, the participants were introduced to the different levels of theraband (Hygenic Corp). The participants began exercises using the yellow nonlatex band at mild tension. The subjects were progressed to the next colour resistive band when they were able to perform required repetitions (Box 1), each with 10 seconds of hold without significant fatigue in the sequence: yellow, red, green, blue, and black. These exercises were individually adjusted and were progressed with higher level theraband and repetitions at the physiotherapist visits during the whole rehabilitation period.

Taping technique used was box taping [45]. Taping material used was non elastic leukotape. Participants were instructed to fully retract and depress their scapula. Two horizontal strips of tape were used to draw the medial border of scapulae together and two vertical strips were used to facilitate thoracic extension. One horizontal strip extended from superior angles of one scapula to superior angle of other scapula and other horizontal strip extended from inferior angle of one scapula to inferior angle of other scapula. The vertical strips overlapped the horizontal strips (Figure 5).

2.6. Statistical Analysis. Descriptive statistics (mean, SD) were computed for each study variable. Data was tested for normality and parametric tests were used for statistical analysis using SPSS version 18.0. The statistical significance was set at alpha < 0.05 at 95% confidence interval. Our study has investigated the effect of intervention on each variable on both sides at 3 different sessions. Each of these variables were analyzed using repeated measures of analysis of variance (ANOVA) with time as within-participant factor at 3 levels (baseline, 7th and 15th session) and group as between participant factor. Mauchly's test of sphericity was used to test homogeneity of variance. In case of significant Mauchly test results for sphericity, Greenhouse-Geisser correction was applied to adjust the tests, as recommended by Portney and Watkins [56]. Where indicated, post hoc multiple pairwise comparisons with Bonferroni correction were used.

3. Results

Nine participants dropped out from both the box taping and standard treatment group, leaving 20 patients for analysis. The groups were comparable before treatment (Table 1). The groups were also similar with respect to scapular alignment at the baseline (Table 2). The CONSORT diagram describing participant recruitment and retention is shown in Figure 6.

At 5% level of significance, ANOVA results revealed that there was a statistically significant improvement for two

Comprehensive exercise treatment program

(i) Stretching of tight anterior shoulder muscles (passive stretching)

Pectoralis minor/major, upper trapezius

1st 5 sessions—5 stretches, each with 30 seconds of hold

Next 10 sessions—10 stretches, each with 30 seconds of hold

(ii) Strengthening exercises for posterior scapular muscles and glenohumeral external rotators with therabands

Posterior scapular muscles—rhomboids, middle and lower trapezius

Glenohumeral external rotators—infraspinatus and teres minor

1st 5 sessions—5 repetition, each with 10 seconds of hold

Next 5 sessions—10 repetition, each with 10 seconds of hold

Last 5 sessions—15 repetition, each with 10 seconds of hold

(iii) Thoracic spine mobilization exercises

Subject was made to lie down supine on a wedge placed at the level of maximum thoracic kyphosis for 5 minutes

(iv) Strengthening of upper back musculature

Subject was made to lie down on a pillow under the chest in prone lying and was instructed to straighten the upper back

1st 5 sessions—5 repetition, each with a hold 10 seconds

Next 10 sessions—10 repetition, each with a hold of 10 seconds

Box 1

Table 1: Characteristics of participants ($N = 20$).

Characteristic	Experiment group ($n = 11$) Mean ± SD	Control group ($n = 9$) Mean ± SD	P value
Age (years)	21.64 ± 1.85	20.44 ± .52	0.06
Weight (kg)	61.63 ± 9.9	61.77 ± 10.8	0.97
Height (cms)	162 ± 6.4	159 ± 5.11	0.30
Male (n)	5	3	
Females (n)	6	6	

of the variables of static scapular alignment that is, NSA ratio (right side) and acromial distance (both sides), but no significant improvement in variables of dynamic scapular alignment in participants of box-taping group (Table 3). Contrarily, in the standard treatment group, statistically significant improvement ($P < 0.05$) was seen only in the NSA ratio bilaterally (Table 4). Over a period of 3 weeks, there was no statistically significant difference between the two groups for any of the static or dynamic scapular alignment variable as the observed P value was more than 0.05. Although, difference between two groups was not statistically significant, the following trend has been seen in measurements for static and dynamic scapular alignment.

3.1. Static Scapular Alignment. Following commencement of treatment, both groups showed improvement (decrease) in NSA ratio, acromial distance, and T 3 distance bilaterally (Tables 3 and 4). However, acromial distance on both sides improved more in taped group than in standard treatment group (Figure 7). Similarly, in post hoc analysis, pair wise comparison indicated that NSA ratio (right side) and acromial distance (both sides) have shown statistically significant

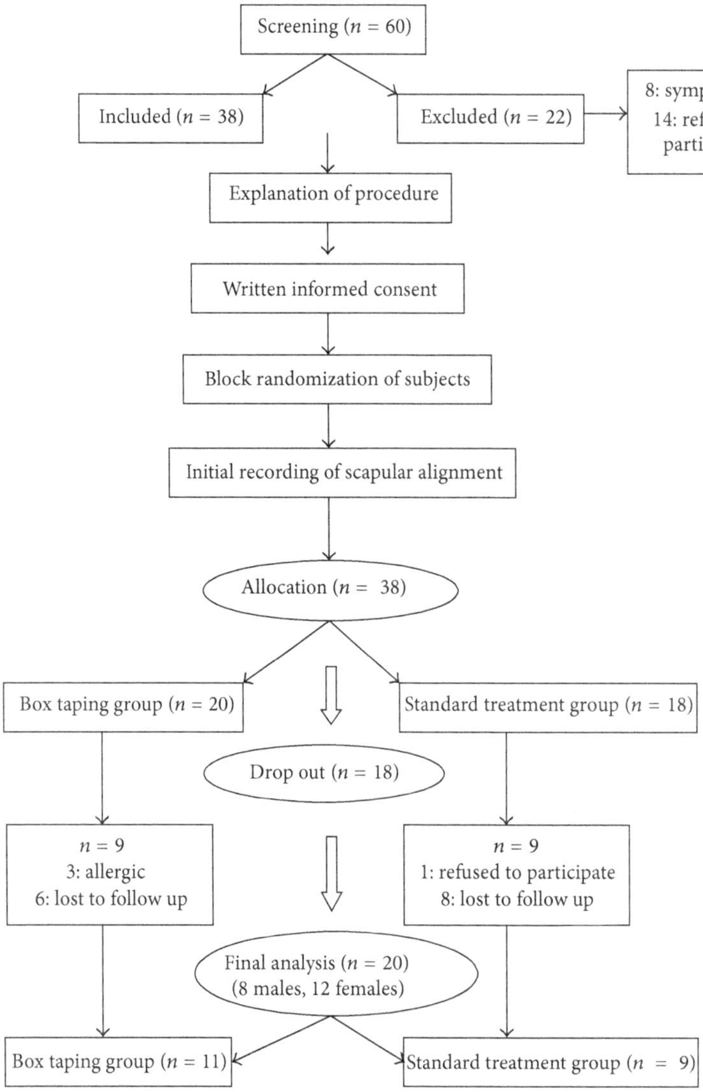

Figure 6: CONSORT diagram describing participant recruitment and retention.

Table 2: Mean difference [95% CI] between two groups at baseline ($n = 20$).

Variable	Left		Right	
	Mean difference [95% CI]	*P* value	Mean difference [95% CI]	*P* value
		Static scapular alignment		
NSA ratio	−0.03 [−0.14, 0.08]	0.59	0.01 [−0.07, 0.10]	0.66
Acromial distance (cm)	1.20 [−0.18, 2.60]	0.08	0.62 [−0.57, 1.81]	0.28
T 3 distance (cm)	0.13 [−0.85, 1.12]	0.78	0.47 [0.50, 1.45]	0.32
		Dynamic scapular alignment (LSST)		
0 degree	0.02 [−1.18, 1.22]	0.97	−0.04 [−1.2, 1.12]	0.94
45 degree	0.44 [−1.85, 0.95]	0.50	0.03 [−1.39, 1.45]	0.96
90 degree	0.15 [−2.00, 1.69]	0.86	0.15 [−2.00,1.69]	0.86

NSA ratio: normalised scapular abduction ratio.
T 3 distance: distance from medial scapular border to 3rd thoracic spine.
LSST: Lateral Scapular Slide Test.

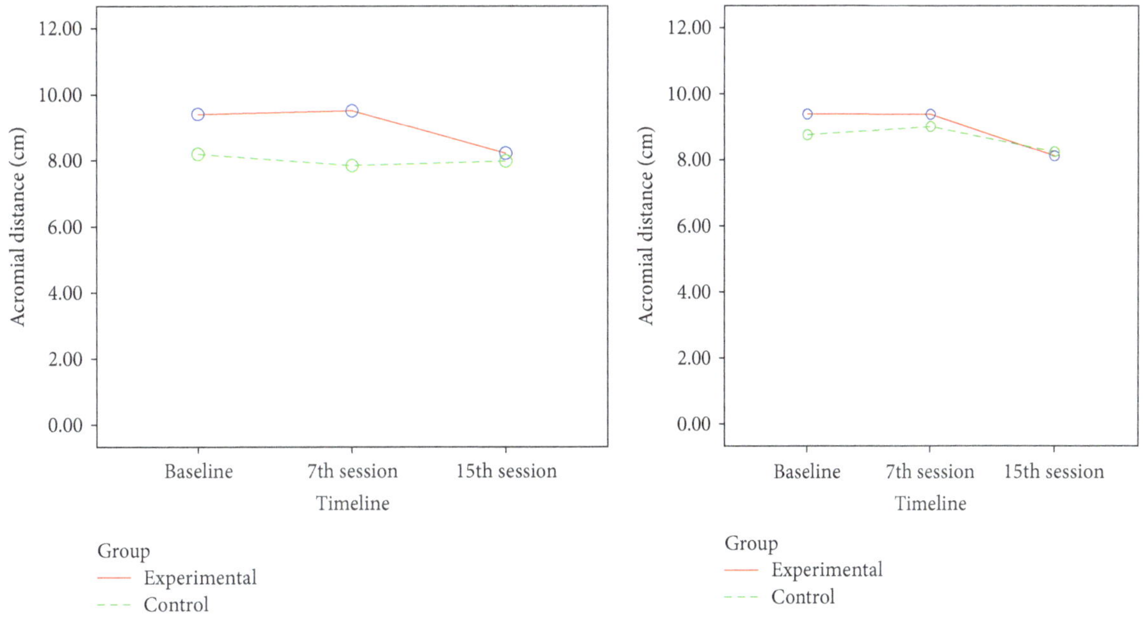

FIGURE 7: Changes in acromial distance: left and righ at baseline (1), 7th session (2), and 15th (3) session.

TABLE 3: Scapular alignment measurements of the Experimental group (mean ± SD) $n = 11$.

Variable	Left			Right		
	Baseline	7th session	15th session	Baseline	7th session	15th session
			Static scapular alignment			
NSA ratio	1.56 ± .15	1.51 ± .12	1.47 ± .07	1.67 ± .10	*1.56 ± .08	†‡1.50 ± .08
Acromial distance (cm)	9.40 ± 1.53	9.51 ± 1.25	†‡8.22 ± 1.32	9.40 ± 1.23	9.39 ± 1.23	†‡8.12 ± 1.46
T 3 distance (cm)	6.30 ± 1.06	6.63 ± 1.36	5.80 ± 1.24	6.86 ± 1.00	6.66 ± 1.09	6.22 ± 1.05
			Dynamic scapular alignment (LSST)			
0 degree	7.90 ± 1.02	8.02 ± 1.09	8.18 ± 1.32	7.68 ± 1.16	8.11 ± .93	8.18 ± 1.36
45 degree	7.77 ± 1.29	8.09 ± 1.64	8.40 ± 1.46	7.86 ± 1.45	8.22 ± 1.57	8.20 ± 1.26
90 degree	8.45 ± 2.09	8.59 ± .76	8.54 ± 1.09	8.54 ± 2.30	8.63 ± 1.05	8.50 ± 1.13

* *P* value significant between baseline and 7th session.
† *P* value significant between 7th and 15th session.
‡ *P* value significant bet baseline and 15th session.
NSA ratio: normalised scapular abduction ratio.
T3 distance: distance from medial scapular border to 3rd thoracic spine.
LSST: Lateral Scapular Slide Test.

decrease and hence improved in box taping group from baseline to last session (Table 3) (Figure 7).

3.2. Dynamic Scapular Alignment. Following commencement of treatment, there is no regular trend towards improvement in distances for LSST at 0 deg, 45 deg, and 90 deg (both sides) in both the groups which could be the reason for no statistical significant difference between as well as within the two groups (Tables 3 and 4).

4. Discussion

Optimal posture provides both mechanical and functional benefits [57]. If body segments are held out of alignment for prolonged periods of time, the soft tissues become shortened or lengthened [14] which inevitably results in altered optimal joint range, force production, and the efficiency of movement. Poor scapular posture and muscle imbalance has been postulated as a mechanism in pathogenesis of various upper quarter dysfunctions. The aim of many conservative rehabilitation programs is to correct posture and muscle imbalance using muscle strengthening, muscle stretching, taping, and joint mobilization techniques [13, 31, 42]. The evidence to support the efficacy of these clinical practices is limited. The application of taping has been hypothesized for many therapeutic reasons such as muscle recruitment [44, 58–60], proprioception [55], pain relief [39, 42, 61], and improvement of function [61] and it was thought to be necessary to demonstrate that one of the effects of taping, as used in this study, is to elicit a change in the static and dynamic posture of the subjects.

Table 4: Scapular alignment measurements of the control group (mean ± SD) $n = 9$.

Variable	Left			Right		
	Baseline	7th session	15th session	Baseline	7th session	15th session
			Static scapular alignment			
NSA ratio	1.59 ± .07	*1.49 ± .08	‡1.47 ± .09	1.65 ± .08	*1.53 ± .08	†‡1.45 ± .08
Acromial distance	8.20 ± 1.40	7.85 ± 2.75	7.98 ± 1.21	8.77 ± 1.30	9.02 ± 1.27	8.25 ± 1.04
T 3 distance (cm)	8.61 ± 1.78	5.77 ± .83	8.33 ± 1.25	8.16 ± 1.58	5.68 ± .80	8.49 ± 1.30
			Dynamic scapular alignment (LSST)			
0 degree	7.88 ± 1.53	7.22 ± 1.60	7.66 ± 1.27	7.72 ± 1.30	7.30 ± 1.43	7.83 ± 1.25
45 degree	8.22 ± 1.69	7.55 ± 1.64	7.61 ± 1.61	7.83 ± 1.58	6.74 ± 2.72	†7.77 ± 1.60
90 degree	8.61 ± 1.78	7.61 ± 1.49	8.33 ± 1.25	8.16 ± 1.58	7.42 ± 1.57	8.49 ± 1.30

*P value significant between baseline and 7th session.
†P value significant between 7th and 15th session.
‡P value significant between baseline and 15th session.
NSA ratio: normalised scapular abduction ratio.
T 3 distance: distance from medial scapular border to 3rd thoracic spine.
LSST: Lateral Scapular Slide Test.

4.1. Static Scapular Alignment. In our study, although we were underpowered to detect significant differences between the two groups at $P < 0.05$, participants of both groups have shown statistically significant change in acromial distance and NSA ratio. Acromial distance is one of the reliable outcome measures for measuring static scapular alignment specifically in healthy forward shoulder posture [53] and has shown a stronger trend towards improvement in box taping group than in standard treatment group (Figure 7). This change in postural measurement can be attributed to a change in static posture of the subject, produced by the subject and further maintained by the tape.

Changes observed in static scapular alignment in our study are similar to results found in a cross-over study done by Lewis et al. [41] where the changes observed were within the wash-out period of one hour and the author recommended future studies to see the long-term effects of scapular taping. In comparison, 15 sessions of taping were given in our study with the tape being applied for 4 hrs/session, which might have resulted in greater correction. This is in accordance with Hall who suggested that up to two or three weeks of scapula taping may be necessary to improve neuromuscular control [62]. The results of our study showing improvement in static scapular alignment were also seen in a study done on effect of stretching and strengthening exercises given for six weeks in competitive swimmers with FSP [44].

The improvement in static scapular alignment was observed in all 20 subjects irrespective of the group in our study which is contradictory to previous studies where 6 weeks (3 times/week) of scapular muscle stretching-strengthening exercises did not find any improvement in static scapular alignment in FSP population [32, 33]. Factors which may have contributed to improvements in this study are the multimodal treatment which included strengthening of upper back musculature and thoracic spine mobilization in addition to scapular muscle stretching-strengthening exercises. Over and above, passive stretches were given with a hold of 30 seconds which is more intensive and preferable to previous studies [33] where stretches were given with only 10 seconds of hold.

4.2. Dynamic Scapular Alignment. The literature has shown that a minimum of six weeks of exercise is needed to show statistically significant strength gains [32, 33, 44]. For improvement in dynamic scapular alignment, the scapular muscles must be strong enough to stabilize scapula on the thorax and must have sufficient motor control to optimize the goal of dynamic stability. Reinforcing coordinated glenohumeral motion should help to improve altered scapulohumeral rhythm. The lack of improvement in dynamic scapular alignment in our study indicates that the exercise programme, though vigorous and supervised and given over a period of three weeks, was insufficient in comparison to unsupervised moderate intensity exercise programme given for six weeks [32, 33]. This highlights that while dosing exercise, we must consider the type, supervision, frequency, and duration of exercise.

The assumption is that taping provides biofeedback and mechanical support for optimal shoulder position. Both the type and duration of biofeedback for optimal posture from taping are different than that provided by advice and exercise. Greater duration of feedback from application of taping should have potential beneficial effect allowing adaptation of neural pathways by consistent correct proprioceptive feedback [63–65]. However, it is possible with repeated applications of scapula taping that the habituation to the feedback from tape may reduce the effectiveness of the feedback. Since increasing the tonic muscle action directed at optimal posture may be a goal of the intervention, then it is important to know whether taping facilitates or inhibits muscle activity in the longer term.

Furthermore, no statistically significant change is observed even when taping was used as an adjunct over a duration of three weeks in overall subject population. This is in support with the literature which has proved that at least 12 weeks of taping may be necessary to affect muscle tension properties in comparison to three weeks of treatment used in the present study [62]. We have used non elastic leukotape for scapular taping. However, other types of taping include kinesiotaping which may have different effects on muscle activity. Future studies with longer duration of high quality tape are needed to see long term effects of box-taping on dynamic scapular alignment.

We conducted measurements of both shoulders in our study. The process revealed interesting data showing more improvement on right side which could be related to hand dominance as all 20 subjects included in the study were right handed or could be due to the fact that subjects included in the study were fourteen right sided, two left sided, and four bilateral FSP subjects. This is a different approach from previous research involving shoulder measurements to evaluate posture, which typically evaluated only one shoulder on each subject, usually the right shoulder [33, 34].

Although this study suggests that the exercise and postural advice program was beneficial in improving posture in the healthy populations who were perceived to be at risk for musculoskeletal problems due to FSP. However, there are a number of limitations that should be considered as limiting our confidence in these findings or their readiness for implementation. There were substantial designs flaws since the trial did not have concealment of treatment allocation, or blinded outcome evaluation. Since blinding of patients was not possible, it would have been preferable if a blinded evaluator had been used to measure the outcomes. However, the measures were at different time points and the treating therapist was unaware of the previous scores. Further, it is unlikely that the treating therapist would have influenced measures like dynamic posture. This potentially reduces the impact of observer bias. There is a need for more research establishing reliable and valid outcome measures for scapular assessment in FSP population.

From an implementation perspective, there were additional concerns which were reflected in a high drop-out rate. Reasons for discontinuing the treatment included allergic reactions with use of leukotape and lack of interest in continuing. The motivation to adhere to treatments that are preventative may be more challenging than those provided to reduce symptoms as the motivation may be low. Finally, since this study recruited a small healthy sample of convenience derived from a single university campus, this precludes generalization of the results beyond the sample population. However, the rate of FSP was high as 50% of those who were screened had FSP. Given that the activities of students involve a lot of sitting, computer work, reading, and so forth they may be considered a young at-risk population and an appropriate target for prevention. Since symptoms may take time to develop, a young population may not have experienced the adverse impacts of this posture. Future studies should focus on populations with higher risk for FSP associated with symptoms such as workers with higher risk occupations, or include a greater education component to explain why prevention is important in asymptomatic groups. Future studies should include measures of adherence, measure reasons for discontinuance, and should include comprehensive outcome assessment measured by a blinded assessor. Importantly, since the link between FSP and future musculoskeletal disorders is tentative, only longer term longitudinal studies will determine whether prevention programs that focus on FSP correction reduce the occurrence, disability, and time lost from work from musculoskeletal disorders.

Implications of the present study are as follows.

(i) Supervised stretching-strengthening exercise program alone or in combination with box-taping were well tolerated in healthy forward shoulder posture subjects for correction of scapular alignment; but adherence may be challenging in asymptomatic young individuals.

(ii) Supervised stretching-strengthening exercise program was effective ($P < 0.05$) in correcting scapular alignment in asymptomatic students presenting with FSP. Thus, supervised stretching-strengthening exercise program may be a useful preventive measure in reducing FSP which is considered an etiological factor in development of upper quarter musculoskeletal disorders.

5. Conclusions

Supervised stretching-strengthening exercise program with or without box-taping resulted in improvement in posture in healthy forward shoulder posture population. There were no significant additive effects of box taping.

Ethical Approval

The research study is approved by institutional review committee of Manipal College of Allied Health Sciences (MCOAHS) towards postgraduation in orthopaedic physical therapy dissertation.

Disclosure

The authors declare that there are no financial gains from the content of this research paper. (i) The research paper is presented as a paper at 9th Triennial Congress of International Federation of Societies for Hand Therapists (IFSHT) and 12th International federation of Societies for Hand Surgeons (IFSSH), New Delhi, India (2013, March 5). (ii) The research paper is presented as a poster at CPA Congress, Montreal (2013, May 25).

Conflict of Interests

The authors declare that they have no conflict of interests.

Acknowledgments

Neha Dewan is supported in part by the Joint Motion Program: "A CIHR Training Program in Musculoskeletal Health Research and Leadership." Dr. Joy C. MacDermid is supported by a CIHR Chair: Gender in Measurement and Rehabilitation of Musculoskeletal Work Disability. The authors would like to thank Dr. Shreemathi Mayya, Mr. Binukumar B, Mr. Jayakrishnan Nair, School of Rehabilitation Sciences graduate students whose advice, at times when needed, contributed a lot for the completion of this paper.

References

[1] Johnson and Borstad, "Project title: Forward shoulder asymmetry: prevalence and pathology," http://www.docstoc.com/docs/103976375/Forward-Shoulder-Asymmetry.

[2] P. Griegel-Morris, K. Larson, K. Mueller-Klaus, and C. A. Oatis, "Incidence of common postural abnormalities in the cervical, shoulder, and thoracic regions and their association with pain in two age groups of healthy subjects," *Physical Therapy*, vol. 72, no. 6, pp. 425–431, 1992.

[3] D. E. Peterson, K. R. Blankenship, J. B. Robb et al., "Investigation of the validity and reliability of four objective techniques for measuring forward shoulder posture," *Journal of Orthopaedic and Sports Physical Therapy*, vol. 25, no. 1, pp. 34–42, 1997.

[4] F. P. Kendall, E. K. McCreary, and P. G. Provance, *Muscles Testing and Function with Posture and Pain*, Lippincott Williams and Wilkins, Baltimore, Md, USA, 4th edition, 2005.

[5] H. O. Kendall, F. P. Kendall, and D. A. Boynton, *Posture and Pain*, Edited by E. Robert, Krieger Publishing Company, Huntington, NY, USA, 1970.

[6] C. K. Wong, D. Coleman, V. diPersia, J. Song, and D. Wright, "The effects of manual treatment on rounded-shoulder posture, and associated muscle strength," *Journal of Bodywork and Movement Therapies*, vol. 14, no. 4, pp. 326–333, 2010.

[7] P. M. Ludewig and J. D. Borstad, "Effects of a home exercise programme on shoulder pain and functional status in construction workers," *Occupational and Environmental Medicine*, vol. 60, no. 11, pp. 841–849, 2003.

[8] P. M. Ludewig and T. M. Cook, "Alterations in shoulder kinematics and associated muscle activity in people with symptoms of shoulder impingement," *Physical Therapy*, vol. 80, no. 3, pp. 276–291, 2000.

[9] J.-S. Roy, H. Moffet, L. J. Hébert, and R. Lirette, "Effect of motor control and strengthening exercises on shoulder function in persons with impingement syndrome: a single-subject study design," *Manual Therapy*, vol. 14, no. 2, pp. 180–188, 2009.

[10] C. A. Thigpen, D. A. Padua, L. A. Michener et al., "Head and shoulder posture affect scapular mechanics and muscle activity in overhead tasks," *Journal of Electromyography and Kinesiology*, vol. 20, no. 4, pp. 701–709, 2010.

[11] P. W. McClure, J. Bialker, N. Neff, G. Williams, and A. Karduna, "Shoulder function and 3-dimensional kinematics in people with shoulder impingement syndrome before and after a 6-week exercise program," *Physical Therapy*, vol. 84, no. 9, pp. 832–848, 2004.

[12] T. Holmgren, H. B. Hallgren, B. Öberg, L. Adolfsson, and K. Johansson, "Effect of specific exercise strategy on need for surgery in patients with subacromial impingement syndrome: randomised controlled study," *British Medical Journal*, vol. 344, no. 7846, article e787, 2012.

[13] C. A. Thigpen, S. S. Lynch, J. P. Mihalik, W. E. Prentice, and D. Padua, "The effects of an exercise intervention on forward head and rounded shoulder postures in elite swimmers," *British Journal of Sports Medicine*, vol. 44, no. 5, pp. 376–381, 2010.

[14] S. Sahrmann, "Movement impairment syndromes of the shoulder girdle," in *Diagnosis and Treatment of Movement Impairment Syndrome*, pp. 193–245, Mosby, St Louis, Mo, USA, 2001.

[15] E. Ayub, "Posture and the upper quadrant," in *Physical Therapy of the Shoulder*, R. A. Donatelli, Ed., chapter 4, p. 81, Churchill Livingstone, New York, NY, USA, 2nd edition, 1997.

[16] J. W. Howell, "Evaluation and management of thoracic outlet syndrome," in *Physical Therapy of the Shoulder*, R. A. Donatelli, Ed., Churchill Livingstone, New York, NY, USA, 2nd edition, 1991.

[17] J. G. Travell and D. G. Simons, *Myofascial Pain and Dysfunction. The Trigger Point Manual*, vol. 1, Williams & Wilkins, Baltimore, Md, USA, 2nd edition, 1999.

[18] H. P. Kopel and W. A. L. Thompson, *Peripheral Entrapment Neuropathies*, Robert E. Krieger, New York, NY, USA, 2nd edition, 1976.

[19] T. S. Ellenbecker and A. Cools, "Rehabilitation of shoulder impingement syndrome and rotator cuff injuries: an evidence-based review," *British Journal of Sports Medicine*, vol. 44, no. 5, pp. 319–327, 2010.

[20] W. Ben Kibler, A. D. Sciascia, T. L. Uhl, N. Tambay, and T. Cunningham, "Electromyographic analysis of specific exercises for scapular control in early phases of shoulder rehabilitation," *American Journal of Sports Medicine*, vol. 36, no. 9, pp. 1789–1798, 2008.

[21] M. L. Voight and B. C. Thomson, "The role of the scapula in the rehabilitation of shoulder injuries," *Journal of Athletic Training*, vol. 35, no. 3, pp. 364–372, 2000.

[22] A. M. Cools, V. Dewitte, F. Lanszweert et al., "Rehabilitation of scapular muscle balance: which exercises to prescribe?" *American Journal of Sports Medicine*, vol. 35, no. 10, pp. 1744–1751, 2007.

[23] J. S. Lewis, A. Green, and C. Wright, "Subacromial impingement syndrome: the role of posture and muscle imbalance," *Journal of Shoulder and Elbow Surgery*, vol. 14, no. 4, pp. 385–392, 2005.

[24] B. Greenfield, P. A. Catlin, P. W. Coats, E. Green, J. J. McDonald, and C. North, "Posture in patients with shoulder overuse injuries and healthy individuals," *Journal of Orthopaedic and Sports Physical Therapy*, vol. 21, no. 5, pp. 287–295, 1995.

[25] S. Raine and L. T. Twomey, "Head and shoulder posture variations in 160 asymptomatic women and men," *Archives of Physical Medicine and Rehabilitation*, vol. 78, no. 11, pp. 1215–1223, 1997.

[26] J. D. Borstad, "Resting position variables at the shoulder: evidence to support a posture-impairment association," *Physical Therapy*, vol. 86, no. 4, pp. 549–557, 2006.

[27] J. S. Lewis, C. Wright, and A. Green, "Subacromial impingement syndrome: the effect of changing posture on shoulder range of movement," *Journal of Orthopaedic and Sports Physical Therapy*, vol. 35, no. 2, pp. 72–87, 2005.

[28] M. P. Bullock, N. E. Foster, and C. C. Wright, "Shoulder impingement: the effect of sitting posture on shoulder pain and range of motion," *Manual Therapy*, vol. 10, no. 1, pp. 28–37, 2005.

[29] C. Hrysomallis and C. Goodman, "A review of resistance exercise and posture realignment," *The Journal of Strength & Conditioning Research*, vol. 15, no. 3, pp. 385–390, 2001.

[30] C. Hrysomallis, "Effectiveness of strengthening and stretching exercises for the postural correction of abducted scapulae: a review," *Journal of Strength and Conditioning Research*, vol. 24, no. 2, pp. 567–574, 2010.

[31] T. Zmierski, S. Kegerreis, and J. Scarpaci, "Scapular muscle strengthening," *Journal of Sport Rehabilitation*, vol. 4, no. 4, pp. 244–252, 1995.

[32] K. Baker-Sawyer, P. McClure, and K. Fitzgerald, "The effect of a scapular retraction exercise program on scapular position and scapular muscle force," *Journal of Orthopaedic & Sports Physical Therapy*, vol. 23, pp. 75–76, 1996.

[33] C.-H. Wang, P. McClure, N. E. Pratt, and R. Nobilini, "Stretching and strengthening exercises: their effect on three- dimensional scapular kinematics," *Archives of Physical Medicine and Rehabilitation*, vol. 80, no. 8, pp. 923–929, 1999.

[34] M. Kluemper, T. Uhl, and H. Hazelrigg, "Effect of stretching and strengthening shoulder muscles on forward shoulder posture in competitive swimmers," *Journal of Sport Rehabilitation*, vol. 15, no. 1, pp. 58–70, 2006.

[35] T. S. Roddey, S. L. Olson, and S. E. Grant, "The effect of pectoralis muscle stretching on the resting position of the scapula in persons with varying degrees of forward head/rounded shoulder posture," *Journal of Manual and Manipulative Therapy*, vol. 10, no. 3, pp. 124–128, 2002.

[36] H. H. Host, "Scapular taping in the treatment of anterior shoulder impingement," *Physical Therapy*, vol. 75, no. 9, pp. 803–812, 1995.

[37] D. Kneeshaw, "Shoulder taping in the clinical setting," *Journal of Bodywork and Movement Therapies*, vol. 6, no. 1, pp. 2–8, 2002.

[38] W. Gilleard, J. McConnell, and D. Parsons, "The effect of patellar taping on the onset of vastus medialis obliquus and vastus lateralis muscle activity in persons with patellofemoral pain," *Physical Therapy*, vol. 78, no. 1, pp. 25–32, 1998.

[39] P. Miller and P. Osmotherly, "Does scapula taping facilitate recovery for shoulder impingement symptoms? A pilot randomized controlled trial," *Journal of Manual & Manipulative Therapy*, vol. 17, no. 1, pp. E6–E13, 2009.

[40] J.-H. Lee and W.-G. Yoo, "Effect of scapular elevation taping on scapular depression syndrome: a case report," *Journal of Back and Musculoskeletal Rehabilitation*, vol. 25, no. 3, pp. 187–191, 2012.

[41] J. S. Lewis, C. Wright, and A. Green, "Subacromial impingement syndrome: the effect of changing posture on shoulder range of movement," *Journal of Orthopaedic and Sports Physical Therapy*, vol. 35, no. 2, pp. 72–87, 2005.

[42] M. D. Thelen, J. A. Dauber, and P. D. Stoneman, "The clinical efficacy of kinesio tape for shoulder pain: a randomized, double-blinded, clinical trial," *Journal of Orthopaedic and Sports Physical Therapy*, vol. 38, no. 7, pp. 389–395, 2008.

[43] B. Ackermann, R. Adams, and E. Marshall, "The effect of scapula taping on electromyographic activity and musical performance in professional violinists," *Australian Journal of Physiotherapy*, vol. 48, no. 3, pp. 197–203, 2002.

[44] M. J. Smith and V. Sparkes, "The immediate effect of scapular taping on surface electromyo-graphic activity of the scapular rotators in swimmers with subacromial impingement symptoms," *Physical Therapy in Sport*, vol. 7, Proceedings of the Physical Therapy in Sport International Conference:Enhancing Recovery and Performance in Sport Birmingham, UK, no. 4, pp. 171–180, 2006.

[45] C. M. Norris, *Sports Injuries, Diagnosis and Management*, Butterworth Heinmann, London, UK, 3rd edition, 2005.

[46] M. H. Gibson, G. V. Goebel, T. M. Jordan, S. Kegerreis, and T. W. Worrell, "A reliability study of measurement techniques to determine static scapular position," *Journal of Orthopaedic and Sports Physical Therapy*, vol. 21, no. 2, pp. 100–106, 1995.

[47] J. DiVeta, M. L. Walker, and B. Skibinski, "Relationship between performance of selected scapular muscles and scapular abduction in standing subjects," *Physical Therapy*, vol. 70, no. 8, pp. 470–476, 1990.

[48] L. Neiers and T. W. Worrell, "Assessment of scapular position," *Journal of Sport Rehabilitation*, vol. 2, no. 1, pp. 20–25, 1993.

[49] J. Nijs, N. Roussel, F. Struyf, S. Mottram, and R. Meeusen, "Clinical assessment of scapular positioning in patients with shoulder pain: state of the art," *Journal of Manipulative and Physiological Therapeutics*, vol. 30, no. 1, pp. 69–75, 2007.

[50] J. S. Lewis and R. E. Valentine, "The pectoralis minor length test: a study of the intra-rater reliability and diagnostic accuracy in subjects with and without shoulder symptoms," *BMC Musculoskeletal Disorders*, vol. 8, article 64, 2007.

[51] J. Nijs, N. Roussel, K. Vermeulen, and G. Souvereyns, "Scapular positioning in patients with shoulder pain: a study examining the reliability and clinical importance of 3 clinical tests," *Archives of Physical Medicine and Rehabilitation*, vol. 86, no. 7, pp. 1349–1355, 2005.

[52] F. Struyf, J. Nijs, J.-P. Baeyens, S. Mottram, and R. Meeusen, "Scapular positioning and movement in unimpaired shoulders, shoulder impingement syndrome, and glenohumeral instability," *Scandinavian Journal of Medicine and Science in Sports*, vol. 21, no. 3, pp. 352–358, 2011.

[53] F. Struyf, J. Nijs, J. De Graeve, S. Mottram, and R. Meeusen, "Scapular positioning in overhead athletes with and without shoulder pain: a case-control study," *Scandinavian Journal of Medicine and Science in Sports*, vol. 21, no. 6, pp. 809–818, 2011.

[54] D. C. Sobush, G. G. Simoneau, K. E. Dietz, J. A. Levene, R. E. Grossman, and W. B. Smith, "The Lennie test for measuring scapular position in healthy young adult females: a reliability and validity study," *Journal of Orthopaedic and Sports Physical Therapy*, vol. 23, no. 1, pp. 39–50, 1996.

[55] D. Morrissey, "Proprioceptive shoulder taping," *Journal of Bodywork and Movement Therapies*, vol. 4, no. 3, pp. 189–194, 2000.

[56] L. G. Portney and M. P. Watkins, *Foundations of Clinical Research: Applications to Practice*, Prentice Hall Health, Upper Saddle River, NJ, USA, 3rd edition, 2009.

[57] I. G. Horsley, J. Pearson, A. Green, and C. Rolf, "A comparison of the musculoskeletal assessments of the shoulder girdles of professional rugby players and professional soccer players.," *Sports Medicine, Arthroscopy, Rehabilitation, Therapy & Technology*, vol. 4, no. 1, article 32, 2012.

[58] A. M. Cools, E. E. Witvrouw, L. A. Danneels, and D. C. Cambier, "Does taping influence electromyographic muscle activity in the scapular rotators in healthy shoulders?" *Manual Therapy*, vol. 7, no. 3, pp. 154–162, 2002.

[59] J.-J. Lin, C.-J. Hung, and P.-L. Yang, "The effects of scapular taping on electromyographic muscle activity and proprioception feedback in healthy shoulders," *Journal of Orthopaedic Research*, vol. 29, no. 1, pp. 53–57, 2011.

[60] G. E. Morin, D. Tiberio, and G. Austin, "The effect of upper trapezius taping on electromyographic activity in the upper and middle trapezius region," *Journal of Sport Rehabilitation*, vol. 6, no. 4, pp. 309–318, 1997.

[61] R. M. Paine and M. Voight, "The role of the scapula," *Journal of Orthopaedic and Sports Physical Therapy*, vol. 18, no. 1, pp. 386–391, 1993.

[62] C. Hall, "The shoulder girdle," in *Therapeutic Exercise. Moving Toward Function*, C. Hall and L. T. Brody, Eds., Lippincott Williams and Wilkins, Philadelphia, Pa, USA, 1999.

[63] C. M. Alexander, M. McMullan, and P. J. Harrison, "What is the effect of taping along or across a muscle on motoneurone excitability? A study using triceps surae," *Manual Therapy*, vol. 13, no. 1, pp. 57–62, 2008.

[64] C. M. Alexander, S. Stynes, A. Thomas, J. Lewis, and P. J. Harrison, "Does tape facilitate or inhibit the lower fibres of trapezius?" *Manual Therapy*, vol. 8, no. 1, pp. 37–41, 2003.

[65] E. Kaya, M. Zinnuroglu, and I. Tugcu, "Kinesio taping compared to physical therapy modalities for the treatment of shoulder impingement syndrome," *Clinical Rheumatology*, vol. 30, no. 2, pp. 201–207, 2011.

Differences in Symptoms among Adults with Canal versus Otolith Vestibular Dysfunction: A Preliminary Report

Lisa Farrell[1,2] and Rose Marie Rine[3]

[1] *Adjunct Clinical Faculty, Nova Southeastern University, 3200 South University Drive, Fort Lauderdale, FL 33328, USA*
[2] *OrthoSport, Inc., 5200 South University Drive, Suite 105, Fort Lauderdale, FL 33328, USA*
[3] *Specialty Therapy Source LLC, 12948 Palmetto Glade Drive, Jacksonville, FL 32246, USA*

Correspondence should be addressed to Lisa Farrell; adventurefour@aol.com

Academic Editors: S. Eyigor and C.-L. Kao

Despite the importance of symptomatology in the diagnosis of vestibular dysfunction, the qualitative nature of the symptoms related to semicircular canal (canal) versus otolith dysfunction is not fully understood. The purpose of this study was to compare symptoms, and their severity, in individuals with canal versus otolith peripheral vestibular dysfunction. A subjective tool, the Descriptive Symptom Index (DSI), was developed to enable categorization of symptoms as rotary, linear, imbalance or falls, and nondistinct. Fourteen adults were recruited and grouped based on vestibular function testing: canal only dysfunction, otolith only dysfunction, or canal and otolith dysfunction. Also, the Dizziness Handicap Inventory (DHI) was used to grade the severity of perceived limitations due to symptoms. The DSI was reliable and differentiated those with canal (rotary symptoms) versus otolith (linear symptoms) dysfunction. Most individuals with otolith only dysfunction did not report rotary symptoms. DHI scores were significantly higher in those with otolith dysfunction, regardless of canal functional status. All who experienced falls had otolith dysfunction and none had canal only dysfunction. Results support the importance of using linear and rotary descriptors of perceived disorientation as part of diagnosing vestibular dysfunction.

1. Introduction

A comprehensive patient history, which includes the qualitative nature of symptoms, is paramount when making the diagnosis of peripheral vestibulopathy (P-VeD) in adults who report dizziness and/or imbalance [1–3]. Rotary vertigo has traditionally been accepted as the primary descriptor related to P-VeD [2, 4–6]. The diagnosis is often confirmed with objective measurement of the functional integrity of the semicircular canals (canals) using calorics, rotational chair, head impulse, and/or Dix-Hallpike testing [4]. However, the clinical diagnostic process has been limited because measurement of otolith function has not been readily available. Also, the qualitative nature of the symptoms of otolith dysfunction has not been formally investigated and determined [7, 8]. Tomanovic and Bergenius [3], who studied the prevalence of different types of dizziness symptoms in subjects with P-VeD, expanded the understanding of subjective descriptors by concluding that in addition to the classic symptoms of vertigo, the presence of "nonclassical" symptoms, such as drop attacks, unsteadiness like walking on a boat, walking on pillows, stepping into a hole, and feeling like being pulled to one side, occur in these individuals. In Tomanovic's study, only tests of canal function, and not otolith function, determined the diagnosis of P-VeD. It is not known whether the otolith organs (e.g., utricle and saccule) were also damaged and may have contributed to the subjects' symptoms, especially the "nonclassical" symptoms.

Advances in vestibular function testing procedures has identified otolith dysfunction [6, 9–11] and several investigations have reported that subjects with otolith dysfunction described their symptoms as feeling like sensations of rocking, tilting, walking on pillows, being pushed or pulled, feeling drunk, and falling [7, 12]. Even though these descriptions were only anecdotally associated with P-VeD, it questions whether the limited focus on symptoms of rotary vertigo impedes the diagnostic process. Consequently, by focusing on rotary vertigo as the symptom associated with P-VeD, successful management, including selection of appropriate vestibular rehabilitation (VR) strategies, may be hindered. The advancement of clinical practice for individuals with complaints of dizziness and/or imbalance requires valid and reliable testing of canal and the otolith end-organ function, confirmation of the selective effect of pathology on canal versus otolith mechanisms, improved understanding of how the unique functional contributions of canal and otolith mechanisms affects perceived orientation and balance ability after substrate damage, and expansion of the descriptors used by individuals with vestibular dysfunction to help with the diagnostic process and with establishing the need for VR.

Recently, there have been improvements in clinical practice with the expansion from testing only canal function (specifically of the horizontal canal) to the emergence of testing of otolith function [5, 6, 13–16]. Tests of utricular function are the subjective visual vertical test (SVV; both static and dynamic) [13] and the ocular vestibular evoked myogenic potential (o-VEMP) [13, 15]. The integrity of the saccule and the inferior branch of the vestibular nerve function is measured by using the cervical vestibular evoked myogenic potential (c-VEMP) [5, 13]. As a consequence of the expansion of vestibular function testing, the understanding of otolith dysfunction is emerging. Traditionally, it has been assumed that canal and otolith mechanisms would not be selectively affected by disease or injury, which would argue against the need for testing all mechanisms of the vestibular system [4]. By utilizing tests of canal and otolith function, results of investigations have shown that involvement of these mechanisms can be discriminative and supports the importance of comprehensive testing. Karlberg et al. [14] presented the cases of two patients diagnosed with superior vestibular neuritis based on abnormal caloric, abnormal SVV, and normal c-VEMP tests, thus indicating both canal and otolith involvement. Halmagyi et al. [17] and Monstad et al. [10] reported that their patients with inferior vestibular neuritis presented with symmetrical calorics, normal head impulse testing of the anterior and horizontal canals, abnormal head impulse tests for the posterior canal, and abnormal c-VEMP results. Similarly, Iwasaki et al. [9] found that patients with Meniere's disease, acoustic neuroma (AN), cerebellopontine angle tumor other than AN, sudden deafness with vertigo, and multiple sclerosis can present with involvement of only the inferior vestibular nerve as measured by normal caloric testing and abnormal c-VEMP testing. According to Kingma and Wit [18], for patients with Meniere's disease, saccular dysfunction is an established pathophysiological feature and explains why abnormal c-VEMP test results are reported. However, other authors report that the results are dependent upon the phase and the stage of the disease [19–21]. Manzari et al. [20] demonstrated that utricular and saccular function is affected differently in patients with Meniere's disease of less than two-year duration. There was a significant increase in o-VEMP response during an active phase as compared to the quiescent phase, but a significant decrease in c-VEMP response during the active phase as compared to quiescence. Young et al. [21] reported that c-VEMP amplitude responses varied depending on the stage of the disease with a significant increase in the asymmetry ratio as the disease progressed. Additionally, de Waele et al. [19] reported that c-VEMP responses were absent in 54% of patients tested in the quiescent period of Meniere's disease (stage not reported) and that c-VEMP results did not correlate with canal paresis. Similar to these reports of saccular pathology, utricular dysfunction has also been reported in patient cases with or without concurrent canal and saccule involvement. Tabak et al. [22] found that a group of patients who had vestibular loss after surgery for acoustic neuroma were deficient in canal and otolith function as measured by calorics and SVV tests. Results of the investigation by Schönfeld et al. [6] also provide evidence of isolated unilateral utricular dysfunction, as demonstrated by asymmetric dynamic SVV results, but symmetric caloric and c-VEMP responses in patients with chronic disease. Despite advances in the development of clinical vestibular function testing and the identification of isolated otolith dysfunction, a comprehensive comparative investigation of the qualitative nature of the symptoms has not been done.

The neurophysiology of the canals and otolith organs is distinct with unique contributions of each to perceived head position and balance abilities. Therefore, adults with dizziness and imbalance due to otolith organ involvement may present with different symptoms as compared to those with canal dysfunction. Both canals and otolith organs contribute to the perception of head orientation, but each responds to unique stimuli [23–25]. The canals are optimally sensitive to angular acceleration, which explains why patients with pathology affecting the canals report symptoms of spinning (rotary vertigo) [7]. The otolith organs, although less thoroughly studied and understood [8, 12], optimally respond to linear and gravitational acceleration due to translational head movements and head tilts [2, 24]. This could explain why anecdotal reports of feeling like rocking, tilting, walking on pillows, being pushed, feeling drunk, and falling have been used by patients with otolith dysfunction [7, 12]. In addition to perceived orientation, canals and otolith organs both contribute to postural control via vestibulospinal pathways. However, it is thought that the contribution of the otoliths is the main vestibular source for postural control [23, 25]. The vestibulospinal pathways that receive canal input terminate on motor neurons of the cervical cord, whereas those of the otolith organs innervate motor neurons from the cervical through the sacral cord [26]. The otolith organ input facilitates activation of antigravity muscles and modulates the tone of neck, trunk, and limb extensor muscles enabling the maintenance of posture [25]. Consequently, it seems logical to conclude that dysfunction of canals versus that of otolith organs would effect perceived orientation and balance differently. In turn, it would seem reasonable that exercise strategies used in rehabilitation would need to be designed specifically to promote stimulation of residual function of these structures.

Vestibular rehabilitation (VR) exercises, which focus on the reduction of complaints of dizziness and imbalance, have been based on diagnoses involving only the canals. VR has emphasized the use of rotational head movement exercises, which optimally stimulates canal function [27]. This may affect the success of intervention because these exercises do not optimally stimulate the otolith organs, and thus, the exercises used may be incomplete or incorrect for individuals with otolith dysfunction. This could explain, at least in part, the variable outcomes of VR that are reported [28, 29]. A prospective, controlled study by Krebs et al. [29] demonstrated that only 60% of patients with unilateral and bilateral P-VeD who performed gaze stability and balance retraining exercises benefited from the VR as indicated by improved gait parameters. Ernst et al. [28] reported that although there was improvement of perceived orientation, gaze stability, and/or postural control following VR in most patients with vestibulopathy, some patients did not have resolution of their symptoms. A prospective study by Enticott et al. [30] found that patients with a mixture of vestibular dysfunctions (canal only, canal and otolith, and otolith only) who performed a variety of head turning and walking tasks over 10 weeks had significant improvement of impairments compared to patients who only performed lower extremity strengthening exercises. Even though perceived disability, balance confidence, and severity of symptoms improved in patients studied by Enticott, patients' perception of the therapy program's impact on their symptoms did not improve significantly in the treatment group compared to the control group. By having a more thorough understanding of the qualitative nature of the symptoms of canal versus otolith dysfunction, the diagnosis could be more specific, which could improve the development of optimal intervention for individuals with vestibulopathy. However, to date, this has not been done.

The primary objective of this investigation was to identify the qualitative nature of dizziness and imbalance and determine the impact of these symptoms on daily activities in adults with canal versus otolith P-VeD. This information can positively impact the selection of diagnostic tests, improve diagnosis, and lead to the development of improved rehabilitation strategies.

2. Methods

Fourteen subjects, aged 36–59 years (mean = 46; sd = 5.8) with complaints of dizziness and/or imbalance due to a diagnosis of P-VeD, were recruited from the patient population seen at the University of Miami Miller School of Medicine's Department of Otolaryngology. Individuals were excluded from the study if they had a cognitive deficit or a confounding diagnosis, such as orthopedic injury or condition involving the spine or lower extremities; neurological, somatosensory, or visual dysfunction due to a CNS lesion; peripheral neuropathy of the legs; or spinal cord injury. Diagnosis was confirmed by history, neurootologic examination, and vestibular function testing (e.g., horizontal head impulse/thrust, rotational chair, calorics, Dix-Hallpike, SVV, and c-VEMP). Diagnoses included acoustic neuroma resection, benign paroxysmal positional vertigo (BPPV), Meniere's disease, superior canal dehiscence, unilateral labyrinthitis, and neuritis. The range of time from symptom onset was 3 weeks to 39 months (mean = 16; sd = 13.5).

Subjects were grouped based on test results: Group 1 had abnormal canal testing and normal otolith testing (n = 3; 21%), Group 2 had abnormal otolith testing and normal canal testing (n = 4; 29%), and Group 3 had abnormal canal and otolith testing (n = 7; 50%). See Table 1 for a summary of subject demographics and group assignment.

3. Instrumentation

A tool, the Descriptive Symptom Index (DSI), was developed to enable examination of symptoms reported. The DSI enabled categorization of subjects' perception of dizziness and imbalance symptoms. To minimize bias, subjects were first asked by an investigator (R.M.R.), who was blinded to vestibular function test results, to describe their symptoms. They were then provided a list of potential symptoms and asked to indicate whether the word did or did not further clarify their symptoms (Table 2). The descriptors provided or selected by subjects were recorded and categorized (rotary sensations for category 1, linear sensations for category 2, symptoms that portray imbalance and falls for category 3, or nondistinct symptoms for category 4). Categorization was used to examine the relationship between the qualitative nature of symptoms and vestibular mechanism involved and to compare symptoms between groups. Retest was completed at the end of initial visit to enable examination of test-retest reliability of the DSI.

To quantify the severity of perceived limitations with daily activities, the Dizziness Handicap Inventory (DHI) was completed. This test is made up of 25 questions that address the emotional, physical, and functional aspects regarding how symptoms of dizziness and/or imbalance impact daily activities. The DHI has been shown to provide high test-retest reliability (r = 0.97) [31], high internal consistency (Cronbach alpha = 0.89) [19], and there is evidence for construct validity with significant correlation between balance confidence and specific measures of balance [32]. Subjects were asked to indicate "yes," "sometimes," or "no" as it pertained to how their dizziness and/or imbalance limited their function. Answers were assigned 4 points for "yes," 2 points for "sometimes," or 0 points for "no." The composite score ranged from 0 (no perceived handicap) to 100 (maximum perceived handicap). Based on the report by Whitney et al. [32], a severity score was assigned based on the composite score: (1) mild handicap ranged from 0 to 30, (2) moderate handicap ranged from 31 to 60, and (3) severe handicap ranged from 61 to 100. The DHI composite and severity scores were used to compare groups' perceived handicap due to dizziness and/or imbalance.

4. Analysis

Statistical analyses were performed using the SPSS software package (SPSS Inc., 233 S. Wacker Drive, Chicago, IL). The reliability of the DSI was calculated using a kappa statistic. Sensitivity, specificity, positive predictive value (PPV), and

Table 1: Subject demographics and group assignment.

Age (yrs)	Gender	Group	Canal function tests				Otolith function tests		Diagnosis(es) established by physician	Onset (months)
			DH	R	C	HT	SVV	VEMP		
36	Female	1	−	−	+	+	−	−	Vestibular labyrinthitis	2
51	Female	1	+	−	−	−	−	−	BPPV	3/4
53	Female	1	−	+	−	+	−	−	Vestibular neuritis	15
44	Male	2	NT	−	NT	−	−	+	Vestibular neuritis	12
44	Female	2	−	−	−	−	+	+	Vestibular neuritis	12
48	Female	2	−	−	−	−	+	−	Vestibular neuritis	36
50	Female	2	−	−	−	−	+	+	Meniere's disease	6
46	Male	3	−	NT	+	+	+	−	Meniere's disease	36
40	Male	3	+	−	+	+	+	+	BPPV and labyrinthitis	18
43	Female	3	+	NT	+	+	+	+	BPPV and acoustic Neuroma resection	1
43	Female	3	+	NT	+	−	−	+	BPPV and vestibular neuritis	39
40	Female	3	NT	+	+	+	+	+	Endolymphatic sac decomp 2° Meniere's	5
59	Female	3	−	+	−	+	+	+	Superior canal dehiscence	24
47	Female	3	+	−	−	−	+	+	BPPV and vestibular neuritis	24

DH: Dix-Hallpike; R: rotary chair; C: calorics; HT: head thrust; SVV: subjective visual vertical; VEMP: vestibular evoked myogenic potential; NT: not tested; BPPV: benign paroxysmal positional vertigo.

Table 2: Descriptive symptom index.

Category 1	Category 2	Category 3	Category 4
Tumbling (self)	Rocking (self)	Off balance	Lightheadedness
Tumbling (world)	Rocking (world)	Unsteady	Floating
Spinning (self)	Tilting (self)	Staggers	Disoriented
Spinning (world)	Tilting (world)	Falls	Swimming
Other	Pulling	Other	Wooziness
	Pushing		Other
	Linear motion (self)		
	Linear motion (world)		
	Other		

negative predictive value (NPV) for the DSI categories 1 (rotary symptoms) and 2 (linear symptoms) were calculated to determine whether these categories were able to discriminate between subjects with canal versus otolith dysfunction. Chi-square statistics were used to compare DSI categories between groups. An ANOVA statistic with Tukey HSD post hoc tests was utilized to compare DHI scores between groups and Kruskal-Wallis statistic was calculated to compare severity rank (mild, moderate, and severe) of DHI scores between groups.

5. Results

An a priori power analysis revealed that, to achieve a power level of 60% with a medium effect size and a significance level of 0.05, a sample size of 23 subjects per group was required. Since this sample size was not achieved, an alpha level of 0.10 was used to determine trends in the data. The fair to excellent sensitivity of DSI categorization supports this approach.

Time from symptom onset did not correlate with severity of symptoms ($P = 0.359$, $r = 0.27$). Although there was no difference in time from symptom onset between groups ($P = 0.29$), there was a trend evident in that Group 3 had the greatest time from symptom onset (Figure 1).

DSI scores had good to excellent test-retest reliability for each symptom category: rotary symptoms $\kappa = 1.0$, linear symptoms $\kappa = 0.63$, imbalance and falls $\kappa = 1.0$, and nondistinct symptoms $\kappa = 1.0$. The good to excellent sensitivity and positive predictive value suggested that the DSI's rotary and linear categorizations (Categories 1 and 2, resp.) were able to

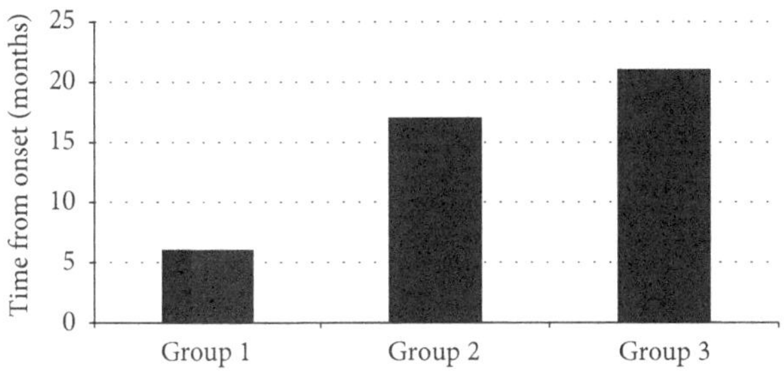

FIGURE 1: Comparison of symptom onset time between groups. Although the difference was not significant, time from symptom onset was greatest in Group 3 (otolith and canal dysfunction), as compared to those in Group 1 (canal only dysfunction) or Group 2 (otolith only dysfunction).

TABLE 3: Sensitivity, specificity, and predictive values for rotary and linear symptoms for subjects with P-VeD.

	Rotary symptoms and canal dysfunction (DSI category 1)	Linear symptoms and otolith dysfunction (DSI category 2)
Sensitivity	80%	100%
Specificity	75%	33%
PPV	89%	85%
NPV	60%	100%

P-VeD: peripheral vestibulopathy; DSI: Descriptive Symptom Index; PPV: positive predictive value; NPV: negative predictive value.

correctly classify individuals' involved vestibular mechanism (Table 3).

It should be noted that one of the four individuals with otolith only dysfunction (Group 2) reported rotary symptoms and one of the three individuals with canal only dysfunction (Group 1) reported linear symptoms. There were group differences in frequency of reported rotary symptoms ($P = 0.01$) with Group 3 reporting rotary symptoms significantly more often than Group 1 ($P = 0.008$) and Group 2 ($P = 0.004$) (Table 4). It was also evident that there was a trend in the difference in frequency of reported linear symptoms between groups ($P = 0.07$) with Group 3 reporting more linear symptoms than Group 1 ($P = 0.05$). Consistent with these findings, when individuals were grouped by the presence or absence of vestibular substrate pathology, those with canal dysfunction (Groups 1 and 3) reported rotary symptoms more often than those without canal dysfunction (Group 2; $P = 0.03$) and those with otolith dysfunction (Groups 2 and 3) reported linear symptoms more often than those without otolith dysfunction (Group 1; $P = 0.02$) (Tables 5 and 6).

Chi-square statistic was not calculated for the imbalance and falls category (category 3) nor for the indistinct category (category 4) of the DSI since all subjects within each group reported these symptoms. The majority of subjects described their balance difficulties as being off balance (100%) and unsteady (100%). Forty-three percent of subjects had a history of falls, and all of the fallers were individuals with otolith dysfunction (Groups 2 and 3) (Figure 2).

TABLE 4: Frequency of reported rotary and linear symptoms for each P-VeD group.

	Group 1 ($n = 3$)	Group 2 ($n = 4$)	Group 3 ($n = 7$)	P value[§]
Rotary (DSI cat. 1)	1 (33.3%)	1 (25%)	7 (100%)	0.01*
Linear (DSI cat. 2)	2 (66.7%)	4 (100%)	7 (100%)	0.07*

P-VeD: peripheral vestibulopathy; Group 1: canal only dysfunction; Group 2: otolith only dysfunction; Group 3: both.
[§]Chi-square statistic.
*$\alpha = 0.10$.

TABLE 5: Frequency of reported rotary and linear symptoms for those with the presence or absence of canal dysfunction.

	Canal dysfunction ($n = 10$)	No canal dysfunction ($n = 7$)	P value[§]
Rotary (DSI cat. 1)	8 (80%)	1 (25%)	0.03*
Linear (DSI cat. 2)	9 (90%)	4 (100%)	0.26

DSI: Descriptive Symptom Index.
[§]Chi-square statistic.
*$\alpha = 0.10$.

TABLE 6: Frequency of reported rotary and linear symptoms for those with the presence or absence of otolith dysfunction.

	Otolith dysfunction ($n = 11$)	No otolith dysfunction ($n = 3$)	P value[§]
Rotary (DSI cat. 1)	8 (73%)	1 (33.3%)	0.10
Linear (DSI cat. 2)	11 (100%)	2 (66.7%)	0.02*

DSI: Descriptive Symptom Index.
[§]Chi-square statistic.
*$\alpha = 0.10$.

Interestingly, the majority of subjects from each of the groups reported being disoriented, woozy, nauseated, and feeling like they were floating, and all, except for one subject with canal dysfunction, had feelings of lightheadedness. Although sensations of feeling fatigued (29%), full headed (14%–25%), floor moving (14%–25%), drunkenness (25%), and uncoordinated (25%) were used by those with otolith dysfunction (Groups 2 and 3), those with canal only dysfunction (Group 1) never used these words to describe their symptoms (Figure 3).

With regards to severity of perceived limitations with daily activities due to symptoms, results of parametric testing revealed that a trend was evident between groups' DHI composite scores ($P = 0.09$) and there were significant differences between groups' physical domain scores ($P = 0.01$; Table 7). Post hoc testing revealed that Group 2 trended toward higher (worse) composite scores compared to Group 1 ($P = 0.10$), and Groups 2 and 3 had significantly higher

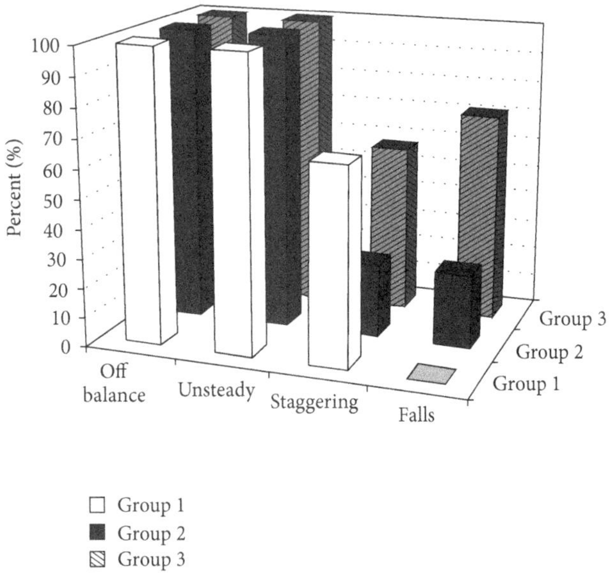

FIGURE 2: Frequency of imbalance and falls symptoms (DSI category 3) between Groups. The percentage of individuals within each Group that reported imbalance symptoms is depicted. All who reported falls had otolith dysfunction (Groups 2 and 3).

TABLE 7: Comparison of groups' DHI scores.

	Group 1 ($n = 3$)	Group 2 ($n = 4$)	Group 3 ($n = 7$)	P value[§]
Composite[†]	43 (14.5)	64 (6.0)	60 (17.6)	0.09*
P-DHI[†]	10 (6.0)	19 (3.0)	20 (4.8)	0.01*
F-DHI[†]	17 (8.3)	24 (4.1)	21 (8.0)	0.28
E-DHI[†]	15 (6.1)	22 (5.3)	19 (8.4)	0.28
Mild[††]	1	0	1	
Moderate[††]	2	1	2	0.18
Severe[††]	0	3	4	

DHI: Dizziness Handicap Inventory; Group 1: canal only dysfunction; Group 2: otolith only dysfunction; Group 3: both.
[†]Mean DHI scores (standard deviation in parentheses).
P-DHI: physical domain; F-DHI: functional domain; E-DHI: emotional domain.
[††]Composite score severity rank frequencies.
[§]ANOVA.
*$\alpha = 0.10$.

(worse) physical domain scores than those in Group 1 (P = 0.04 and P = 0.01, resp.; Figure 4(a)).

If subjects were grouped by the presence or absence of otolith dysfunction, individuals with otolith dysfunction (Groups 2 and 3) did have higher (worse) composite and physical domain DHI scores as compared to those without otolith dysfunction (Group 1; P = 0.03, P = 0.004, resp.; Table 8; Figure 4(b)).

Examination of the frequency of mild, moderate, or severe ranking of DHI scores did not differ between the three groups (Table 7). However, when grouped by those with and without otolith dysfunction, there was a trend for individuals with otolith dysfunction (Groups 2 and 3) to have

TABLE 8: Comparison of those with and without otolith dysfunctionDHI scores.

	Otolith dysfunction ($n = 11$)	Normal otolith function ($n = 3$)	P value[§]
Composite[†]	61 (14.1)	43 (14.5)	0.03*
P-DHI[†]	20 (4.2)	10 (6.0)	0.004*
F-DHI[†]	22 (6.7)	17 (8.3)	0.17
E-DHI[†]	19 (7.2)	17 (6.1)	0.17
Mild[††]	1	1	
Moderate[††]	3	2	0.07*
Severe[††]	7	0	

DHI: Dizziness Handicap Inventory.
[†]Mean DHI scores (standard deviation in parentheses).
P-DHI: physical domain; F-DHI: functional domain; E-DHI: emotional domain.
[††]Composite score severity rank frequencies.
[§]ANOVA.
*$\alpha = 0.10$.

DHI rankings that were more severe as compared to those without otolith dysfunction (Group 1; P = 0.07; Table 8). All individuals with otolith dysfunction (Groups 2 and 3), except one, had DHI rankings that were categorized as either moderate or severe, whereas those without otolith dysfunction (Group 1) had DHI rankings that were categorized as either mild or moderate.

6. Discussion

Evidence from this preliminary investigation confirmed that the qualitative nature of dizziness and the severity of perceived limitations with daily activities due to these symptoms vary in adults with report of dizziness and/or imbalance depending upon the involved pathological vestibular mechanism. Symptoms reported by those with canal dysfunction (Groups 1 and 3) were predominantly rotary in nature. These individuals used words like "spinning" and "tumbling" to describe their symptoms, whereas those with otolith dysfunction (Groups 2 and 3) reported symptoms that were predominantly linear in nature by using words like "tilting," "pulling," "pushing," "floor falling away," and/or "rocking to and fro" or "rocking back and forth" to describe their symptoms. These types of symptoms were also reported anecdotally in studies by Brandt [7] and Basta et al. [12]. The results reported here, that most individuals with only otolith dysfunction did not report rotary-type symptoms, argue for the inclusion of linear descriptors of symptoms in the diagnostic process. Furthermore, not only did most individuals with isolated pathology (Group 1 and Group 2) report distinct symptomology that was expected for their pathology, all individuals with both canal and otolith dysfunction (Group 3) reported both rotary-type and linear-type symptoms. This information is invaluable since patient history remains of the utmost importance when determining whether symptoms of dizziness and/or imbalance are due to P-VeD [2]. It can also improve the diagnostic process

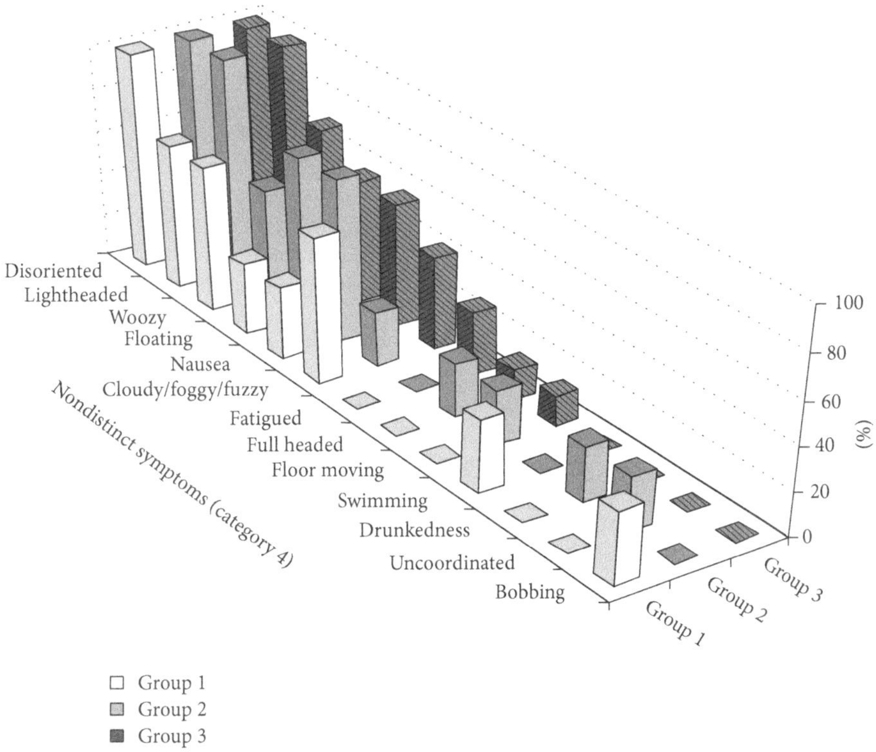

FIGURE 3: Frequency of nondistinct symptoms (DSI category 4) between Groups. Interestingly, most subjects in each of the groups (Group1 = canal only dysfunction; Group 2 = otolith only dysfunction; Group 3 = otolith and canal dysfunction) reported nondistinct symptoms, such as lightheaded, disorientation, and feeling woozy, but several were unique to those with otolith only dysfunction (e.g., full headed, floor moving, feeling drunk, and uncoordinated) and a couple were unique to those with canal only dysfunction (e.g., swimming, bobbing).

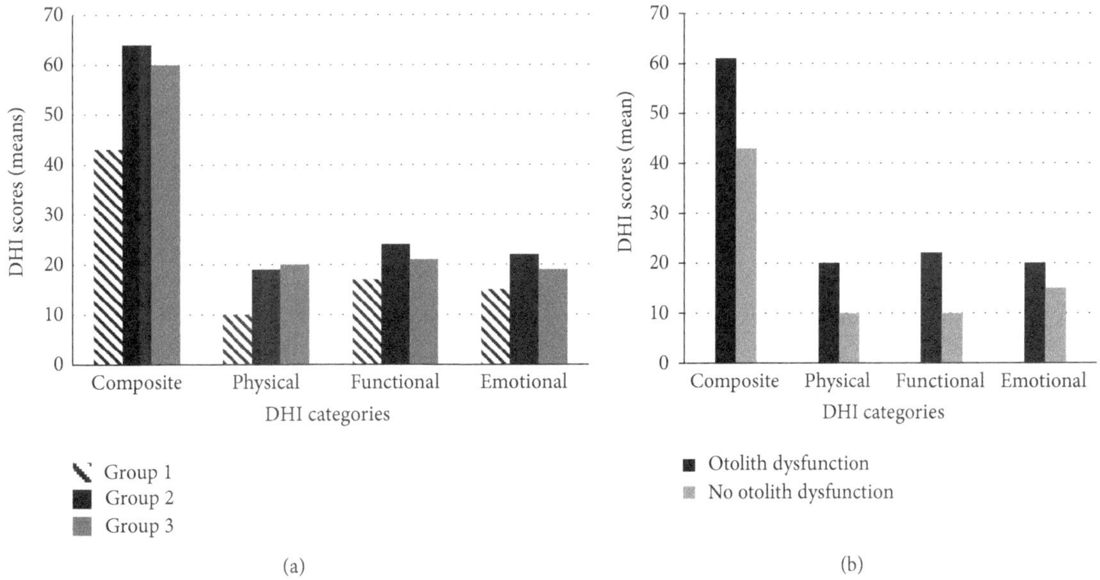

FIGURE 4: (a) Comparison of Dizziness Handicap Inventory (DHI) scores between groups. All DHI scores were higher (worse) for Groups 2 (otolith only dysfunction) and 3 (otolith and canal dysfunction) as compared to Group 1 (canal only dysfunction), most notably on the composite scores ($P = 0.09$) and physical domain scores ($P = 0.01$). (b) Comparison of DHI scores between those with and without otolith dysfunction. Comparison of composite and physical scores revealed that those with otolith dysfunction (Groups 2 and 3) had significantly worse scores as compared to those with canal only dysfunction (Group 1) ($P = 0.03$ and $P = 0.004$, resp.). This suggests that those with otolith dysfunction perceive their symptoms to be more disruptive of their life style as compared to those with canal only dysfunction.

by guiding the physical examination and aid in deciding which vestibular function tests are needed to confirm the diagnosis [1]. Improvement of the diagnostic process can lead to better management of adults with complaints of dizziness and imbalance by referring them to VR.

Whereas specific symptoms related to rotary- and linear-type symptoms (DSI categories 1 and 2) were associated with the involved vestibular mechanism, symptoms related to those of imbalance (DSI category 3) and those that were nondistinct (category 4) did not help distinguish the type of involved vestibular mechanism. All individuals reported that they felt "off balance," "unsteady," and "disoriented." Although imbalance and nondistinct descriptors were not helpful in identifying involved P-VeD mechanism, the information should not be disregarded. This information identifies the need for further assessment, particularly evaluation of possible postural control impairments. Although ambiguous reports of imbalance did not identify the involved vestibular mechanisms, reports of falls in DSI category 3 did demonstrate apparent differences between P-VeD groups. No individuals with canal only dysfunction reported falls. This may be attributed to the neurophysiological role that the otolith organs play in modifying tone in antigravity muscles for postural control. Additional support for this theory was demonstrated with the greater severity of perceived limitations with daily activities, as measured by DHI, in individuals who had otolith dysfunction, regardless of the presence of canal dysfunction (Groups 2 and 3). In particular, the physical domain scores were significantly higher (worse) scores when all individuals were grouped based on presence of otolith dysfunction, regardless of whether or not the individuals had canal dysfunction (Groups 2 and 3), as compared to those with canal only dysfunction (Group 1). Walking in the market, walking down a sidewalk, and bending over were the items within the physical domain of the DHI that demonstrated the most differences. The findings of greater subjective reports of falls and the limitations with daily activities in this study are supported by evidence of objective impairments of postural control in those with reduced otolith function. Basta et al. [12] demonstrated that sensory organization testing and trunk sway measures during stance and gait activities were impaired in those with otolith only dysfunction as compared to healthy controls. Serrador et al. [33] demonstrated that with age there is a reduction of utricular function as measured by ocular counter rolling, and as a result, individuals can have increased postural sway and be at increased risk of falling. Interestingly, the difference in the severity of perceived limitations with daily activities reported in this study is in contrast to that reported by Murray et al. [34]. These investigators found no difference in DHI scores between subjects who had canal only dysfunction (positive calorics) as compared to those who had canal and otolith dysfunction (positive calorics, positive VEMP, and/or SVV). Although this study and the Murray et al. [34] study were similar by using the same vestibular function tests to confirm the diagnosis of subjects with chronic complaints of dizziness and/or imbalance, differences in the subject sampling may explain the differences in DHI findings. In the current study, several subjects with otolith only dysfunctions were included and they were not in the Murray et al. [34] article. This study provides support for the predominant functional contribution of the otolith organs to postural control, as was reported by Markham [25]. However, further objective comparison of postural control and balance impairments between those with canal versus otolith dysfunction needs to confirm these findings.

Although it was not the primary objective of this investigation, comprehensive vestibular function testing confirmed the selective effect of pathology on vestibular mechanisms, which resulted in distinct canal and otolith pathology or a combination of the two [4, 16]. In this investigation, seven (50%) of individuals had both canal and otolith dysfunction (Group 3), four (29%) of individuals had otolith only dysfunction (Group 2), and three (21%) of individuals had canal only dysfunction (Group 1). These findings contribute to the growing body of knowledge that has found that involvement of different vestibular mechanisms occurs with P-VeD [6, 9, 10, 14]. This information was paramount to the current investigation because it provided the foundation for the investigation's primary objective. Confirmation of the selective effect of pathology on canal and otolith mechanisms led to the expansion of the descriptors used by individuals with vestibular dysfunction and improved our understanding of how the unique functional contributions of canal and otolith mechanisms affects perceived orientation and balance ability after substrate damage.

In summary, when individuals report symptoms of dizziness due to suspected P-VeD, the qualitative nature can assist in deciding which vestibular mechanisms are involved. From the history, the focus should not only be on recognizing rotary vertigo as the descriptor related to P-VeD, but should also include words that reflect linear-type sensations. Expanding the descriptors to accept both rotary- and linear-type symptoms can facilitate identification of individuals that need vestibular function testing that includes measurement of both canal and otolith function. Furthermore, improved understanding of the involved vestibular mechanism may impact the implementation and success of rehabilitation. The distinct impairments found in individuals with canal versus otolith dysfunction also support further investigation to identify whether use of exercises strategies that optimally stimulate residual function specific to the involved vestibular mechanism would improve outcomes in VR.

There are several limitations and improvements that can be made with this preliminary report. Although there has been recent expansion of vestibular function testing, which includes testing of otoliths, there are limitations with all current available testing [5, 16]. While caloric testing is a widely accepted as the "gold standard" for detecting unilateral vestibular loss and strongly recommended technique, it only tests a very low frequency range of vestibular function and there can also be a variability of response if there is inadequate irrigation [35]. The rotational chair uses head movement as the stimulus and provides stimulus frequencies that are higher as compared to caloric testing; however, the frequencies are on the lower end of normal head motion and the chair is less helpful in detecting unilateral lesions [35]. According to Schubert et al. [36], the horizontal head thrust (head impulse) test, which is used for identifying VOR dysfunction, has a sensitivity of 71% and specificity of 82%. The authors questioned whether the variability of the sensitivity could be due to proficiency in performing the testing technique. With SVV testing there has been limited benefit from testing patients beyond the acute stage of P-VeD because the results tend to normalize over time. However, when SVV is measured while applying vibration to the mastoid bone, as was used in this study, the sensitivity has been calculated as 91% and the specificity as 92% [37]. With VEMP testing, reliability and validity of the responses is dependent on delivery of an adequate stimulus and with a consistent tonic contraction of the sternocleidomastoid muscle; however, the response can vary depending on the methodology used [16, 38]. To address these potential problems, this study performed monitoring of electromyography (EMG) concurrently with the auditory stimulus and provided visual feedback to subjects to maintain uniform EMG during testing. Also, if an abnormal response to the auditory stimulus occurred, a bone stimulus to the mastoid process was performed to prevent a false positive due to possible stimulus conduction issues. The limitations with these vestibular function tests may have caused misclassification of vestibular dysfunction of some individuals. As the validity and reliability of testing improves, future studies can verify this study's findings. Also, to improve the DSI's usefulness in the clinic, future examination of the validity and reliability of this instrument should be performed on individuals with and without P-VeD who report dizziness and imbalance.

The small sample size of this study limits the generalizability of conclusions drawn from these results. Additional investigations with larger sample sizes that include individuals with dysfunction of canal only, otolith only, and canal and otolith substrate are needed. Information from this type of study would support investigations that examine the use of exercise strategies that may optimally rehabilitate impairments of canal versus otolith dysfunction.

Conflict of Interests

The authors declare that there is no conflict of interests regarding the publication of this paper.

Acknowledgments

This work was supported by Florida Physical Therapy Association's Linda Crane Research Grant. The authors thank Dr. Simon Angeli, M.D., and Dr. Fred Telischi, M.D., from the Ear Institute of the University of Miami Miller School of Medicine, Miami, FL, for their referral of subjects.

References

[1] A. H. Clarke, "Laboratory testing of the vestibular system," *Current Opinion in Otolaryngology and Head and Neck Surgery*, vol. 18, no. 5, pp. 425–430, 2010.

[2] J. A. Goebel, "Practical anatomy and physiology," in *Practical Management of the Dizzy Patient*, pp. 3–16, Lippincott, Williams & Wilkins, Philadelphia, Pa, USA, 2001.

[3] T. Tomanovic and J. Bergenius, "Different types of dizziness in patients with peripheral vestibular diseases their prevalence and relation to migraine," *Acta Oto-Laryngologica*, vol. 130, no. 9, pp. 1024–1030, 2010.

[4] T. Brandt and M. Strupp, "General vestibular testing," *Clinical Neurophysiology*, vol. 116, no. 2, pp. 406–426, 2005.

[5] G. M. Halmagyi, "Garnett Passe and Rodney Williams memorial lecture: new clinical tests of unilateral vestibular dysfunction," *Journal of Laryngology and Otology*, vol. 118, no. 8, pp. 589–600, 2004.

[6] U. SchÖnfeld, K. Helling, and A. H. Clarke, "Evidence of unilateral isolated utricular hypofunction," *Acta Oto-Laryngologica*, vol. 130, no. 6, pp. 702–707, 2010.

[7] T. Brandt, "Otolithic vertigo," *Advances in Oto-Rhino-Laryngology*, vol. 58, pp. 34–47, 2001.

[8] J. G. Colebatch, G. M. Halmagyi, and N. F. Skuse, "Myogenic potentials generated by a click-evoked vestibulocollic reflex," *Journal of Neurology Neurosurgery and Psychiatry*, vol. 57, no. 2, pp. 190–197, 1994.

[9] S. Iwasaki, Y. Takai, K. Ito, and T. Murofushi, "Abnormal vestibular evoked myogenic potentials in the presence of normal caloric responses," *Otology and Neurotology*, vol. 26, no. 6, pp. 1196–1199, 2005.

[10] P. Monstad, S. Økstad, and A. Mygland, "Inferior vestibular neuritis: 3 cases with clinical features of acute vestibular neuritis, normal calorics but indications of saccular failure," *BMC Neurology*, vol. 6, article 45, 2006.

[11] B. S. Shin, S. Y. Oh, J. S. Kim et al., "Cervical and ocular vestibular-evoked myogenic potentials in acute vestibular neuritis," *Clinical Neurophysiology*, vol. 123, no. 2, pp. 369–375, 2012.

[12] D. Basta, I. Todt, H. Scherer, A. Clarke, and A. Ernst, "Postural control in otolith disorders," *Human Movement Science*, vol. 24, no. 2, pp. 268–279, 2005.

[13] S. C. A. Hegemann and A. Palla, "New methods for diagnosis and treatment of vestibular diseases," *F1000 Medicine Reports*, vol. 2, no. 1, article 60, 2010.

[14] M. Karlberg, M. Annertz, and M. Magnusson, "Acute vestibular neuritis visualized by 3-T magnetic resonance imaging with high-dose gadolinium," *Archives of Otolaryngology—Head and Neck Surgery*, vol. 130, no. 2, pp. 229–232, 2004.

[15] Y. Valko, S. C. A. Hegemann, K. P. Weber, D. Straumann, and C. J. Bockisch, "Relative diagnostic value of ocular vestibular evoked potentials and the subjective visual vertical during tilt and eccentric rotation," *Clinical Neurophysiology*, vol. 122, no. 2, pp. 398–404, 2011.

[16] F. L. Wuyts, J. Furman, R. Vanspauwen, and P. van de Heyning, "Vestibular function testing," *Current Opinion in Neurology*, vol. 20, no. 1, pp. 19–24, 2007.

[17] G. M. Halmagyi, S. T. Aw, M. Karlberg, I. S. Curthoys, and M. J. Todd, "Inferior vestibular neuritis," *Annals of the New York Academy of Sciences*, vol. 956, pp. 306–313, 2002.

[18] C. M. Kingma and H. P. Wit, "Asymmetric vestibular evoked myogenic potentials in unilateral Menière patients," *European Archives of Oto-Rhino-Laryngology*, vol. 268, no. 1, pp. 57–61, 2011.

[19] C. de Waele, P. T. B. Huy, J. Diard, G. Freyss, and P. P. Vidal, "Saccular dysfunction in Meniere's disease," *The American Journal of Otology*, vol. 20, no. 2, pp. 223–232, 1999.

[20] L. Manzari, A. R. Tedesco, A. M. Burgess, and I. S. Curthoys, "Ocular and cervical vestibular-evoked myogenic potentials to

bone conducted vibration in Ménière's disease during quiescence versus during acute attacks," *Clinical Neurophysiology*, vol. 121, no. 7, pp. 1092–1101, 2010.

[21] Y. H. Young, T. W. Huang, and P. W. Cheng, "Assessing the stage of Ménière's disease using vestibular evoked myogenic potentials," *Archives of Otolaryngology—Head and Neck Surgery*, vol. 129, no. 8, pp. 815–818, 2003.

[22] S. Tabak, H. Collewijn, and L. J. J. M. Boumans, "Deviation of the subjective vertical in long-standing unilateral vestibular loss," *Acta Oto-Laryngologica*, vol. 117, no. 1, pp. 1–6, 1997.

[23] J. H. J. Allum and N. T. Shepard, "An overview of the clinical use of dynamic posturography in the differential diagnosis of balance disorders," *Journal of Vestibular Research: Equilibrium and Orientation*, vol. 9, no. 4, pp. 223–252, 1999.

[24] R. W. Baloh and V. Honrubia, "The peripheral vestibular system," in *Clinical Neurophysiology of the Vestibular System*, pp. 20–43, F.A. Davis, Philadelphia, Pa, USA, 1990.

[25] C. H. Markham, "Vestibular control of muscular tone and posture," *Canadian Journal of Neurological Sciences*, vol. 14, no. 3, pp. 493–496, 1987.

[26] V. J. Wilson and B. W. Peterson, "Peripheral and central substrates of vestibulospinal reflexes," *Physiological Reviews*, vol. 58, no. 1, pp. 80–105, 1978.

[27] S. J. Herdman, "Vestibular rehabilitation," *CONTINUUM Lifelong Learning in Neurology*, vol. 12, no. 4, pp. 151–167, 2006.

[28] A. Ernst, D. Basta, R. O. Seidl, I. Todt, H. Scherer, and A. Clarke, "Management of posttraumatic vertigo," *Otolaryngology—Head and Neck Surgery*, vol. 132, no. 4, pp. 554–558, 2005.

[29] D. E. Krebs, K. M. Gill-Body, S. W. Parker, J. V. Ramirez, and M. Wernick-Robinson, "Vestibular rehabilitation: useful but not universally so," *Otolaryngology—Head and Neck Surgery*, vol. 128, no. 2, pp. 240–250, 2003.

[30] J. C. Enticott, J. J. Vitkovic, B. Reid, P. O'Neill, and M. Paine, "Vestibular rehabilitation in individuals with inner-ear dysfunction: a pilot study," *Audiology and Neurotology*, vol. 13, no. 1, pp. 19–28, 2007.

[31] G. P. Jacobson and C. W. Newman, "The development of the dizziness handicap inventory," *Archives of Otolaryngology—Head and Neck Surgery*, vol. 116, no. 4, pp. 424–427, 1990.

[32] S. L. Whitney, D. M. Wrisley, K. E. Brown, and J. M. Furman, "Is perception of handicap related to functional performance in persons with vestibular dysfunction?" *Otology and Neurotology*, vol. 25, no. 2, pp. 139–143, 2004.

[33] J. M. Serrador, L. A. Lipsitz, G. S. Gopalakrishnan, F. O. Black, and S. J. Wood, "Loss of otolith function with age is associated with increased postural sway measures," *Neuroscience Letters*, vol. 465, no. 1, pp. 10–15, 2009.

[34] K. J. Murray, K. D. Hill, B. Phillips, and J. Waterston, "The influence of otolith dysfunction on the clinical presentation of people with a peripheral vestibular disorder," *Physical Therapy*, vol. 87, no. 2, pp. 143–152, 2007.

[35] T. D. Fife, R. J. Tusa, J. M. Furman et al., "Assessment: vestibular testing techniques in adults and children—report of the therapeutics and technology assessment subcommitte of the American academy of neurology," *Neurology*, vol. 55, no. 10, pp. 1431–1441, 2000.

[36] M. C. Schubert, R. J. Tusa, L. E. Grine, and S. J. Herdman, "Optimizing the sensitivity of the head thrust test for identifying vestibular hypofunction," *Physical Therapy*, vol. 84, no. 2, pp. 151–158, 2004.

[37] M. Karlberg, S. T. Aw, G. M. Halmagyi, and R. A. Black, "Vibration-induced shift of the subjective visual horizontal: a sign of unilateral vestibular deficit," *Archives of Otolaryngology—Head and Neck Surgery*, vol. 128, no. 1, pp. 21–27, 2002.

[38] F. W. Akin, O. D. Murnane, P. C. Panus, S. K. Caruthers, A. E. Wilkinson, and T. M. Proffitt, "The influence of voluntary tonic EMG level on the vestibular-evoked myogenic potential," *Journal of Rehabilitation Research and Development*, vol. 41, no. 3, pp. 473–480, 2004.

5

Supportive Care Needs following Cancer Treatment: A Comparison of Breast and Brain Cancer in an Australian Cohort

Bhasker Amatya,[1] Fary Khan,[1,2,3] Louisa Ng,[1,2] and Mary Galea[1,2]

[1] *Department of Rehabilitation Medicine, Royal Melbourne Hospital, 34-54 Poplar Road, Parkville, Melbourne, Victoria 3052, Australia*
[2] *Department of Medicine (Royal Melbourne Hospital), The University of Melbourne, Parkville, Victoria 3052, Australia*
[3] *School of Public Health and Preventive Medicine, Monash University, Clayton, Victoria 3800, Australia*

Correspondence should be addressed to Bhasker Amatya; bhasker.amatya@mh.org.au

Academic Editors: H. Jia, K. Nas, and C. Zwingmann

Objective. To assess and identify patient-reported supportive care needs following definitive treatment in persons with breast cancer (BC) and primary brain tumours (gliomas) (BT) in an Australian community cohort and to assess the commonalities and/or discrepancies of the reported needs in these oncological populations. *Methods.* A prospective cross-sectional survey of persons with BC (n = 85) and BT (n = 106) using questionnaires for supportive care needs, psychological morbidity, and quality of life. *Results.* BT participants were younger than BC patients (mean ages 51 and 57 years). The median time since diagnosis for both groups was over 2 years. The level of psychological morbidity, mainly depression, was high in both groups: BC (22%) and BT (20%). Participants in both groups reported at least one need ("met" or "unmet"). The BC patients reported higher numbers of "needs" and "unmet" needs compared with BT patients (mean 13.7 versus 11.6 needs; "unmet" needs mean 6.0 versus 4.1). The common "met" and "unmet" needs highlighted by both groups were comparable; the domain for most "met" needs included comprehensive cancer care, while "unmet" needs related to existential survivorship issues. *Conclusion.* Despite successful treatment many cancer survivors experience unmet supportive care needs in longer term. Understanding the impact of these beyond the acute phase is important as care shifts to community settings. More research in existential survivorship issues is needed.

1. Introduction

Cancer is a leading cause of death worldwide [1]. Breast cancer (BC) is the most common malignancy in women [1], comprising up to 16% of all cancers in women [2]. Primary brain tumours (BT), a comparatively rare and diverse group of neoplasms, account for 2% of all cancers [3] and affect 7 per 100,000 population annually worldwide [4]. The overall incidence of BC and BT is on increase worldwide [2]. In Australia, by 2015, 1 in 9 women will develop BC [5]. It is estimated that in 2009, there were 22,070 new cases of BT in United States [6, 7]. In Australia, a similarly high incidence rate is reported, with approximately 1400 new cases and more than 1200 deaths annually [8]. The World Health Organisation (WHO) promotes the integration of prevention, early detection, diagnosis and treatment [9], rehabilitation and palliative care [2] in the management of. BC and BT within the national cancer control programs.

With recent therapeutic advances, survival rates of persons with cancers have improved [10–12]. However, recovery and treatment options after BC or BT can be challenging, and many survivors experience transient and/or persistent physical, functional, and psychosocial morbidities impacting everyday activities, participation (work, social activities), and quality of life (QoL) [12–14]. In the community, various issues may surface during transition: adjustment (self-worth, self-image), coping with new demands associated with increased care needs, inability to return to driving and work, financial constraints, marital stress, and restriction in participation. Further, treatment regimens can be associated with complications and/or side-effects [14–16]. After treatment, many BC and BT patients report a range of psychological sequalae across the survivorship continuum (e.g., anxiety, depression, and sexual dysfunction) [17–19]. These disabilities can have a cumulative effect over time and cause considerable distress to the cancer survivors and their families and reduce QoL.

There are significant costs and socioeconomic implications of increased demand for health care, social and vocational services, and caregiver burden [15].

A number of studies assessed QoL, psychosocial variables and patient satisfaction in cancer cohorts [20, 21]. These studies largely evaluated problems experienced by these patients but not whether help is required to manage these problems and if patients actually received the help required. This has resulted in the development of specific measures to more broadly assess cancer patients' needs and unmet needs by directly measuring the gap between a person's experience of a service and the actual service required [22]. Some studies have attempted to use this needs-based research approach in various oncological conditions, such as BC, gynaecological, prostate, and colorectal cancers, to evaluate the problems and "needs" cancer survivors experience [23–26]. These studies were conducted in the acute care settings (hospital oncology clinics) and none address the extent of assistance/need experienced by the cancer survivors living in the community in Australian context. To our knowledge no studies compare the care needs amongst diverse cancer populations such as BC and BT. The *primary objectives* of this study therefore were to assess and identify supportive care needs in patients following definitive treatment for BC and BT in an Australian community cohort and to assess the commonalities and/or discrepancies of the reported needs in these oncological populations. The findings from this study will identify the needs from patients' perspective and will inform healthcare providers for potentially important factors impacting patients' everyday activities to facilitate optimal delivery of limited health care resources.

2. Methods

2.1. Participants and Setting. This cross-sectional study was part of a prospective rehabilitation outcomes oncological research program at the Royal Melbourne Hospital (RMH), a tertiary referral centre in Victoria, Australia and approved by its Human Research Ethics Committee (numbers 2010.203 and 2010.216). The recruitment process has been reported previously [27–29]. All consecutive patients with BC or BT (main diagnosis, *first* admission only) discharged to the community following acute treatment at RMH between 2007 and 2011 were identified. The RMH Access Database was used for cross-indexing of diseases from the Patient Administrator System of Hospital Information Systems, Department of Health, Victoria, Australia. Information in the database was from a pool of persons residing in the community, referred to the RMH from public and private medical clinics across greater Melbourne in Victoria. All participants were aged >18 years and fulfilled standard diagnostic criteria for BC as defined by the American Joint Committee on Cancer [30] and for BT using the grading system (grades I–IV) for gliomas as outlined by the WHO for Central Nervous System Tumours [31] and assessed by a surgeon/oncologist. Exclusion criteria included survival rate less than 4 months, benign and metastatic tumours, significant comorbidities or medically unstable, or psychiatric disorders (such as uncontrolled schizophrenia, actively suicidal/self-harm or physical aggressiveness (based on clinical judgment)) limiting participation in rehabilitation, and bed-bound and/or institutionalized in nursing homes.

2.2. Procedure. All 450 patients identified on the RMH Database (n = 298 BC and 152 BT patients) were invited by mail to participate in the study and a total of 191 participants (n = 85 BC and 106 BT patients) who consented were recruited. These participants undertook rehabilitation program, which provided acute surgical/oncological and rehabilitative care for inpatients and in ambulatory setting to minimize activity limitation and enhance participation.

2.2.1. Assessment. All assessments were completed in hospital clinics (or participants' homes) in a 6-week period, using a structured format, by three independent assessors. These assessors (two physicians, one research officer) were trained in cognitive and functional ability assessments (examined and accredited by a national body—the Australian Rehabilitation Outcomes Centre). They were not in contact with the acute surgical/oncological services or the rehabilitation treating teams and received separate clinical record forms. They completed demographic, functional assessments and health-related QoL measures using standardized instruments (see measures). These assessment interviews took approximately 30 minutes. The assessors did not prompt participants but provided assistance for those who had difficulty completing the questionnaires. All assessments were secured and filed and opened only at the time of entry into the database by an independent data entry officer.

2.3. Measurement

2.3.1. Demographic Characteristics. A self-reported questionnaire was used to gather basic demographic information and disease related data (surgery, pathology, treatments received, signs and symptoms, etc.).

2.3.2. Supportive Care Needs. Cancer survivor unmet needs measure (CaSUN) [22] assessed and identified needs experienced by cancer survivors within the preceding month. This included 35 need items: 6 positive change items and one open-ended question. Need items were scored as: no need (0), "met" need (1), or "unmet" need (2); "unmet" needs were further rated as weak, moderate, or strong. The total scores were derived by summing responses in that category. The "needs" items were in five domains: existential survivorship (14 items), comprehensive care (6 items), information (3 items), QoL (2 items), and relationships (3 items), as well as six positive change items. This scale has good acceptability, internal consistency, and validity [22].

2.3.3. Measures for Participation and Quality of Life. The cancer rehabilitation evaluation system—short form (CARES-SF) [32], a self-administered 59-item questionnaire, the cancer specific rehabilitation needs, and QoL. Global scores indicate QoL with summary scores for 5 domains (physical, psychosocial, medical interaction, and marital and sexual function). The participant rated the degree to which a given problem applied during the 4 weeks before the survey. Scoring was based on a four-point Likert scale, with higher scores indicating more difficulty or impairment.

The depression anxiety stress scale-21 (DASS) [33], a set of three 7-item self-report scales, measured the negative emotional states of depression, anxiety, and stress. Participants rated the extent to which they experienced each state over the past week on a 4-point Likert rating scale. Subscale scores were derived by totalling and multiplying by two to ensure consistent interpretation with the longer DASS 42-item version, as per the manual.

2.4. Statistical Analysis. All statistical analysis was conducted using SPSS for Windows software version 16 (SPSS, Chicago, IL). Kolmogorov-Smirnov tests were used to test for normality. For the CaSUN measure all 35 items were included in the calculation of the sum of total "met," total "unmet" and total needs. Factor analysis for each domain of the CaSUN was conducted. The responses format of the positive change items was interpreted descriptively. A complete case analysis strategy was used; hence, cases with missing values on a variable were excluded from the analyses of that particular variable.

3. Results

3.1. Sample Characteristics. Mean age of BC participants was 57 years (all female), with median time since definitive diagnosis of 2.2 years (IQR 1.4, 4.9), while mean age of the BT participants was 51 years (range 21–77 years), and the majority were female (56%) with median time since diagnosis of 2.1 years. More than a third (39%) of the BT patients had high grade gliomas (grade IV) and underwent surgery; two-thirds had radiotherapy (64.2%) and less than half had chemotherapy (43%). Over half of the BC patients had Bloom-Richardson-Elston (BRE) grade 3 tumours (54%), were estrogen-receptor positive (85%) and with lymph node involvement (66%). More than a third (37%) of BC patients had breast conservation surgery (lumpectomy) with axillary clearance (Table 1).

3.2. Current Symptoms. Both patient groups reported various condition-related symptoms. The main symptoms in BT patients were pain/headache (56%), ataxia (44%), seizures (43%), paresis (37%), cognitive dysfunction (36%), and visual impairment (35%). Three quarters of the BC patients reported some degree of breast related pain (75%), with 39% (n = 24) rating the pain as >5 on a 10-point scale. Other symptoms in BC patients included upper limb weakness (32%), pain limiting shoulder movement (31%), and lymphedema (29%) (Table 1).

3.3. Current Level of Psychological Wellbeing and QoL. Compared with a normative sample of the Australian population (13%) [33], a substantial number of participants reported high levels of depression: BC (22%); BT (20%) (measured by DASS). Although the stress scores were almost similar (12% each), higher level of anxiety was expressed only by BC participants (19%) (Table 2).

The highest median scores (indicating greatest distress or disability) in the CARES-SF for BT participants were found on subscales for "physical" (median (Md) = 1.0, IQR = 0.5, 1.5) (evaluating problems with daily activity) and "psychological" factors (evaluating communication and relationship) (Md = 0.6, IQR = 0.4, 1.1), while for BC participants highest scores were in "marital" (Md = 1.0, IQR = 0, 2) and "physical" factors (Md = 0.5, IQR = 0.3, 1.3) (Table 2).

3.4. Supportive Care Needs. Except for one participant in each group, both BT (99.1%, n = 105) and BC groups (98.8%, n = 84) reported at least one need ("met" or "unmet"). BC patients had slightly higher numbers of reported needs ("met" or "unmet"): mean 13.7 needs (range 0–31) compared to mean 11.6 needs (range 0–29) in BT patients (Table 2).

3.4.1. "Unmet" Needs. The majority of participants in the BC group (85%, n = 72) endorsed at least one "unmet" need, with an average of 6.0 ± 6.3 "unmet" needs (range 0–28). More than one-third of these participants (41.2%) rated their "unmet" needs as severe. The ten most frequently endorsed "unmet" needs by BC patients are shown in Table 3.

Compared to BC participants slightly fewer BT participants endorsed at least one "unmet" need (n = 81, 76%), with an average of 4.1 ± 4.9 (range 0–26) "unmet" needs. Similar to the BC group, more than one-third of the participants (41.2%) rated their "unmet" needs as severe. The ten most frequently endorsed "unmet" needs by BT patients are shown in Table 4.

Both patient groups had similar "unmet" needs with the highest needs related to dealing with fears of cancer spreading, making decision about life, stress, need for complementary medicine, and hospital parking. Additional "unmet" needs in the BC group included adjusting the body image, managing ongoing side effects, and concern about the coordinated care from treating clinicians. The BT group's additional "unmet" needs included communication with health care professionals, peers, finance, and family support.

3.4.2. "Met" Needs. Of the total BC participants, 96.5% (n = 82) reported at least one "met" need, with an average of 7.7 ± 4.6 (range 0–27) "met" needs. Similarly, most of the BT participants 98.1% (n = 104) reported at least one "met" need, with an average of 7.3 ± 4.0 (range 0–24) "met" needs. The ten most frequently endorsed "met" needs by BC patients are shown in Table 5 and by BT patients in Table 6.

Most common "met" needs were similar in both patient groups, the highest number of "met" needs relating to medical care, information, local health services, communications with treating medical team and healthcare professionals, and emotional support. Additional "met" needs in the BC group included communication with peers and overall help and support. The BT group's additional "met" needs included managing side effects and financial support.

Table 1: Sociodemographic characteristics of participants ($n = 85$).

	n, (%) (unless otherwise stated)	
	Breast cancer ($n = 85$)	Brain tumour ($n = 106$)
Demographic factors		
Age (years)		
(Mean (SD), range)	57.6 (10.6), 34.8–81.8	52.6 (13.6), 22.1–78.5
Sex		
Female	85 (100)	61 (57.5)
Marital status		
Married/partner	53 (62.4)	81 (76.4)
Living with		
Partner/family	68 (80.0)	81 (76.4)
Education		
Secondary	37 (43.5%)	55 (51.9)
Tertiary	43 (50.6%)	47 (44.3)
Smokers	13 (15.3%)	17 (16.0)
Consumes alcohol	46 (54.1%)	45 (42.5)
Clinical characteristics		
Disease duration (years)		
(Md, (IQR))	2.2 (1.4–4.9)	2.1 (0.8, 4.0)
Tumour grading	BRE* ($n = 83$)	WHO** ($n = 96$)
Grade 1	10 (12.0%)	14 (14.6)
Grade 2	28 (33.7%)	30 (31.3)
Grade 3	45 (54.2%)	15 (15.6)
Grade 4	N/A	37 (38.5)
Surgery	85 (100%)	105 (99.1)
≥2 surgery episodes	36 (42.4%)	33 (31.4)
Chemotherapy	63 (74.1%)	45 (42.5)
Multiple episode	54 (96.4%)	19 (42.2)
Side effects	60 (70.6%)	31 (68.9)
Radiotherapy	63 (74.1%)	68 (64.2)
Multiple episode	48 (76.2%)	44 (64.7)
Side effects	47 (55.3%)	45 (66.2)
Currently on treatment	55 (64.7%)	
Comorbidities		
Hypertension	27 (31.8%)	30 (28.3)
Diabetes	5 (5.9%)	5 (4.7)
Depression	28 (32.9%)	12 (11.3)
Pain	63 (74.1%)	59 (55.7)
VAS pain score (0: no pain; 10: extreme pain)		
Mean (SD), range	3.8 (2.1), 1–8	3.0 (2.0, 5.0)

IQR: interquartile range, Md: median, n: total number, SD: standard deviation, VAS: visual analogue scale.
*BRE: Bloom-Richardson-Elston grading.
**WHO: World Health Organisation classification of brain tumours (gliomas).

TABLE 2: Descriptive statistics for subscales of the depression anxiety stress scale, cancer rehabilitation evaluation system-short form and cancer survivor unmet needs measure.

Scales	Statistics	
	Breast cancer (n = 85)	Brain tumour (n = 106)
DASS (Md, IQR)		
Depression (0–42)	2 (0, 12)	4 (0, 10)
Anxiety (0–42)	4 (2, 8)	2, (0, 6)
Stress (0–42)	8 (4, 14)	6 (2, 14)
DASS group: (n, %)		
Depression		
Normal/mild (0–13)	66 (77.6%)	85 (80.2)
Moderate/severe/extreme severe (≥14)	19 (22.4%)	21 (19.8)
Anxiety		
Normal/mild (0–9)	69 (81.2%)	93 (87.7)
Moderate/severe/extreme severe (≥10)	16 (18.8%)	13 (12.3)
Stress		
Normal/mild (0–18)	75 (88.2%)	93 (87.7)
Moderate/severe/extreme severe (≥19)	10 (11.8%)	13 (12.3)
CARES-SF (global scores) (Md, IQR)		
Physical (0–4)	0.5 (0.3, 1.3)	1.0, (0.5, 1.5)
Psychological (0–4)	0.4 (0.3, 1)	0.6 (0.4, 1.1)
Medical (0–4)	0 (0, 0.5)	0 (0, 1.0)
Martial (0–4)	1 (0, 2)	0.2 (0, 0.8)
Sexual (0–4)	0.3 (0.1, 0.6)	0.3 (0, 1.5)
Overall (0–4)	0.5 (0.4, 1)	0.6 (0.4, 1.0)
CaSUN (mean (SD), range)		
Total needs	13.7 (6.5), 0–31	11.6 (5.9), 0–29
Total "unmet" needs	6.0 (6.3) 0–28	4.1 (4.9), 0–26
Total "met" needs	7.7 (4.6), 0–27	7.3 (4.0), 0–24

CARES-SF: cancer rehabilitation evaluation system-short form; CaSUN: cancer survivor unmet needs measure; DASS: depression anxiety stress scale; n: total number; Md: median; IQR: interquartile range.

TABLE 3: Breast cancer survivors' most frequently endorsed ten "unmet" needs (n = 85).

Rank*	CaSUN need items	n	%
1	I need help to manage my concerns about the cancer coming back	35	41.2
2	I need help to adjust to changes to the way I feel about my body	29	34.1
3	I need help to reduce stress in my life	29	34.1
4	I need help to manage ongoing side effects and/or complications of treatment	29	34.1
5	I need access to complementary and/or alternative therapy services	26	30.6
6	I need to know that all my doctors talk to each other to coordinate my care	22	25.9
7	I need more accessible hospital parking	21	24.7
8	I need to feel like I am managing my health together with the medical team	18	21.2
9	I need any complaints regarding my care to be properly addressed	18	21.2
10	I need help to try to make decisions about my life in the context of uncertainty	18	21.2

CaSUN: cancer survivors' unmet needs measure; n: total number.
*All items also reported by BT participants are bolded.

TABLE 4: Brain tumour survivors' most frequently endorsed ten "unmet" needs (n = 106).

Rank*	CaSUN need items	n	%
1	I need help to try to make decisions about my life in the context of uncertainty	28	26.4
2	I need help to manage my concerns about the cancer coming back	26	24.5
3	I need help to reduce stress in my life	25	23.5
4	I need to talk to others who have experienced cancer	25	23.5
5	I need more accessible hospital parking	23	21.7
6	I need an ongoing case manager to whom I can go to find out about services whenever they are needed	22	20.8
7	I need access to complementary and/or alternative therapy services	18	17.0
8	I need help to know how to support my partner and/or family	18	17.0
9	I need help to find out about financial support and/or government benefits to which I am entitled	17	16.0
10	I need help to adjust to changes in my quality of life as a result of my career	16	15.1

CaSUN: cancer survivors' unmet needs measure; n: total number.
*All items also reported by BC participants are bolded.

3.4.3. Domains of Needs. The domains of highest "met" needs for both BC and BT patients were very similar. The most frequently endorsed "met" needs by the BC group were in "comprehensive cancer care" (mean 2.6 ± 1.3), followed by "existential survivorship" (mean 2.5 ± 2.6). Likewise, the most frequently endorsed "unmet" needs in the BC group were in "existential survivorship domain" (mean 2.7 ± 3.5, range 0–13) followed by "comprehensive cancer care" domain (mean 1.1 ± 1.4, range 0–6) (Table 7, Figure 1).

The most frequently endorsed total "met" needs by the BT patients were also in "comprehensive cancer care" (mean 2.8 ± 1.3), followed by "information" domain (mean 1.7 ± 1.2) and existential survivorship (mean 1.6 ± 1.9). Similar to the BC group, the most frequently endorsed "unmet" needs by BT group were in "existential survivorship" (mean 1.9 ± 2.6) followed by "comprehensive cancer care" (mean 0.8 ± 1.1) (Table 7, Figure 1).

4. Discussion

To our knowledge, this cross-sectional study is the first to report comparative ongoing "needs" in two diverse groups of cancer populations (BC and BT) in the community following successful completion of their treatment. The BT and BC survivors in this study are similar to those in other studies in terms of age, gender, disease severity, and treatment [10, 34–38]. The median time since diagnosis was just over 2 years with established impairments and functional disability. Although most cancer survivors in this study seem to have adjusted well, a significant proportion experienced transient and/or persistent physical and psychosocial morbidities which necessitated some form of care. Almost all participants from both BC and BT groups reported at least one need ("met" or "unmet") and over two-thirds reported that one or more of their needs were unmet. BC patients reported a slightly higher number of "unmet" needs compared to BT patients (85% versus 76%). Of these "unmet" needs, over 40% in both groups reported that their "unmet" needs were severe.

As expected, there were commonalities and overlap amongst the supportive care needs endorsed by BT and BC survivors. Highest levels of "met" needs across the survivorship continuum reported by both groups were in the "comprehensive care," "existential survivorship," and "information" domains, consistent with those in other oncological cohorts such as gynaecology, prostrate, and colorectal cancers [24, 26]. Remarkably, the highest levels of the "unmet" needs in both groups were similar, in the domains of "existential survivorship" and "comprehensive care." Further, a substantial number of participants in both groups reported high levels of depression, anxiety, and stress (measured by DASS), compared with only 13% in an Australian normative sample [33].

Advanced medical management in cancer has significantly improved survival rate both in BC and BT populations, and there is growing recognition of these conditions as a long-term illnesses impacting psychological functioning and QoL [39, 40]. However, the physical and psychological morbidity and needs associated with these impairments, as in other cancer patients, can be underestimated [15, 41]. Understanding the long-term posttreatment impact of cancer and the needs of these patients is important as followup moves from acute settings to community health services.

This study provides an overview of the commonalities and discrepancies of the needs from the perspective of BC and BT patients across the survivorship trajectory. The findings of this study not only validate the ongoing challenges of survivorship reported by studies in other oncological groups [24–26, 42–44], but also are an important step towards understanding the problems with which a growing number of cancer survivors require assistance in the community. This information will assist in evidence-based planning and management and can improve clinical service delivery in identified areas for improved patient outcomes [26, 45].

This study has some potential limitations. First, this is a cross-sectional study, which limits the ability to draw causal relationships between the many domains of reported needs

Table 5: Breast cancer survivors' most frequently endorsed "met" needs (n = 85).

Rank*	CaSUN need items	n	%
1	I need the very best medical care	71	83.5
2	I need up-to-date information	50	58.8
3	I need to feel like I am managing my health together with the medical team	50	58.8
4	I need information provided in a way that I can understand	46	54.1
5	I need local health care services that are available when I require them	45	52.9
6	I need to know that all my doctors talk to each other to coordinate my care	43	50.6
7	I need emotional support to be provided for me	42	49.4
8	I need to talk to others who have experienced cancer	32	37.6
9	My family and/or partner needs information relevant to them	27	31.8
10	I need help to move on with my life	24	28.2

CaSUN: cancer survivors' unmet needs measure; n: total number.
*All items also reported by BT participants are bolded.

Table 6: Brain tumour survivors' most frequently endorsed "met" needs (n = 106).

Rank*	CaSUN need items	n	%
1	I need the very best medical care	89	84.0
2	I need local health care services that are available when I require them	70	66.0
3	I need to feel like I am managing my health together with the medical team	67	63.2
4	I need up-to-date information	62	58.5
5	I need information provided in a way that I can understand	61	57.5
6	My family and/or partner needs information relevant to them	57	53.8
7	I need to know that all my doctors talk to each other to coordinate my care	57	53.8
8	I need help to manage ongoing side effects and/or complications of treatment	38	35.8
9	I need emotional support to be provided for me	36	34.0
10	I need help to find out about financial support and/or government benefits to which I am entitled	33	31.1

CaSUN: cancer survivors' unmet needs measure; n: total number.
*All items also reported by BC participants are bolded.

Table 7: Participants' endorsement of the cancer survivor unmet needs measure ranked by total "met" needs.

Rank	CaSUN factor	Brain tumour (n = 106)				Breast cancer (n = 85)			
		Total met need		Total unmet need		Total met need		Total unmet need	
		Mean (SD)	Range	Mean (SD)	Range	Mean (SD)	Range	Mean (SD)	Range
1	Comprehensive cancer care	2.8 (1.4)	0–5	0.8 (1.1)	0–5	2.6 (1.3)	0–5	1.1 (1.4)	0–6
2	Existential survivorship	1.6 (1.9)	0–11	1.9 (2.6)	0–12	2.5 (2.6)	0–13	2.7 (3.5)	0–13
3	Information	1.7 (1.2)	0–3	0.3 (0.7)	0–3	1.5 (1.1)	0–3	0.4 (0.7)	0–3
4	Quality of life	0.5 (0.6)	0–2	0.3 (0.6)	0–2	0.3 (0.6)	0–2	0.5 (0.7)	0–2
5	Relationship	0.1 (0.4)	0–2	0.4 (0.8)	0–3	0.2 (0.6)	0–3	0.5 (0.9)	0–3

CaSUN: cancer survivor unmet needs measure; n: total number; SD: standard deviation.

and functional improvements. Second, as this study utilized relatively small selective cohorts listed on a database held at single tertiary institution, with strict inclusion criteria who volunteered to participate, which may limit generalizability of findings. The study cohorts, however, are similar to cohorts reported in other studies and represent a wide sample of BT and BC survivors in the community. Participants in this study were complex in terms of disease severity, symptoms, and comorbidities (reflective of those seen in clinical practice). In an attempt to reduce recall and information bias, the assessors worked individually with each participant and all questions were limited to the person's current situation. Thirdly, we acknowledge that we were not able to capture and evaluate various other needs and problems (such as spiritual and religious needs) beyond those included within the domains of the CaSUN, this was beyond the scope of this study. The CaSUN measure, however, was broad and expansive.

5. Conclusions

BT and BC are complex and challenging conditions, with multifaceted physical, psychological, and cognitive disabilities and participatory limitations that require an integrated interdisciplinary approach [39, 40]. Understanding the impact of BT and BC in the longer term (beyond the acute phase) is important, as current medical advances have

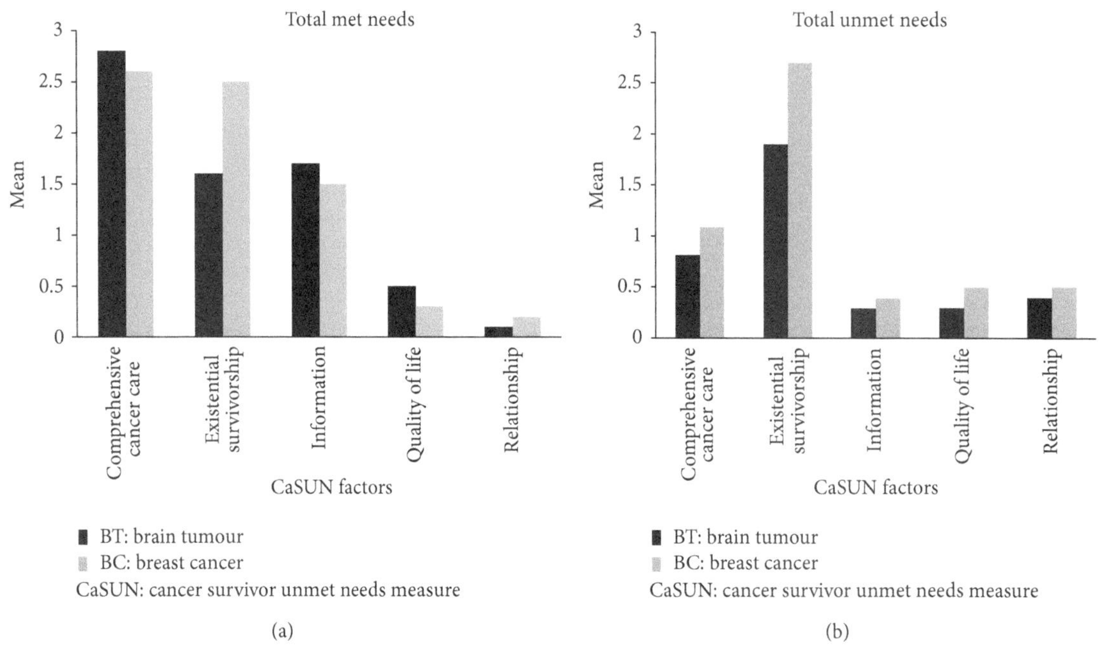

FIGURE 1: Participants' endorsement of the cancer survivor unmet needs measure factors. BT = brain tumour; BC = breast cancer; CaSUN = cancer survivor unmet needs measure.

improved patient survival and shifted care patient management to the ambulatory care sector. Supportive care needs were frequently reported by both BT and BC survivors in the longer term along the disease-survivorship continuum, with over two-thirds reporting one or more of their needs not unmet. The most frequently reported needs were in domains of "existential survivorship" and "comprehensive care." The specific needs experienced by these survivors were similar many years after apparently successful cancer treatment. Findings from this study highlight the multifaceted needs and problems reported by these complex patient populations, which needs to be assessed and addressed by all healthcare professionals involved in the follow-up care. These findings, however, need to be confirmed in robust clinical trials with larger study samples in multiple settings.

Abbreviations

BC:	Breast cancer
BT:	Brain tumour
BRE:	Bloom-Richardson-Elston grading
CaSUN:	Cancer survivor unmet needs
CARES-SF:	Cancer rehabilitation evaluation system—short form
DASS:	Depression anxiety stress scale
IQR:	Interquartile range
VAS:	Visual analogue scale
WHO:	World Health Organisation.

Ethical Approval

The study was approved by the Royal Melbourne Hospital Ethical Committee and informed consent was obtained from all the subjects.

Disclosure

The corresponding author has the right to grant on behalf of all authors and does grant on behalf of all authors an exclusive license to the ISRN Rehabilitation.

Conflict of Interests

The authors declare that there is no conflict of interests regarding the publication of the paper.

Acknowledgments

The authors are grateful to all participants with breast cancer in this study. The authors particularly wish to thank Ms. L. Oscari and Drs. N. Zhang and I. Rajapaksa for patient assessments and T. Khan for data entry. The authors also acknowledge Professor B. Mann and Associate Professor Kate Drummond of Cancer Services at the Royal Melbourne Hospital.

References

[1] Australian Institute of Health and Welfare (AIHW) and Australasian Association of Cancer Registries (AACR), *Cancer in Australia: An Overview, 2012*, Cancer Series no. 74. Cat. No. CAN 70, AIHW, Canberra, Australia, 2012.

[2] World Health Organisation, *The Global Burden of Disease: 2004 Update*, WHO, Geneva, Switzerland, 2008.

[3] A. Arber, S. Faithfull, M. Plaskota et al., "A study of patients with a primary malignant brain tumour and their carers: symptoms and access to services," *International Journal of Palliative Nursing*, vol. 16, no. 1, pp. 24–30, 2010.

[4] D. M. Parkin, S. L. Whelan, and J. Ferlay, *Cancer Incidence in Five Continents*, vol. 1–8, no. 7 of *IARC Cancerbase*, Lyon, France, 2005.

[5] Australian Institute of Health and Welfare (AIHW), *Breast Cancer in Australia: An Overview. National Breast and Ovarian Cancer Centre*, Cancer Series no 50. Cat no CAN 46, AIHW, Canberra, Australia, 2009.

[6] A. Flowers, "Brain tumors in the older person," *Cancer Control*, vol. 7, no. 6, pp. 523–538, 2000.

[7] A. Jemal, R. Siegel, E. Ward, Y. Hao, J. Xu, and M. J. Thun, "Cancer statistics, 2009," *CA Cancer Journal for Clinicians*, vol. 59, no. 4, pp. 225–249, 2009.

[8] Brain Foundation, "Brain tumour and braincancer," 2011, http://brainfoundation.org.au/medical-info/brain-tumour.

[9] C.-H. Yip, R. A. Smith, B. O. Anderson et al., "Guideline implementation for breast healthcare in low- and middle-income countries: early detection resource allocation," *Cancer*, vol. 113, no. 8, pp. 2244–2256, 2008.

[10] M. E. Huang, J. E. Wartella, and J. S. Kreutzer, "Functional outcomes and quality of life in patients with brain tumors: a preliminary report," *Archives of Physical Medicine and Rehabilitation*, vol. 82, no. 11, pp. 1540–1546, 2001.

[11] G. Poggi, M. Liscio, V. Pastore et al., "Psychological intervention in young brain tumor survivors: the efficacy of the cognitive behavioural approach," *Disability and Rehabilitation*, vol. 31, no. 13, pp. 1066–1073, 2009.

[12] B. Thewes, P. Butow, A. Girgis, and S. Pendlebury, "The psychosocial needs of breast cancer survivors; a qualitative study of the shared and unique needs of younger versus older survivors," *Psycho-Oncology*, vol. 13, no. 3, pp. 177–189, 2004.

[13] K. L. Campbell, A. L. Pusic, D. S. Zucker et al., "A prospective model of care for breast cancer rehabilitation: function," *Cancer*, vol. 118, no. 8, pp. 2300–2311, 2012.

[14] V. Tang, M. Rathbone, J. Park Dorsay, S. Jiang, and D. Harvey, "Rehabilitation in primary and metastatic brain tumours: impact of functional outcomes on survival," *Journal of Neurology*, vol. 255, no. 6, pp. 820–827, 2008.

[15] D. J. Franklin, "Cancer rehabilitation: challenges, approaches, and new directions," *Physical Medicine and Rehabilitation Clinics of North America*, vol. 18, no. 4, pp. 899–924, 2007.

[16] N. M. Aziz and J. H. Rowland, "Trends and advances in cancer survivorship research: challenge and opportunity," *Seminars in Radiation Oncology*, vol. 13, no. 3, pp. 248–266, 2003.

[17] J. S. Carpenter, M. A. Andrykowski, P. Sloan et al., "Post mastectomy/post lumpectomy pain in breast cancer survivors," *Journal of Clinical Epidemiology*, vol. 51, pp. 1285–1292, 1998.

[18] T. Ownsworth, A. Hawkes, S. Steginga, D. Walker, and D. Shum, "A biopsychosocial perspective on adjustment and quality of life following brain tumor: a systematic evaluation of the literature," *Disability and Rehabilitation*, vol. 31, no. 13, pp. 1038–1055, 2009.

[19] F. A. Tager, P. S. McKinley, F. R. Schnabel et al., "The cognitive effects of chemotherapy in post-menopausal breast cancer patients: a controlled longitudinal study," *Breast Cancer Research and Treatment*, vol. 123, no. 1, pp. 25–34, 2010.

[20] F. Fehlauer, S. Tribius, A. Mehnert, and D. Rades, "Health-related quality of life in long term breast cancer survivors treated with breast conserving therapy: impact of age at therapy," *Breast Cancer Research and Treatment*, vol. 92, no. 3, pp. 217–222, 2005.

[21] K. K. Ness, E. B. Morris, V. G. Nolan et al., "Physical performance limitations among adult survivors of childhood brain tumors," *Cancer*, vol. 116, no. 12, pp. 3034–3044, 2010.

[22] K. Hodgkinson, P. Butow, G. E. Hunt et al., "The development and evaluation of a measure to assess cancer survivors' unmet supportive care needs: TheCaSUN (Cancer Survivors' Unmet Needs measure)," *Psycho-Oncology*, vol. 16, no. 9, pp. 796–804, 2007.

[23] H. S. Campbell, R. Sanson-Fisher, D. Turner, L. Hayward, X. S. Wang, and J. Taylor-Brown, "Psychometric properties of cancer survivors' unmet needs survey," *Supportive Care in Cancer*, vol. 19, no. 2, pp. 221–230, 2010.

[24] S. E. Harrison, E. K. Watson, A. M. Ward et al., "Primary health and supportive care needs of long-term cancer survivors: a questionnaire survey," *Journal of Clinical Oncology*, vol. 29, no. 15, pp. 2091–2098, 2011.

[25] K. Hodgkinson, P. Butow, G. E. Hunt, S. Pendlebury, K. M. Hobbs, and G. Wain, "Breast cancer survivors' supportive care needs 2–10 years after diagnosis," *Supportive Care in Cancer*, vol. 15, no. 5, pp. 515–523, 2007.

[26] K. Hodgkinson, P. Butow, A. Fuchs et al., "Long-term survival from gynecologic cancer: psychosocial outcomes, supportive care needs and positive outcomes," *Gynecologic Oncology*, vol. 104, no. 2, pp. 381–389, 2007.

[27] F. Khan and B. Amatya, "Factors associated with long-term functional outcomes, psychological sequelae and quality of life in persons after primary brain tumour," *Journal of Neuro-Oncology*, vol. 111, no. 3, pp. 355–366, 2013.

[28] F. Khan, B. Amatya, J. F. Pallant, and I. Rajapaksa, "Factors associated with long-term functional outcomes and psychological sequelae in women after breast cancer," *Breast*, vol. 21, no. 3, pp. 314-320, 2012.

[29] F. Khan, B. Amatya, J. F. Pallant et al., "Multidisciplinary rehabilitation in women following breast cancer treatment: a randomized controlled trial," *Journal of Rehabilitation Medicine*, vol. 44, no. 9, pp. 788–794, 2012.

[30] American Joint Committee on Cancer (AJCC), *Breast, in AJCC Cancer Staging Manual*, Springer, New York, NY, USA, 2002.

[31] P. Kleihues, P. C. Burger, and B. W. Scheithauer, "The new WHO classification of brain tumours," *Brain Pathology*, vol. 3, no. 3, pp. 255–268, 1993.

[32] P. A. Ganz, C. A. C. Schag, J. J. Lee, and M.-S. Sim, "The CARES: a generic measure of health-related quality of life for patients with cancer," *Quality of Life Research*, vol. 1, no. 1, pp. 19–29, 1992.

[33] S. H. Lovibond and P. F. Lovibond, *Manual for the Depression, Anxiety, Stress Scales*, The Psychology Foundation of Australia Inc, Sydney, Australia, 1995.

[34] C. Clayforth, L. Fritschi, S. P. McEvoy et al., "Five-year survival from breast cancer in Western Australia over a decade," *Breast*, vol. 16, no. 4, pp. 375–381, 2007.

[35] N. Devoogdt, M. Van Kampen, I. Geraerts et al., "Physical activity levels after treatment for breast cancer: one-year follow-up," *Breast Cancer Research and Treatment*, vol. 123, no. 2, pp. 417–425, 2010.

[36] J.-G. Han, Y.-D. Jiang, C.-H. Zhang et al., "Clinicopathologic characteristics and prognosis of young patients with breast cancer," *Breast*, vol. 20, no. 4, pp. 370–372, 2011.

[37] M. E. Huang, D. X. Cifu, and L. Keyser-Marcus, "Functional outcomes in patients with brain tumor after inpatient rehabilitation: comparison with traumatic brain injury," *American Journal of Physical Medicine and Rehabilitation*, vol. 79, no. 4, pp. 327–335, 2000.

[38] M. Bartolo, C. Zucchella, A. Pace et al., "Early rehabilitation after surgery improves functional outcome in inpatients with

brain tumours," *Journal of Neuro-Oncology*, vol. 107, no. 3, pp. 537–544, 2012.

[39] F. Khan, B. Amatya, L. Ng et al., "Multidisciplinary rehabilitation for follow-up of women treated for breast cancer," *Cochrane Database of Systematic Reviews*, no. 12, Article ID CD009553, 2012.

[40] F. Khan, B. Amatya, L. Ng et al., "Multidisciplinary rehabilitation after primary brain tumour treatment," *Cochrane Database of Systematic Reviews*, no. 1, Article ID CD009509, 2013.

[41] N. A. Hutchison, "Cancer rehabilitation," *Minnesota Medicine*, vol. 93, no. 10, pp. 50–52, 2010.

[42] J. Armes, M. Crowe, L. Colbourne et al., "Patients' supportive care needs beyond the end of cancer treatment: a prospective, longitudinal survey," *Journal of Clinical Oncology*, vol. 27, no. 36, pp. 6172–6179, 2009.

[43] V. Beesley, E. Eakin, S. Steginga, J. Aitken, J. Dunn, and D. Battistutta, "Unmet needs of gynaecological cancer survivors: implications for developing community support services," *Psycho-Oncology*, vol. 17, no. 4, pp. 392–400, 2008.

[44] S. L. Sanders, E. O. Bantum, J. E. Owen, A. A. Thornton, and A. L. Stanton, "Supportive care needs in patients with lung cancer," *Psycho-Oncology*, vol. 19, no. 5, pp. 480–489, 2010.

[45] S. H. Campbell, M. Carey, R. Sanson-Fisher et al., "Measuring the unmet supportive care needs of cancer support persons: the development of the Support Person's Unmet Needs Survey—short form," *European Journal of Cancer Care*, 2013.

6

Metronome-Cued Stepping in Place after Hemiparetic Stroke: Comparison of a One- and Two-Tone Beat

Rachel L. Wright,[1] Afia Masood,[1] Elinor S. MacCormac,[1] David Pratt,[2] Catherine M. Sackley,[3] and Alan M. Wing[1]

[1] *School of Psychology, University of Birmingham, Edgbaston, Birmingham B15 2TT, UK*
[2] *West Midlands Rehabilitation Centre, Birmingham Community Healthcare Trust, Birmingham B29 6HZ, UK*
[3] *School of Allied Health Professions, University of East Anglia, Norwich NR4 7TJ, UK*

Correspondence should be addressed to Rachel L. Wright; r.wright.1@bham.ac.uk

Academic Editors: G. N. Lewis and C. I. Renner

Hemiparetic gait is characterised by temporal asymmetry and variability, and these variables are improved by auditory cueing. Stepping in place incorporates aspects of gait and may be a useful tool for locomotor training. The aim of this pilot study was to investigate the use of a single-tone and dual-tone metronome to cue stepping in place after hemiparetic stroke. Eight participants completed an uncued baseline stepping condition and two cued stepping conditions utilising a single-tone and a dual-tone metronome. Step times were determined from force plate data, and asymmetry and variability were calculated for the three conditions. Step time asymmetry was significantly reduced in the single-tone condition compared to baseline, and paretic step time variability was significantly reduced in both cued conditions. The single-tone metronome appeared to be preferred to the dual-tone metronome based on participant feedback. The results of this pilot study suggest that metronome cueing produces similar benefits on stepping in place to previously reported findings in walking. Further research on whether stepping in place to a metronome can be used for locomotor training is needed.

1. Introduction

Hemiparetic gait is characterised by several specific deficits, including decreased walking speed [1], increased variability [2], and asymmetrical stepping [3, 4]. Understanding and rehabilitating these features of hemiparetic gait are of paramount importance as walking affords a considerable level of independence and thus a better quality of life for many stroke survivors [5].

Temporal asymmetry is a common characteristic of hemiparetic walking, even amongst independent ambulators [6], is very resistant to rehabilitation efforts [7], and appears to progress in later stages after stroke [8]. Temporal asymmetry is associated with increased vertical ground reaction forces through the nonparetic limb [9], and repeated higher forces over prolonged periods increase the risk of joint pain [10] and degeneration [11]. Temporal asymmetry is associated with decreased performance on clinical balance tests [12] and therefore may be linked to the increased risk of falling observed after stroke.

Increases in the variability of gait parameters is of concern as only a small increase in stride time variability is associated with a risk of future falls [13]. Greater intraindividual variability in step length and double support time is linearly associated with increased risk of multiple falls in older adults, with a nonlinear association for step time variability [14]. Gait variability is higher after stroke than in healthy controls, and there is a direct association between underlying paretic limb impairment and step variability [2]. It is possible that this increased variability is linked to inferior dynamic balance after stroke.

The use of an auditory rhythm, such as a metronome, has been investigated as a means to improve hemiparetic gait [15]. Immediate effects of a metronome have been reported, with chronic stroke patients able to synchronise to a metronome during treadmill walking [14]. Improvements in temporal symmetry were observed with acoustic pacing, as was the ability to make gait adjustments in response to auditory cues [16]. Auditory cueing has also resulted in a decrease in swing time variability and muscle activation variability in the paretic limb during gait [17].

Cueing of each step has demonstrated stronger auditory-motor synchronisation as opposed to cueing only the paretic or nonparetic step [18], indicating that cueing both footfalls is important in metronome studies. The most beneficial metronome cueing rate for auditory-motor synchronisation is at the preferred cadence of the individual participant [19], and this is likely to be the most effective at improving gait symmetry. Gait has been cued with a different pitch for left and right footfalls [19], however it is unknown whether this approach has benefits over the use of a single pitch for both footfalls.

Stepping in place is a skill which requires reciprocal flexion and extension of the lower limbs by timely coordination and synchronisation to create a single limb support phase, a swing phase and a step frequency [20]. These components are also found in gait, and suggest stepping in place is an appropriate form of locomotor training. The temporal asymmetries typically seen in hemiparetic walking are also shown in stepping in place [20]. Therefore, it is possible that stepping in place to an auditory cue may provide an alternative to gait training, allowing stepping to be conducted in environments where space is restricted for walking training or as a precursor to overground walking training.

The first aim of this pilot study was to assess whether immediate improvements in step timing and variability observed in metronome-cued walking could be elicited by metronome-cued stepping in place. The second aim was to investigate whether the use of a single-tone to cue both limbs or a separate tone to cue each limb provided any additional advantage.

2. Materials and Methods

2.1. Participants. Ten community-dwelling adults (four female) with chronic hemiparesis (see Table 1), gave written informed consent to participate. Favourable ethical opinion was granted by the Local Research Ethics Committee and was carried out in accordance with the principles laid down by the Declaration of Helsinki. Participants were recruited through local media publicity. Inclusion criteria were at least 6 months afterstroke, walking disability but retained ability to stand and transfer, and a Rivermead Motor Assessment Gross Function (RMA GF) scale score [21] of 6–12. Participants were excluded if they had cognitive impairments preventing understanding of the task or hearing impairments reducing ability to hear the metronome.

2.2. Data Collection. All testing occurred during a single session and consisted both of uncued and cued stepping in place. Participants stepped on two force plates (Bertec 4060 H, Ohio, USA), placed side by side, with one foot on each force plate. Participants were asked to step in place at their comfortable speed to obtain baseline measures. Their average step time at baseline was determined and used to determine the interresponse interval (IRI) for the metronome. In the cued trials, participants were instructed to listen to the first 5 tones before initiating their first step response. Participants were instructed to time their footfalls to the metronome beep. In the dual-tone condition, they were instructed to time their left footfall to the high beep and their right footfall to the low beep (see Figure 1). Each baseline and cued trial lasted 30 s, and participants were given breaks between trials to minimise fatigue.

Table 1: Demographic information.

Demographic information	
Age	61 ± 16 years
Time since stroke	6 ± 2 years
Gender	6 male, 4 female
Paretic side	6 right, 4 left
RMA GF (maximum 13)	10 ± 1

Participants synchronised their footfalls to the pulse of a metronome programme running on a PC which played at a regular IRI. The single-tone metronome and the first pitch of the dual-tone metronome were set to a frequency of 700 Hz, whereas the second pitch of the dual-tone metronome was set to 1400 Hz. The tone duration was 100 ms. The IRI of the metronome pulse was created based on the participants' individual uncued stepping times (average of left and right step time) and presented using the MatTAP toolbox [22].

Five baseline stepping trials were conducted, followed by 5 stepping trials in each cued condition. A crossover design was adopted so that half the participants were randomly assigned condition 1 followed by condition 2 and vice versa. A familiarisation period of 30 s stepping to the cue was utilised prior to data collection in the cued conditions. The Timed Up and Go (TUG) test [23, 24] was conducted after each stepping condition as a functional mobility test. A rest period of 10 minutes was given between the two cueing conditions to minimise crossover effects.

2.3. Data Analysis. Data were sampled at 2000 Hz and filtered using a 2nd-order, multipass Butterworth filter with a cut-off frequency of 15 Hz. Paretic and nonparetic step timings were determined from initial footfall contact on the force plates using a custom analysis script in MatLab (MathWorks, Natick, MA, USA). Paretic step time was defined as the time between a nonparetic foot contact to the next paretic foot contact, whereas nonparetic step time was defined as the time between a paretic foot contact to the next nonparetic foot contact. The first 5 step times were discounted from analysis. Step time asymmetry was determined using a step time ratio, where paretic step time was divided by nonparetic step time. The coefficient of variation (CoV) was calculated as a measure of variability for step time for the paretic and nonparetic sides. Over 24 steps of data were collected for each condition, meeting the recommendations for gait variability studies [25].

Differences between cued and baseline conditions were examined using a Friedman test. Posthoc analysis using

TABLE 2: Step time asymmetry and variability and Timed Up and Go times for the three conditions.

	Baseline	Single tone	Dual tone	P
Step time asymmetry	1.24 ± 0.24	1.16 ± 0.15	1.19 ± 0.18	0.048
Paretic step time variability (%)	11.31 ± 0.05	9.04 ± 0.03	9.53 ± 0.03	0.034
Nonparetic step time variability (%)	12.02 ± 0.07	7.89 ± 0.03	8.62 ± 0.03	0.135
Timed Up and Go (s)	23.8 ± 15.2	20.8 ± 12.1	24.5 ± 16.2	0.089

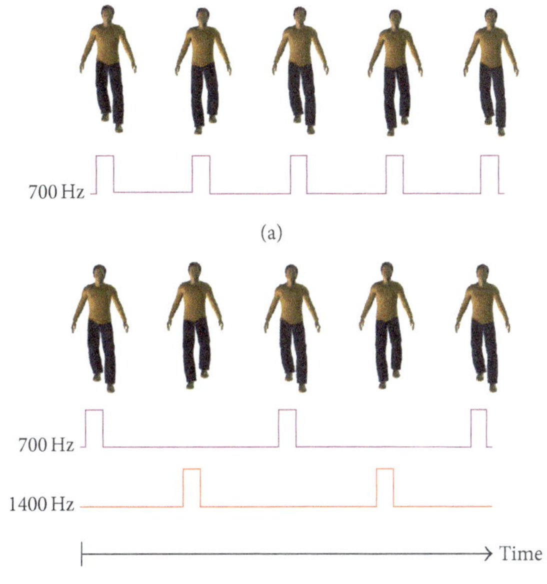

FIGURE 1: Illustration of metronome-cued stepping in (a) the single-tone condition and (b) the dual-tone condition.

Wilcoxon signed-rank tests identified the location of any differences from baseline. A Bonferroni adjustment for multiple testing was also investigated, resulting in $\alpha = 0.025$ for the post hoc analysis.

3. Results

One participant withdrew due to lacking confidence in stepping in place, whilst another participant withdrew due to a dislike of the dual-tone metronome; therefore, 8 participants completed the study.

Six of the eight participants displayed mild asymmetry (step time ratio 1.10–1.50) and two displayed severe asymmetry at baseline (>1.50). For these two participants with severe asymmetry, the use of a metronome reduced their asymmetry to <1.50. There was a significant main effect for condition ($\chi^2(2) = 6.077$, $P = 0.048$) for step time asymmetry (see Table 2). Post hoc analysis revealed this difference to be between baseline and the single-tone condition ($Z = -2.207$, $P = 0.027$); however, this was not significant with the application of a Bonferroni adjustment.

There was a significant main effect of condition for paretic step time variability ($\chi^2(2) = 6.750$, $P = 0.034$). Post hoc analysis showed these differences to be between baseline and both the single- ($Z = -2.240$, $P = 0.025$) and dual-tone conditions ($Z = -2.173$, $P = 0.030$). However, only the difference between baseline and the single-tone condition remained significant with the application of a Bonferroni adjustment. Nonparetic step time variability was lower in the two cued conditions compared to baseline; however, there was no significant main effect for this variable ($\chi^2(2) = 4.000$, $P = 0.135$). There was a trend for quicker TUG times after the single-tone condition, but this did not reach significance ($\chi^2(2) = 4.839$, $P = 0.089$).

4. Discussion

The aim of this pilot study was to examine the use of a single- and dual-tone metronome to cue stepping in place. The results indicate a trend towards better symmetry of step time during cueing and significantly reduced paretic step time variability, with the improvements being slightly more pronounced for the single- than the dual-tone cue. There was also a trend towards improved TUG times after the single-tone cueing condition. This provides an early indication that a single-tone cue may be more efficient than a dual-tone cue at eliciting improvements when stepping in place in a stroke population.

Temporal asymmetry has a high prevalence after stroke [6], shows resilience to rehabilitation [7], and progresses over time [8]. Temporal asymmetry is associated with poorer results in clinical balance tests [12]; therefore, any improvement might be expected to have benefits for balance after stroke. The reduction in step time asymmetry observed here with the single-tone metronome is of a similar magnitude to that previously observed with auditory-cued treadmill walking [14]; however, the mean temporal asymmetry in the current study is milder at baseline than the mean asymmetry for the study population in [14]. Two of the participants in the current study would be classified as having severe asymmetry at baseline, and for both participants, the asymmetry was reduced with the metronome cue. This suggests that cueing is effective and immediate even in those with a high level of asymmetry. Future research is needed to see if these improvements in temporal asymmetry can be elicited in a larger sample stroke population with severe temporal asymmetry.

The variability in step time on both the paretic and nonparetic steps was reduced in both cueing conditions compared to baseline, although this was only statistically significant for the paretic step. This reduction in variability with auditory cueing is consistent with gait studies involving participants with stroke [17] and Parkinson's disease [26]. Increased step time variability is associated with a risk of multiple future falls in older adults [13], and stroke survivors are over twice as likely to experience at least one fall than population controls [27]. Therefore, these reductions in variability may have benefits for balance control after stroke.

Some of the participants commented on how the dual tone metronome did not sound like a regular beat, and one participant withdrew from the study because he/she did not like the dual-tone. It is possible that there was superior detection of gaps between stimuli in the single-tone condition compared to the dual-tone condition where the tones were dissimilar, which may cause a slight illusion in the perception of the gaps between stimuli [28]. Caution needs to be employed when using a different tone to cue the footfall of the left and right limbs that the tones themselves do not cause a distortion in the perception of the timing intervals.

Stepping in place incorporates many of the aspects of walking gait. Temporal asymmetries displayed during stepping are consistent with those present during walking [20]. Step time variability during stepping in a virtual reality environment has also been found to be similar to stride time variability during gait, although that was for a Parkinson's disease population [29]. The immediate improvements in both asymmetry and variability, when stepping was cued to a metronome, were consistent with those previously reported for cued walking [14]. In addition, the trend for improved TUG times after the single-cue condition suggests that there may be an immediate carry-over effect on functional mobility. Therefore, auditory-cued stepping may be a useful tool for locomotor training in rehabilitation.

Individuals with chronic stroke perform notably reduced amounts of daily stepping than sedentary older adults, even in those receiving physiotherapy [30]. This suggests that individuals after stroke are not performing enough repetitions for optimal benefits in locomotor training, and sedentary behaviour is associated with multiple adverse health outcomes [31]. Intensive locomotor training has shown improvements in walking performance after discharge from rehabilitation for reaching a "recovery plateau," and this was likely to be related to the dose of training [32]. If a metronome could be adapted for step training at home, then this could be a rehabilitation tool that could be utilised daily and therefore provides a much higher dosage of step training than clinic-based training alone.

The 10-minute break between cueing conditions may not have been sufficiently long enough to exclude an effect of the first condition on the second one. However, the use of a crossover design should have reduced the tendency for any carryover or fatigue that could influence the findings. Although improvements were seen in stepping during the cued conditions, we did not find a significant improvement in the TUG, and we did not specifically examine the transfer of these skills to everyday, community walking. Therefore, future study is required to examine whether improvements in stepping in place are carried into functional walking improvement in hemiparetic stroke.

5. Conclusions

Early evidence from this pilot study suggests that the use of a metronome for stepping in place has benefits for step time asymmetry and variability after hemiparetic stroke. These modifications in the step pattern are immediate and not the result of a training effect. Caution needs to be applied if a dual tone is used for cueing, as this may not optimise rehabilitation as the effects do not appear as strong as for a single-tone metronome; plus, not all participants liked the dual tone as they thought that it did not sound like a regular beat. This may have an effect on compliance if used as a training tool in rehabilitation. Further research is needed to assess whether auditory-cued step training results in significant improvements in functional walking and whether any improvements are maintained after a follow-up period.

Acknowledgment

This study was funded through a project grant from the Stroke Association (Grant code TSA2009/06).

References

[1] S. J. Olney and C. Richards, "Hemiparetic gait following stroke. Part I: characteristics," *Gait & Posture*, vol. 4, no. 2, pp. 136–148, 1996.

[2] C. K. Balasubramanian, R. R. Neptune, and S. A. Kautz, "Variability in spatiotemporal step characteristics and its relationship to walking performance post-stroke," *Gait & Posture*, vol. 29, no. 3, pp. 408–414, 2009.

[3] A. L. Hsu, P. F. Tang, and M. H. Jan, "Analysis of impairments influencing gait velocity and asymmetry of hemiplegic patients after mild to moderate stroke," *Archives of Physical Medicine and Rehabilitation*, vol. 84, no. 8, pp. 1185–1193, 2003.

[4] G. Chen, C. Patten, D. H. Kothari, and F. E. Zajac, "Gait differences between individuals with post-stroke hemiparesis and non-disabled controls at matched speeds," *Gait & Posture*, vol. 22, no. 1, pp. 51–56, 2005.

[5] C. L. Richards, F. Malouin, S. Wood-Dauphinee, J. I. Williams, J. P. Bouchard, and D. Brunet, "Task-specific physical therapy for optimization of gait recovery in acute stroke patients," *Archives of Physical Medicine and Rehabilitation*, vol. 74, no. 6, pp. 612–620, 1993.

[6] K. K. Patterson, I. Parafianowicz, C. J. Danells et al., "Gait asymmetry in community-ambulating stroke survivors," *Archives of Physical Medicine and Rehabilitation*, vol. 89, no. 2, pp. 304–310, 2008.

[7] M. H. Thaut, G. C. McIntosh, and R. R. Rice, "Rhythmic facilitation of gait training in hemiparetic stroke rehabilitation," *Journal of the Neurological Sciences*, vol. 151, no. 2, pp. 207–212, 1997.

[8] K. K. Patterson, W. H. Gage, D. Brooks, S. E. Black, and W. E. McIlroy, "Changes in gait symmetry and velocity after stroke: a cross-sectional study from weeks to years after stroke," *Neurorehabilitation and Neural Repair*, vol. 24, no. 9, pp. 783–790, 2010.

[9] D. C. Norvell, J. M. Czerniecki, G. E. Reiber, C. Maynard, J. A. Pecoraro, and N. S. Weiss, "The prevalence of knee pain and symptomatic knee osteoarthritis among veteran traumatic amputees and nonamputees," *Archives of Physical Medicine and Rehabilitation*, vol. 86, no. 3, pp. 487–493, 2005.

[10] L. Nolan, A. Wit, K. Dudziñski, A. Lees, M. Lake, and M. Wychowañski, "Adjustments in gait symmetry with walking speed in trans-femoral and trans-tibial amputees," *Gait & Posture*, vol. 17, pp. 142–151, 2003.

[11] J. M. Hausdorff, D. A. Rios, and H. K. Edelberg, "Gait variability and fall risk in community-living older adults: a 1-year prospective study," *Archives of Physical Medicine and Rehabilitation*, vol. 82, no. 8, pp. 1050–1056, 2001.

[12] M. D. Lewek, C. E. Bradley, C. J. Wutzke, and S. M. Zinder, "The relationship between spatiotemporal gait asymmetry and balance in individuals with chronic stroke," *Journal of Applied Biomechanics*. In press.

[13] M. L. Callisaya, L. Blizzard, M. D. Schmidt et al., "Gait, gait variability and the risk of multiple incident falls in older people: a population-based study," *Age and Ageing*, vol. 40, no. 4, pp. 481–487, 2011.

[14] M. Roerdink, C. J. C. Lamoth, G. Kwakkel, P. C. W. van Wieringen, and P. J. Beek, "Gait coordination after stroke: benefits of acoustically paced treadmill walking," *Physical Therapy*, vol. 87, no. 8, pp. 1009–1022, 2007.

[15] M. H. Thaut, A. K. Leins, R. R. Rice et al., "Rhythmic auditory stimulation improves gait more than NDT/Bobath training in near-ambulatory patients early poststroke: a single-blind, randomized trial," *Neurorehabilitation and Neural Repair*, vol. 21, no. 5, pp. 455–459, 2007.

[16] T. A. Pelton, L. Johannsen, H. Y. Chen, and A. M. Wing, "Hemiparetic stepping to the beat: asymmetric response to metronome phase shift during treadmill gait," *Neurorehabilitation and Neural Repair*, vol. 24, no. 5, pp. 428–434, 2010.

[17] M. H. Thaut, G. C. McIntosh, S. G. Prassas, and R. R. Rice, "Effect of rhythmic auditory cuing on temporal stride parameters and EMG. Patterns in hemiparetic gait of stroke patients," *Neurorehabilitation and Neural Repair*, vol. 7, pp. 9–16, 1993.

[18] M. Roerdink, C. J. C. Lamoth, J. van Kordelaar et al., "Rhythm perturbations in acoustically paced treadmill walking after stroke," *Neurorehabilitation and Neural Repair*, vol. 23, no. 7, pp. 668–678, 2009.

[19] M. Roerdink, P. J. M. Bank, C. L. E. Peper, and P. J. Beek, "Walking to the beat of different drums: practical implications for the use of acoustic rhythms in gait rehabilitation," *Gait & Posture*, vol. 33, no. 4, pp. 690–694, 2011.

[20] R. K. Garcia, A. J. Nelson, W. Ling, and C. van Olden, "Comparing stepping-in-place and gait ability in adults with and without hemiplegia," *Archives of Physical Medicine and Rehabilitation*, vol. 82, pp. 36–42, 2001.

[21] F. M. Collen, D. T. Wade, G. F. Robb, and C. M. Bradshaw, "The Rivermead mobility index: a further development of the Rivermead motor assessment," *International Disability Studies*, vol. 13, no. 2, pp. 50–54, 1991.

[22] M. T. Elliott, A. E. Welchman, and A. M. Wing, "MatTAP: a MATLAB toolbox for the control and analysis of movement synchronisation experiments," *Journal of Neuroscience Methods*, vol. 177, no. 1, pp. 250–257, 2009.

[23] D. Podsiadlo and S. Richardson, "The timed "up and go": a test of basic functional mobility for frail elderly persons," *Journal of the American Geriatrics Society*, vol. 39, no. 2, pp. 142–148, 1991.

[24] S. S. Ng and C. W. Hui-Chan, "The timed up & go test: its reliability and association with lower-limb impairments and locomotor capacities in people with chronic stroke," *Archives of Physical Medicine and Rehabilitation*, vol. 86, no. 8, pp. 1641–1647, 2005.

[25] S. Lord, T. Howe, J. Greenland, L. Simpson, and L. Rochester, "Gait variability in older adults: a structured review of testing protocol and clinimetric properties," *Gait & Posture*, vol. 34, no. 4, pp. 443–450, 2011.

[26] J. M. Hausdorff, J. Lowenthal, T. Herman, L. Gruendlinger, C. Peretz, and N. Giladi, "Rhythmic auditory stimulation modulates gait variability in Parkinson's disease," *European Journal of Neuroscience*, vol. 26, no. 8, pp. 2369–2375, 2007.

[27] V. Weerdesteyn, M. de Niet, H. J. R. van Duijnhoven, and A. C. H. Geurts, "Falls in individuals with stroke," *Journal of Rehabilitation Research and Development*, vol. 45, no. 8, pp. 1195–1214, 2008.

[28] P. J. Fitzgibbons, A. Pollatsek, and I. B. Thomas, "Detection of temporal gaps within and between perceptual tonal groups," *Perception & Psychophysics*, vol. 16, no. 3, pp. 522–528, 1974.

[29] M. Gilat, J. M. Shine, S. J. Bolitho et al., "Variability of stepping during a virtual reality paradigm in Parkinson's disease patients with and without freezing of gait," *PLoS ONE*, vol. 8, Article ID e66718, 2013.

[30] C. E. Lang, J. R. MacDonald, D. S. Reisman et al., "Observation of amounts of movement practice provided during stroke rehabilitation," *Archives of Physical Medicine and Rehabilitation*, vol. 90, no. 10, pp. 1692–1698, 2009.

[31] A. A. Thorp, N. Owen, M. Neuhaus, and D. W. Dunstan, "Sedentary behaviors and subsequent health outcomes in adults: a systematic review of longitudinal studies, 1996–2011," *The American Journal of Preventive Medicine*, vol. 41, no. 2, pp. 207–215, 2011.

[32] J. L. Moore, E. J. Roth, C. Killian, and T. G. Hornby, "Locomotor training improves daily stepping activity and gait efficiency in individuals poststroke who have reached a "plateau" in recovery," *Stroke*, vol. 41, no. 1, pp. 129–135, 2010.

7

Horizontal and Declined Squats in Healthy Individuals: A Study of Kinematic and Muscle Patterns

Valdeci Carlos Dionisio,[1] Bruna Maria Silva Azevedo,[2] and Daniela Abrahão Siqueira[2]

[1] *Physical Therapy Course, Federal University of Uberlândia, Benjamin Constant Street No. 1286, 38400-678 Uberlândia, MG, Brazil*
[2] *Physical Therapy Course of the University Center of Triângulo, Nicomedes Alves dos Santos Avenue No. 4545, 38411-106 Uberlândia, MG, Brazil*

Correspondence should be addressed to Valdeci Carlos Dionisio; vcdionisio@gmail.com

Academic Editors: K.-H. Lin and A. Ozcan Edeer

Squats are frequently incorporated in physiotherapy programmes and performed in different ways. Accordingly, muscle and kinematic patterns also differ. The objective was to compare the kinematics and EMG patterns of the major muscles of knee and ankle joints during different squat exercises on horizontal (HP) and 25° decline (DP) boards. Seventeen healthy individuals performed squats on HP and DP with bilateral support and restriction of trunk movements in the sagittal plane. The knee and ankle angular displacements in the sagittal plane and the EMG activities of the major muscles of the lower limb in four subphases of movement were recorded and analyzed. For the descending phase of the HP squats, the angular excursion, as well as the initial and final positions, was smaller for the knee ($P < 0.05$) but larger for the ankle ($P = 0.01$). For the ascending phase of the HP squats, the initial and final positions were larger for the ankle ($P < 0.02$) and the final position was smaller for the knee ($P = 0.05$). All muscles remained activated and showed similarity between the tasks ($P > 0.44$), except for the tibialis anterior in both squat exercises ($P < 0.03$). The HP and DP squats produced different kinematics (knee and ankle joints) but did not modify the EMG strategy for both movement phases.

1. Introduction

Injuries of the knee joint account for numerous lesions that affect the lower extremities [1]. In any lesion involving the knee, a reflex inhibition of the quadriceps is observed, accompanied by hypotrophy [2, 3], which causes knee instability [4]. This instability contributes to chronic pain, increasing the inhibition process and weakening the quadriceps and, in turn, leading to dysfunctions of the extensor mechanism [5]. Under these circumstances, quadriceps strengthening is essential to stabilize and minimize or reverse the process of inhibition and muscle weakening; such strengthening is therefore the main challenge that confronts the rehabilitation process [4].

Several protocols have been suggested for recovering quadriceps force, but multijoint exercises are the preferred form of therapy for dysfunctions of the extensor mechanism [6, 7]. Multijoint exercises are regarded as advantageous because they simulate functional activities [6, 8], exert minimal stress on the patellofemoral joint during the functional range of movements [6], and enable muscle cocontraction, which contributes to joint stability [9]. An effective multijoint exercise extensively used in clinical practice by physiotherapists is the squat [7, 10]. Some studies have demonstrated the usefulness of performing squats during knee rehabilitation [7, 10]—an effectiveness that may be attributed to the fact that such exercises increase the muscle activities of the hip, knee joints, and ankle joints; this increase is supported by the high electromyographic (EMG) activities of the hamstrings, quadriceps, and gastrocnemius muscles [11]. Some researchers have suggested that squats performed on a 25° decline plane (DP) more effectively treat patellar tendinitis than do traditional squats performed on a horizontal plane (HP) [12–14]. The DP squat is performed on a platform sufficiently large to enable positioning the feet at an incline 25° to the surface (heel elevation). The tibia is positioned vertically and strong plantar flexion of the ankle is observed. The literature discusses several indications that quadriceps muscles produce more force in DP than in HP given greater quadriceps EMG activity [13–15], greater effort (tension) of the patellar tendon [15–17], and greater knee joint torque [14, 17]. In all these studies [14–17], however, squatting tasks were performed with unipodal (single leg) support and without any type of trunk control (displacement in the sagittal plane). Trunk position and bipodal (both legs) support can modify the position of the centre of mass (COM), as well as the pattern and magnitude of EMG activity of the major muscles of the lower limb, thereby enabling individuals to maintain balance and perform tasks [18]. During the initial phase of a rehabilitation programme, multijoint exercises are performed with bipodal support and, sometimes, with control over the trunk position (e.g., trunk upright). DP and HP squats have not been tested under these conditions, and the related kinematics and EMG patterns remain uncertain. If EMG activities are higher under DP squats than under HP squats (similar to that observed in previous studies, in which exercises were performed under unipodal support), using DP squats would be the therapy of preference for recovering quadriceps force across all the phases of a rehabilitation programme.

Clarifying this issue is an important consideration for coaches and physiotherapists, especially those focusing on rehabilitating quadriceps force. The present study aimed to compare the kinematics and EMG patterns of the major muscles of knee and ankle joints during the descending and ascending phases of HP and DP squats. Bipodal support and restriction of trunk movements in the sagittal plane were applied.

2. Methods

Seventeen healthy individuals (8 men, 9 women) aged 18–35 years participated in the study. The means and standard deviations of age, weight, and height were 22.8 ± 3.14 years, 65.4 ± 13.18 kg, and 169 ± 0.08 cm, respectively. All the individuals are right-handed and weekend athletes who do not exercise regularly. The exclusion criteria were a history of pain that suggests joint or muscle disorder and surgery or musculoskeletal disorders in the lower limbs, spine, or shoulders. The individuals signed an informed consent form approved by the Research Ethics Committee (protocol 634853/2007).

After shaving and skin asepsis with alcohol, active bipolar surface electrodes (DataHominis Tecnologia Ltda) were positioned on the vastus medialis obliquus (VMO), vastus lateralis (VL), biceps femoris (BF), tibialis anterior (TA), soleus (SO), and erector spinae (EE) muscles. For the VMO, surface electrode was placed on the belly muscle along the direction of the fibres (about 54°). To identify the motor point, the participants were asked to perform an isometric contraction of the quadriceps so that the VMO activity could be observed [19]. Then, an electrode was placed 2 cm distal from the motor point. For the other muscles, electrodes were placed in accordance with the guidelines of the Surface Electromyography for the Noninvasive Assessment of Muscles project of the European Union's Biomedical Health and Research Program (BIOMED II) [20]. Each electrode consists of two parallel silver plates measuring 1 cm long and 1 mm wide, positioned 1 cm apart. The electrodes had a gain of 20 (amplification), an impedance of 10 GΩ, and a common mode rejection ratio of 84 dB. They were connected to computer-aided EMG equipment (DataHominis Tecnologia Ltda) capable of 100-time amplification (2000-time total amplification). It had a 15 Hz to 1 kHz bandpass filter and an acquisition frequency of 2000 Hz. A 3 cm^2 ground electrode was also attached to the right iliac crest and daubed with electroconductive gel to improve signal transfer. An auxiliary channel was also used with a DataHominis electrogoniometer with flexible poles and 360° rotation. It was placed on the knee and ankle joints (lateral epicondylus femoris and 2 cm below the lateral malleolus). Before the assessment, the electrogoniometer channels were calibrated to determine the maximum range (i.e., 180°). For total knee extension, this range was 0° and for flexion, the range was any value greater than 0°. The maximum range for the ankle was the same (0° to 180°), but the initial position was estimated at around 90°. A range greater than 90° indicates dorsiflexion, whereas a range less than 90° reflects plantar flexion.

The individuals performed HP and DP squats, both in the ascending and descending phases separately. They were positioned with feet parallel and shoulder-width apart, but the angle of the feet relative to the boards was chosen according to individual preference. In general, this angle varied from 5° to 8° of external rotation. The participants were also advised to keep their arms flexed at 90° in relation to the shoulders and use it as a single rigid body (without moving the elbow, wrist, and hand) to guide movement (Figure 1). This position was considered partly restrictive of trunk movements in the sagittal plane (trunk upright), thereby allowing for the same strategy in performing the squats; in previous studies, this position was also adopted for HP squats [19, 21, 22] and sit-to-stand exercises [22]. The EMG signals were recorded only from the right-hand side. The electrical activity of the muscles was captured during horizontal and 25° decline squats in both descending and ascending phases. The ranges of motion for the descending and ascending phases were 0° to 70° and 70° to 0° of knee flexion, respectively. For the decline squats, a platform declined at an angle of 25° was used for the ankle positioned in plantar flexion. An adjustable support was placed behind the participants to restrain the final movement of the descending phase and to mark the onset of the ascending phase movement. The support served as a guide, but the participants were prohibited from resting on support (Figure 1).

Each individual was allowed two repetitions for him/her to learn the movements and to verify whether any electrode wire limited his/her movements. The individuals performed 10 repetitions of the HP squats, with five of the repetitions executed in the ascending phase and five in the ascending phase. Then, they performed 10 repetitions of the DP squats,

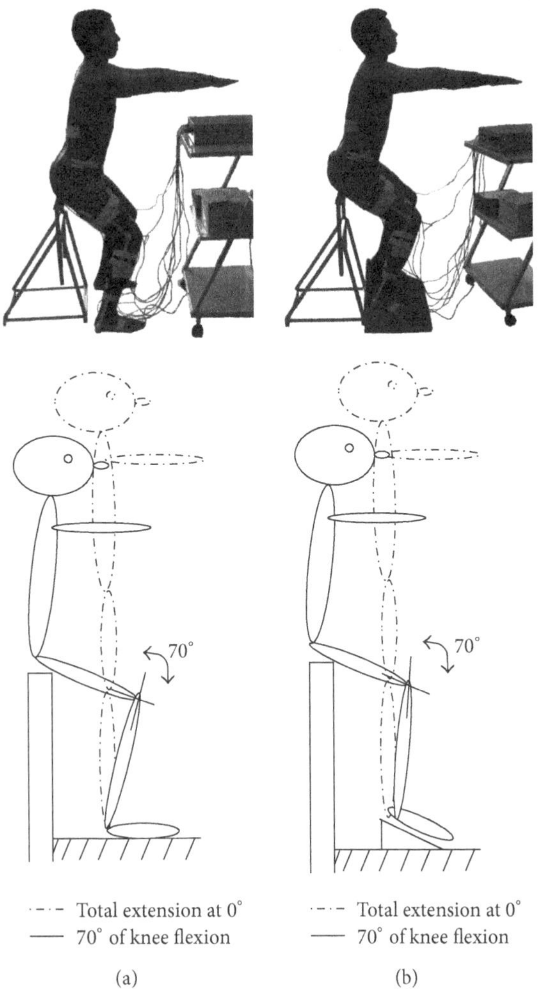

FIGURE 1: Task model for squats performed in HP (a) and DP (b). During the descending phase, movement ranged from 0° to 70° of the knee flexion, and, during the ascending phase, the movement ranged from 70° to 0° of the knee flexion.

with five of the repetitions executed in the ascending phase and five in the ascending phase. Between each set of five repetitions, an interval of 1 minute was allocated. For each squat (HP and DP), the participants were given a 3-minute rest period to avoid muscle fatigue.

A verbal instruction from the researcher signalled the onset of each movement. The individuals were instructed to perform the movements as quickly as possible and to maintain the final position (FP) until the end of data collection, which lasted 2 seconds.

Electrogoniometric signals were obtained in degrees, filtered at 50 Hz, and calculated as the velocities of the knee and ankle joints. The EMG signals, obtained in microvolt (μV), were rectified (full wave), filtered at 25 Hz, and normalized by maximal voluntary isometric contraction (MVIC). For all MVIC tests, the participants were seated in a comfortable chair [19]. The MVICs of all portions of the quadriceps were tested with the knee of the participant fixed manually at 20° of flexion (0° equal to full extension), and resistance was applied to the tibia just above the ankle in the flexion direction. The MVIC of the biceps femoris was tested with the knee of the participant fixed manually at 90°, and resistance was applied to the tibia just above the ankle in the extension direction. For the MVIC of the tibialis anterior, the knee was at full extension and the ankle was fixed manually at 90°; resistance was applied to the forefoot in the plantar flexion direction. The MVIC of the soleus was tested with the knee flexed at 90° and the foot positioned on the ground; resistance was applied over the knee in the ground direction to avoid knee movements in the superior direction. Finally, for MVIC of the erector spinae, the knees were flexed at 40°, the feet were flat on the ground, the arms were positioned over the chest, and the trunk was fixed manually on the scapulas [23]; resistance was applied in the anterior direction. On the basis of knee velocity, the EMG signals were analyzed from four subphases of movement: (1) subphase 1, 100 ms just before the knee velocity first achieved 5% of its peak (the beginning of movement); (2) subphase 2, defined as the acceleration time of the squat, that is, the interval between the end of subphase 1 and the time at which knee velocity achieved its peak; (3) subphase 3, defined as the deceleration time of the squat, and the interval between the end of subphase 2 and the time at which knee velocity returned to 5% of its peak; and (4) subphase 4, defined as the time point during which the body remained at the target squat position for 100 ms following the end of subphase 3. The mean of the five repetitions of each individual for each of the phases (ascending and descending) of the tasks (HP and DP squats) was obtained. The integral of each muscle for each subphase of movement was calculated on the basis of the mean of each individual. These procedures were carried out in Excel (Microsoft Office XP 2003) and KaleidaGraph (Synergy, version 3.08).

To evaluate the kinematic variables (angular displacement and maximal velocity of the knee and ankle joints), we employed the t-test for dependent samples. To evaluate the effect of the tasks (HP and DP squats), we used two-way factorial ANOVA for repeated measures (task (HP and DP) $\times$ muscle (curve integral of each muscle separately)). As a post hoc test, we used Tukey's honestly significant difference method to test significant differences between specific subphases. The data were analyzed in a personal computer using Statistica for Windows (Statsoft, Inc., version 5.0). For all evaluations, the significance level (α) was set at 0.05, with 90% power.

3. Results

For the descending phase of the movements, the t-test revealed that during the DP squats, the ankle exhibited a larger plantar flexion in the initial position (IP) and a lower range in the FP and angular excursion (AE) than during the HP squats. For the knee, the DP squats produced a larger knee flexion in IP, FP, and AE than did the HP squats (Table 1). Moreover, maximal ankle velocity was greater during the HP squats than during the DP squats. The maximal knee velocity was similar in both squatting movements (Table 1).

TABLE 1: Kinematic variables across all subjects for phases of the squats.

Variable (dg)[a]	Descent phase				Ascent phase			
	HP[b] mean (SD)[d]	DP[c] mean (SD)	*t* value	*P* value	HP mean (SD)	DP mean (SD)	*t* value	*P* value
Knee IP[e]	2.30 (5.13)	3.84 (5.23)	−2.15	0.04*	65.00 (10.19)	67.32 (11.06)	−1.61	0.12
Knee FP[f]	61.89 (9.97)	67.82 (10.15)	−4.86	0.01*	2.25 (5.41)	5.12 (6.61)	−2.08	0.05*
Knee AE[g]	59.58 (10.77)	63.98 (10.86)	−3. 54	0.01*	62.74 (10.57)	62.19 (10.71)	0.41	0.68
Ankle IP	85.38 (5.59)	75.42 (5.21)	9.68	0.01*	94.98 (8.24)	89.28 (5.95)	3.22	0.01*
Ankle FP	101.75 (6.58)	89.40 (6.56)	12.65	0.01*	79.71 (7.78)	75.57 (7.69)	2.58	0.02*
Ankle AE	16.37 (3.23)	13.97 (5.13)	3.26	0.01*	15.26 (4.61)	13.71 (5.10)	1.93	0.07
Maximal knee velocity (dg/s)[h]	295.63 (89.93)	283.94 (78.93)	0.59	0.55	62.74 (53.37)	54.00 (54.67)	0.73	0.47
Maximal ankle velocity (dg/s)	75.04 (20.24)	58.84 (24.20)	4.60	0.01*	15.03 (7.9)	12.67 (9.82)	1.07	0.29

[a]Degrees: dg; [b]horizontal plane: HP; [c]decline plane: DP; [d]standard deviation: SD; [e]initial position: IP (measured in degrees); [f]final position: FP; [g]angular excursion: AE; [h]degrees by second (dg/s); *statistical significance.

For the ascending phase of the movements, the *t*-test revealed no difference between the squats for the IP and AE of the knee joint. The FP of this joint exhibited a difference between squats. The IP and FP of the ankle joint also exhibited a difference, but the AE was similar between squats (Table 1). With regard to the maximal knee and ankle velocities, no difference was observed between the squatting movements (Table 1).

For the descending phase of the movements (Figure 2), ANOVA revealed no effect of the squats on EMG activity ($P > 0.44$), except for TA ($P = 0.03$). However, ANOVA revealed a difference in the subphases of movement for all the muscles ($P < 0.01$); interaction between the squats and subphases was observed only in TA ($P = 0.02$). The post hoc analysis showed that this difference occurred in subphase 3 (deceleration), with higher activity in the HP squats than in the DP squats ($P < 0.01$). The other subphases were similar between squats ($P > 0.91$).

For the ascending phase of the movements (Figure 3), ANOVA again revealed no effect of the squats on EMG activity ($P > 0.46$), but differences were found in all the muscles with regard to the subphases ($P < 0.01$); interaction between the squats and subphases was found only in TA ($P = 0.02$). The post hoc analysis revealed that this difference occurred during subphase 1, with higher activity in the HP squats than in the DP squats ($P < 0.02$). The other subphases were similar between squats ($P > 0.75$).

4. Discussion

The primary aim of the study was to evaluate the kinematics and EMG patterns of the main muscles that produce movements in the knee and ankle joints during bipodal squats in HP and DP, with restriction of trunk movements in the sagittal plane. The control of trunk movements in the sagittal plane was reported in previous studies, showing that different individuals can perform squats [19, 21] or sit-to-stand exercises [22] in a similar manner through repetitions. The performance of the participants revealed the use of a common strategy, in which the knee and ankle joints direct movement and exhibit large joint torques.

During the descent phase of the movements, differences in kinematic variables were found (Table 1). The strong plantar flexion in the DP squats influenced the position of the other joints during the standing position (IP) and the squat position (FP). This influence was reflected in AE. Although some researchers did not find differences in various declination angles—that is, 0°, 8°, 16°, and 24° [17]—the limitation imposed on the ankle joint in DP (strong plantar flexion) resulted in a small ankle velocity, compensated for by strong knee flexion. The same results were also derived in previous studies [15, 16]. Dorsiflexion is greater during HP squats than during DP squats, thereby producing greater AE and ankle velocity, which leads to a more horizontal position (anterior displacement) of the tibia [17, 24].

Coactivation of the muscles that act on the ankle was reported by many studies on squatting movements [18, 25]. This coactivation was also observed in the present study, specifically between TA and SO muscles, with greater activation during the HP squats than in the DP squats (Figures 2(b) and 2(d)). The more horizontal position of the tibia [24] increased the dorsiflexion of the ankle [17] and the demand on the TA muscles in the HP squats. On the other hand, during the DP squats, the position of the ankle increased the TA length, leading to a length-tension relationship that is inappropriate for good activation [25]. To counter the anterior displacement of the tibia caused by the action of the TA muscles and gravitational force, the SO muscles are activated to decelerate during the descending phase of the squats, aiding the anteroposterior stability of the ankle and maintenance of balance [25].

Despite these differences in kinematics and in TA EMG activity, the quadriceps did not present a difference between tasks. During acceleration (subphase 2), the gravitational force led to knee flexion, and the VMO, VL, and BF muscles (Figures 2(a), 2(c), and 2(e)) maintained low activities [19, 25]. Conversely, during subphase 3, the quadriceps showed increased EMG activity, being coactivated with the BF muscles (Figures 2(a), 2(c), and 2(e)), as well as with the EE muscles [19] for knee [19, 26] and pelvis stabilization, respectively; this coactivation avoids excessive hip flexion [19, 21] whilst maintaining control over the trunk. The eccentric action of the quadriceps (VMO and VL) was necessary in

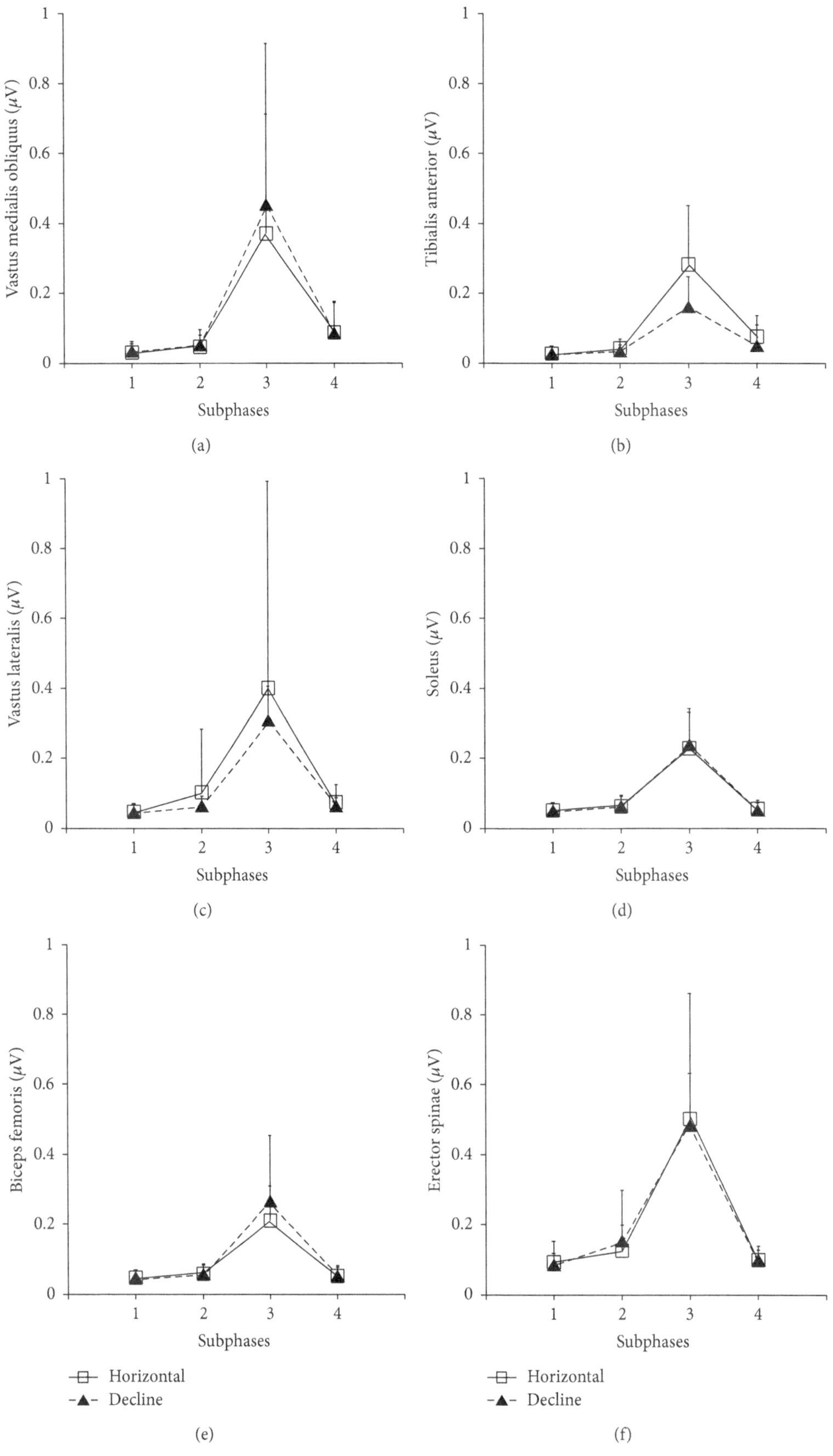

FIGURE 2: Mean values and standard deviation across all individuals to all muscles (VMO, VL, BF, TA, SO, and EE) during the descending phase for both squats (HP, open squares; DP, closed triangles) in all subphases of the movement.

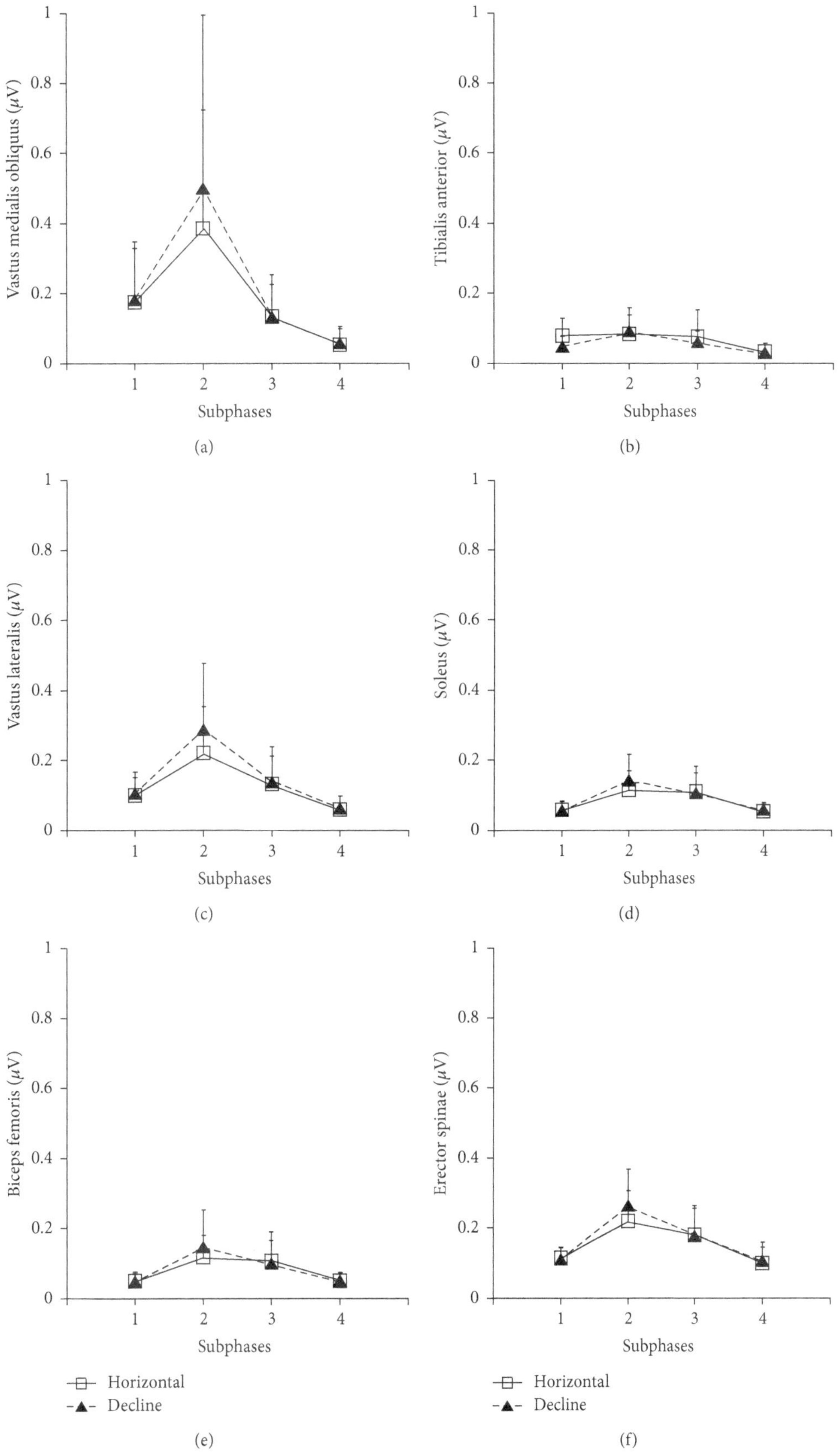

FIGURE 3: Mean values and standard deviation across all individuals to all muscles (VMO, VL, BF, TA, SO, and EE) during the ascending phase for both squats (HP, open squares; DP, closed triangles) in all subphases of the movement.

both tasks for decelerating gravitational action [19, 25, 26] and for identifying the target position (70° flexion). However, some studies demonstrated that DP squats presented greater demand on the extensor knee mechanism than did HP squats, but these studies were carried out with unipodal support. With unipodal support, joint demand is accentuated (gravitational force), which increases the need for a stronger activation of the quadriceps to decelerate movement [25]. This activation can produce up to a 30% increase in eccentric work, mean and peak patellar tendon force, and angle at peak force relative to those derived under bipodal support [15]. In the current work, similar mechanical demands on the joints involved characterized the similarities in action of the quadriceps muscles between the squat movements.

Another important aspect is the anteroposterior displacement of the trunk, which influences COM displacement [19]. The anterior displacement of the COM favoured the decrease in the EMG activity demand on the quadriceps in the HP squats. In the DP squats, on the other hand, the COM was further displaced toward the posterior direction, consequently increasing the demand on the quadriceps [14]. This displacement was due to the plantar flexion of the ankle. In previous studies, unipodal support was applied without control over the trunk position and a higher EMG activity of the quadriceps was found [14, 15, 17]. In the present study (with bipodal support), trunk movements in the sagittal plane were controlled, thereby avoiding anterior trunk displacement. This control also explained the similar activation of the quadriceps in both tasks. However, Alves et al. [25] who also studied squats with bipodal support, did not control trunk movements and observed a similarity between tasks. This result suggests that type of support (unipodal or bipodal) is more important than trunk control in influencing the EMG activities under different types of squats (HP and DP). Nevertheless, further studies should be conducted to confirm this hypothesis.

For the ascent phase of the squats, the HP squats presented greater IP and FP of the ankle but lower FP of the knee than did the DP squats. The other variables, including knee and ankle velocities, were not influenced by ankle position. For this phase of the squat, the knee and ankle velocities were small because acceleration depends on muscular activation to overcome inertial forces for the generation of movement [21]. For the TA muscles, however, a difference between squats was found; this difference required greater activity in the HP squats than in the DP squats (Figure 3(b)). It was also influenced by the position of the ankle, which needs more stability given the anterior displacement of the tibia. To overcome inertia and enable the body to perform ascending movements, all the muscles increased their EMG activities in both tasks during acceleration (Figure 3). The VMO and VL muscles were activated to enable knee extension, and the BF muscles were activated to enable pelvis pushing movements and maintain hip extension [26, 27]. The EE muscles were also activated (Figure 3(f)), thereby aiding the BF muscle in controlling trunk flexion and maintaining its extension [25]. In this ascent phase of the squat, the TA and SO muscles were coactivated in a similar manner between the tasks (Figures 5(b) and 5(d)), which provided ankle stability.

In summary, we showed that DP and HP squats have the same EMG patterns in the quadriceps, indicating that DP squats are not necessarily more effective than HP squats. Therefore, in the early stages of a rehabilitation programme for recovering quadriceps force, both DP and HP squats can be performed under bipodal support. Nonetheless, our results should be interpreted with caution because the movements studied do not fully correspond to the exercises used for knee rehabilitation. In particular, the participants were instructed to execute the moves as quickly as possible; thus, such movements cannot be extrapolated to the recommendations of the American College of Sports Medicine with regard to squats.

5. Conclusion

DP and HP squats with bipodal support and control of trunk movements in the sagittal plane produced different kinematics (ankle and knee joints) but did not modify the EMG activities in HP and DP squats, as well as in descending and ascending phases of the movements.

Conflict of Interests

The authors declare that there is no conflict of interests.

References

[1] J. Yang, S. W. Marshall, J. M. Bowling, C. W. Runyan, F. O. Mueller, and M. A. Lewis, "Use of discretionary protective equipment and rate of lower extremity injury in high school athletes," *American Journal of Epidemiology*, vol. 161, no. 6, pp. 511–519, 2005.

[2] Y. Okada, "Histochemical study on the atrophy of the quadriceps femoris muscle caused by knee joint injuries of rats," *Hiroshima Journal of Medical Sciences*, vol. 38, no. 1, pp. 13–21, 1989.

[3] R. M. Palmieri, J. A. Tom, J. E. Edwards et al., "Arthrogenic muscle response induced by an experimental knee joint effusion is mediated by pre- and post-synaptic spinal mechanisms," *Journal of Electromyography and Kinesiology*, vol. 14, no. 6, pp. 631–640, 2004.

[4] C. M. Powers, "Rehabilitation of patellofemoral joint disorders: a critical review," *Journal of Orthopaedic and Sports Physical Therapy*, vol. 28, no. 5, pp. 345–354, 1998.

[5] D. A. Rice and P. J. McNair, "Quadriceps arthrogenic muscle inhibition: neural mechanisms and treatment perspectives," *Seminars in Arthritis and Rheumatism*, vol. 40, no. 3, pp. 250–266, 2010.

[6] L. A. Steinkamp, M. F. Dillingham, M. D. Markel, J. A. Hill, and K. R. Kaufman, "Biomechanical considerations in patellofemoral joint rehabilitation," *American Journal of Sports Medicine*, vol. 21, no. 3, pp. 438–444, 1993.

[7] S. F. Tang, C. K. Chen, R. Hsu, S. W. Chou, W. H. Hong, and H. L. Lew, "Vastus medialis obliquus and vastus lateralis activity in open and closed kinetic chain exercises in patients with patellofemoral pain syndrome: an electromyographic study," *Archives of Physical Medicine and Rehabilitation*, vol. 82, no. 10, pp. 1441–1445, 2001.

[8] J. Nyland, T. Brosky, D. Currier, A. Nitz, and D. Caborn, "Review of the afferent neural system of the knee and its contribution to motor learning," *Journal of Orthopaedic and Sports Physical Therapy*, vol. 19, no. 1, pp. 2–11, 1994.

[9] J. T. Podraza and S. C. White, "Effect of knee flexion angle on ground reaction forces, knee moments and muscle co-contraction during an impact-like deceleration landing: implications for the non-contact mechanism of ACL injury," *Knee*, vol. 17, no. 4, pp. 291–295, 2010.

[10] E. Witvrouw, R. Lysens, J. Bellemans, K. Peers, and G. Vanderstraeten, "Open versus closed kinetic chain exercises for patellofemoral pain: a prospective, randomized study," *American Journal of Sports Medicine*, vol. 28, no. 5, pp. 687–694, 2000.

[11] R. F. Escamilla, "Knee biomechanics of the dynamic squat exercise," *Medicine and Science in Sports and Exercise*, vol. 33, no. 1, pp. 127–141, 2001.

[12] C. R. Purdam, P. Johnsson, H. Alfredson, R. Lorentzon, J. L. Cook, and K. M. Khan, "A pilot study of the eccentric decline squat in the management of painful chronic patellar tendinopathy," *British Journal of Sports Medicine*, vol. 38, no. 4, pp. 395–397, 2004.

[13] M. A. Young, J. L. Cook, C. R. Purdam, Z. S. Kiss, and H. Alfredson, "Eccentric decline squat protocol offers superior results at 12 months compared with traditional eccentric protocol for patellar tendinopathy in volleyball players," *British Journal of Sports Medicine*, vol. 39, no. 2, pp. 102–105, 2005.

[14] M. Kongsgaard, P. Aagaard, S. Roikjaer et al., "Decline eccentric squats increases patellar tendon loading compared to standard eccentric squats," *Clinical Biomechanics*, vol. 21, no. 7, pp. 748–754, 2006.

[15] A. Frohm, K. Halvorsen, and A. Thorstensson, "Patellar tendon load in different types of eccentric squats," *Clinical Biomechanics*, vol. 22, no. 6, pp. 704–711, 2007.

[16] J. Zwerver, S. W. Bredeweg, and A. L. Hof, "Biomechanical analysis of the single-leg decline squat," *British Journal of Sports Medicine*, vol. 41, no. 4, pp. 264–268, 2007.

[17] J. Richards, D. Thewlis, J. Selfe, A. Cunningham, and C. Hayes, "A biomechanical investigation of a single-limb squat: implications for lower extremity rehabilitation exercise," *Journal of Athletic Training*, vol. 43, no. 5, pp. 477–482, 2008.

[18] K. Hase, M. Sako, J. Ushiba, and N. Chino, "Motor strategies for initiating downward-oriented movements during standing in adults," *Experimental Brain Research*, vol. 158, no. 1, pp. 18–27, 2004.

[19] V. C. Dionisio, G. L. Almeida, M. Duarte, and R. P. Hirata, "Kinematic, kinetic and EMG patterns during downward squatting," *Journal of Electromyography and Kinesiology*, vol. 18, no. 1, pp. 134–143, 2008.

[20] H. J. Hermens, B. Freriks, C. Disselhorst-Klug, and G. Rau, "Development of recommendations for SEMG sensors and sensor placement procedures," *Journal of Electromyography and Kinesiology*, vol. 10, no. 5, pp. 361–374, 2000.

[21] V. C. Dionisio, N. Marconi, I. D. Santos, and G. L. Lmeida, "Upward squatting in individuals with and without patellofemoral pain syndrome: abiomechanical study," *Journal of Strength and Conditioning Research*, vol. 25, no. 5, pp. 1437–1446, 2011.

[22] L. A. de Souza, M. D. B. Curtarelli, M. Mukherjee, and V. C. Dionisio, "The effect of the partially restricted sit-to-stand task on biomechanical variables in subjects with and without Parkinson's disease," *Journal of Electromyography and Kinesiology*, vol. 21, no. 5, pp. 719–726, 2011.

[23] P. Konrad, *The ABC of EMG: A Practical Introduction to Kinesiological Electromyography*, Noraxon, Boston, Mass, USA, 2005.

[24] W. Mathiyakom, J. L. McNitt-Gray, P. Requejo, and K. Costa, "Modifying center of mass trajectory during sit-to-stand tasks redistributes the mechanical demand across the lower extremity joints," *Clinical Biomechanics*, vol. 20, no. 1, pp. 105–111, 2005.

[25] F. Alves, F. Oliveira, C. Junqueira, B. Azevedo, and V. C. Dionísio, "Analysis of electromyographic patterns during standard and declined squats," *Revista Brasileira de Fisioterapia*, vol. 13, no. 2, pp. 164–172, 2009.

[26] R. F. Escamilla, G. S. Fleisig, N. Zheng, S. W. Barrentine, K. E. Wilk, and J. R. Andrews, "Biomechanics of the knee during closed kinetic chain and open kinetic chain exercises," *Medicine and Science in Sports and Exercise*, vol. 30, no. 4, pp. 556–569, 1998.

[27] J. C. Ninos, J. J. Irrgang, R. Burdett, and J. R. Weiss, "Electromyographic analysis of the squat performed in self-selected lower extremity neutral rotation and 30∘of lower extremity turn-out from the self-selected neutral position," *Journal of Orthopaedic and Sports Physical Therapy*, vol. 25, no. 5, pp. 307–315, 1997.

8

Elder Chinese Martial Art Practitioners Have Higher Radial Bone Strength, Hand-Grip Strength, and Better Standing Balance Control

Shirley S. M. Fong,[1] X. Guo,[2] Alice P. M. Cheung,[2] Alex T. L. Jo,[2] Gary K. W. Lui,[2] Dennis K. C. Mo,[2] Shamay S. M. Ng,[2] and William W. N. Tsang[2]

[1] *Institute of Human Performance, The University of Hong Kong, Pokfulam, Hong Kong*
[2] *Department of Rehabilitation Sciences, The Hong Kong Polytechnic University, Hung Hom, Hong Kong*

Correspondence should be addressed to Shirley S. M. Fong; smfong@hku.hk

Academic Editors: A. Danielsson, B. Dugue, J. J. Sosnoff, and C. Zwingmann

This study explored the feasibility of using Ving Tsun (VT) martial art as a fall-prevention exercise for male seniors. We compared the radial bone strength, hand-grip strength, and standing balance control of senior VT practitioners and nonpractitioners under various sensory environments. Sixteen male VT practitioners (mean age ± SD: 51.3 ± 7.8 years) and 17 sex- and age-matched control adults (mean age ± SD: 53.7 ± 5.9 years) participated in the study. The bone strength of the distal radius, hand-grip strength, and standing balance control were assessed using an ultrasound bone sonometer, a Jamar dynamometer, and sensory organization test (SOT) on the NeuroCom Balance Master, respectively. A multivariate analysis of variance (MANOVA) was used to compare the outcome variables between the two groups. Results revealed that VT practitioners had significantly higher radial bone strength (T-score) on the dominant side ($P = 0.015$), hand-grip strength (dominant side, $P = 0.034$; nondominant side, $P = 0.026$), and standing balance control (SOT composite equilibrium score, $P = 0.005$) than the control participants. Male elder VT practitioners had higher radial bone strength, hand-grip strength, and better standing balance control than nonpractitioners. Our findings shed light on the use of VT exercise to prevent falls and fall-related fractures of the distal radius in male elders.

1. Introduction

Falls among the elderly are common and a global cause of morbidity and mortality. It has been reported that there are over 400 potential risk factors for falling [1]. Among these risk factors, the physical deteriorations associated with advancing age such as decreased bone mass [2], decreased muscular strength [3, 4], and balance deficits [5], along with physical inactivity [6–8], have been found to be the major determinants of falls among seniors [1]. Improving bone and muscular strength and postural stability using exercises could reduce fall risks and fall-related injuries (e.g., the fracture of the distal radius) [9, 10], improving the quality of life experienced by the elderly [8, 11].

To date, ample studies have investigated the effects of fall-prevention programs (e.g., Tai Chi) on improving physical impairments (e.g., decreased bone and muscular strength), functioning (e.g., body balance) and reducing falls or fall risk among elderly women [12–15]. However, elderly men are an underexamined group that also suffers from falls and subsequent osteoporotic fractures. Studies have been called for to design treatment strategies specifically for elderly men [16].

Ving Tsun (VT) is a traditional Chinese martial art characterized by rapid and forceful punching techniques and stable yet agile footwork. Owing to its simplicity and functionality as self-defense, VT is popular among male adults all over the world. The most well-known practitioners of VT were Bruce Lee and Ip Man [17–19]. VT practitioners are considered physically strong because they undergo high-impact training such as wooden dummy training (Figure 1), sticking-hand exercise (Figure 2), and sandbag workout with "one-inch punch" [18, 19]. We hypothesized that VT practitioners' forearm bone and muscle strength and body balance might be superior to those of nonpractitioners. However,

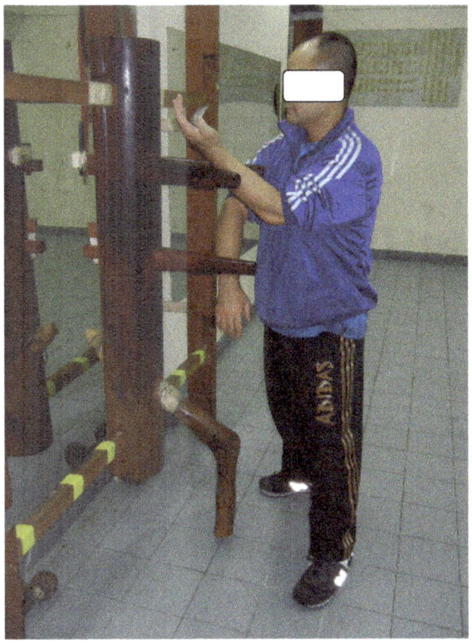

Figure 1: Ving Tsun wooden dummy training.

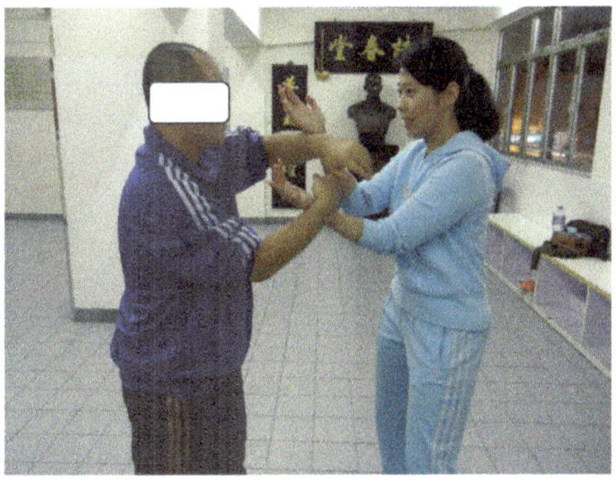

Figure 2: Ving Tsun sticking-hand drills.

to our knowledge, no study has investigated the beneficial effects of VT training in male seniors thus far.

The aims of this pilot study were to (1) compare the radial bone strength, hand-grip strength, and standing balance control between senior male VT practitioners and nonpractitioners under various sensory conditions and (2) examine whether there were any side-to-side differences in forearm bone and muscle strength among VT practitioners.

2. Materials and Methods

2.1. Participants. Thirty-three male older adults participated in the study, 16 of whom were advanced VT practitioners. They were recruited from three local VT schools by convenience sampling, and each had over three years of VT experience, trained for two to eight hours per week, and had attained the instructor level. The other 17 participants were healthy seniors recruited from the community. The participant characteristics are described in Table 1. None of the participants engaged in any regular physical training

Table 1: Participants' characteristics.

	VT group (mean ± SD) (n = 16)	Control group (mean ± SD) (n = 17)	P value
Age, years	51.3 ± 7.8	53.7 ± 5.9	0.315
Sex, n	16 males	17 males	
Height, m	1.69 ± 0.05	1.68 ± 0.06	0.585
Weight, kg	73.0 ± 9.3	72.0 ± 8.1	0.747
Ving Tsun experience, years	16.1 ± 9.6	0	

(except VT training for the VT group participants), and any who exhibited significant cognitive, musculoskeletal, cardiopulmonary, visual, vestibular, or neurological disorders that might affect physical performance were excluded. This study was approved by the Human Subjects Ethics Review Subcommittee of the Hong Kong Polytechnic University. The testing procedures were fully explained to the participants, and written consent was obtained before data collection.

2.2. Procedures and Measures. Data collection was performed by a physiotherapist and four physiotherapy students between June 2012 and February 2013 following Declaration of Helsinki guidelines. All of the assessments took place in the Sports Training and Rehabilitation Laboratory of the Hong Kong Polytechnic University. Relevant information such as general health and exercise habits was obtained by interviewing the participants face to face. The body height and weight of each participant were first measured by a mechanical scale equipped with a height rod (420KL Physician Scale, Health-O-Meter, Bridgeview, IL, USA). Participants then underwent the following assessments in random order.

2.2.1. Bone Strength of Distal Radius. The bone strength of the distal radius was assessed using the Sunlight Mini-Omni Ultrasound Bone Sonometer (Sunlight, BeamMed Ltd., Israel) because it is radiation free and the measurement is independent of body height and weight [20]. Ultrasound gel was applied to the skin surface at the measurement site to facilitate acoustic coupling. Placement of the handheld probe was at the distal third of the radius (i.e., midpoint between the olecranon process of the ulna and the tip of the distal phalanx of the third digit). The transducers within the probe were rotated around the radius slowly by the assessor without lifting the probe from the skin surface. The measurement was repeated at least three times. The velocity of the ultrasound wave ("speed of sound" or "SOS" in m/s) traveling through a few centimeters of radial bone parallel to its axis within the outer 2 mm to 6 mm was measured [21]. The SOS values were then converted into a T-score using inbuilt computer software. The SOS T-score represents the units of standard deviations relative to population reference values of healthy young adults of the same ethnicity. It reflects the bone's fragility and is highly correlated with bone strength [21, 22]. However, unlike the T-score obtained by using dual-energy X-ray absorptiometry, SOS measurements cannot predict forearm bone mineral density [22], and hence the standard World Health Organization's (WHO) definition of osteoporosis cannot be applied in this case. Instead, SOS T-score thresholds for diagnosis of osteoporosis and osteopenia at the distal radius are suggested to be −2.6 and −1.4, respectively [23]. The average SOS T-scores of the three trials (obtained from both dominant and nondominant arms) were used for analysis. The Sunlight ultrasound systems have been reported to be reliable (intraoperator precision at distal radius: 0.36%) and precise (in vivo precision: 0.4%–0.8%) in previous studies [23–25].

2.2.2. Hand-Grip Strength. All of the participants were assessed for maximal hand-grip strength using a Jamar dynamometer (Sammons Preston, Mississauga, ON, Canada). Standard assessment procedures were followed [26]. In brief, participants were in a standing position with the testing shoulder adducted and neutrally rotated, elbow flexed at 90°, forearm in midprone, and wrist in a neutral position. Before the actual tests, the participants were allowed to squeeze the dynamometer twice to familiarize themselves with the testing procedure. This was followed by a 10-second rest. Participants were then instructed to squeeze the dynamometer using maximal effort. A total of three trials were performed on each side, and the highest grip-strength value of each hand was recorded [26]. The interrater reliability (ICC: 0.98) and intrarater reliability (ICC: 0.94–0.98) of this hand-grip strength test were reported to be good to excellent [26].

2.2.3. Postural Control. Standing balance was assessed using the sensory organization test (SOT) performed on the NeuroCom Balance Master (Smart Equitest, NeuroCom International Inc., Clackamas, OR, USA). This machine quantifies the participants' ability to maintain standing balance under reduced or conflicting sensory conditions. The participants stood barefoot on the movable platform of the machine and wore a security harness to prevent falling. They were then instructed to maintain bipedal standing balance under six sensory conditions that provide inaccurate or absent somatosensory, visual, or vestibular information to the participant. Each condition consisted of three trials and each trial lasted for 20s. The six conditions included (1) eyes open, stable visual surround and platform; (2) eyes closed, stable visual surround and platform; (3) eyes open, sway-referenced visual surround and stable platform; (4) eyes open, stable visual surround and sway-referenced platform; (5) eyes closed, stable visual surround and sway-referenced platform; and (6) eyes open, sway-referenced visual surround and platform. All of the participants were given a familiarization trial before the actual test [27].

The platform (dual-force plates) recorded the trajectory of the participant's center of pressure (COP) during postural sway. The NeuroCom computer program then generated an equilibrium score (ES) for each of the six sensory conditions based on the COP movements in standing. Moreover, a composite ES, which characterized the overall level of performance, was calculated from the weighted average of the ES of conditions 1 through 6. Higher ES (close to 100) represents little sway in standing, whereas lower ES (close to 0) represents excessive sway that may exceed the limit of stability [27, 28]. The ES of each sensory condition and the composite ES were used for analysis. A previous study showed that the ICC values of the six sensory conditions ranged from 0.72 to 0.93, indicating moderate-to-good test-retest reliability of SOT in older adults [15].

2.3. Statistical Analysis. The normal distribution of outcome variables was first checked using the Kolmogorov-Smirnov test. Independent t-tests were used to compare the age, body height, and weight between the VT and control groups. To compare the bone strength of the distal radius and the hand-grip strength between the two groups, a single multivariate analysis of variance (MANOVA) incorporating all relevant outcomes (i.e., SOS T-scores of bilateral radii and bilateral hand-grip strength values) was performed. Another separate MANOVA was conducted to compare the SOT-derived outcomes (i.e., equilibrium scores of conditions 1 to 6) between the two groups. Because the composite ES is the average of all of the equilibrium scores, an independent t-test was used to identify whether there was any significant between-group difference for this outcome parameter. The results from the MANOVA showed the effects of the group on all outcomes simultaneously and the corresponding Bonferroni-adjusted P values, hence avoiding the increased probability of type I errors. Effect sizes (i.e., partial eta-squared for MANOVA and Cohen's d for independent t-test) are also reported for each outcome variable. By convention, Cohen's d values of 0.2, 0.5, and 0.8 are considered small, medium, and large effect sizes, respectively. For partial eta-squared values, 0.01, 0.06, and 0.14 represent small, medium, and large effect sizes, respectively [29]. Secondary data analysis was carried out to further examine whether there were any side-to-side differences in SOS T-score and hand-grip strength values in the VT group. All of the previous statistical analyses were performed using the IBM Statistical Package for Social Sciences 20.0 software. A significance level of 0.05 was set for the statistical tests (two tailed).

Because the sample size was relatively small, it was necessary to determine whether our study was underpowered to detect significant differences between groups. Post hoc power analyses were performed to examine the statistical power of the comparisons of radial bone strength, hand-grip strength, and SOT-derived scores between the VT and control groups. The G Power computer program (Faul & Erdfelder, Bonn University, Germany) was used.

3. Results

There was no significant difference between the two groups in age, body height, or weight (Table 1). Regarding the bone strength of the distal radius, the SOS T-score obtained from the dominant side was significantly higher in the VT participants than in the control participants by 53.8% ($P = 0.015$). However, the SOS T-score obtained from the nondominant side showed no significant difference between the two groups ($P = 0.093$) (Table 2). Secondary analysis demonstrated

Table 2: Between-group comparison of radial bone strength, hand-grip strength, and balance control.

	VT group (mean ± SD) (n = 16)	Control group (mean ± SD) (n = 17)	P value	Effect size
Bone strength of distal radius (SOS T-score)				
Dominant side	−0.6 ± 0.8[†]	−1.3 ± 0.8	0.015[*]	0.176
Nondominant side	−1.0 ± 1.0	−1.6 ± 1.0	0.093	0.088
Hand-grip strength				
Dominant side, kg	42.1 ± 7.0[†]	37.1 ± 6.0	0.034[*]	0.136
Nondominant side, kg	39.7 ± 4.5	35.7 ± 5.2	0.026[*]	0.149
Sensory organization test				
Condition 1 ES	94.9 ± 1.3	92.5 ± 4.1	0.037[*]	0.137
Condition 2 ES	91.4 ± 4.2	91.9 ± 2.3	0.703	0.005
Condition 3 ES	92.0 ± 3.5	89.4 ± 4.9	0.083	0.097
Condition 4 ES	81.9 ± 8.1	75.9 ± 9.8	0.067	0.107
Condition 5 ES	62.6 ± 12.8	53.9 ± 16.8	0.108	0.084
Condition 6 ES	68.7 ± 10.7	54.7 ± 14.2	0.004[*]	0.247
Composite ES	78.7 ± 5.4	71.7 ± 7.5	0.005[*]	0.233

[*]Denotes a significant between-group difference ($P < 0.05$).
[†]Denotes a difference significant at $P < 0.05$ when compared to the nondominant side.

that the SOS T-score of the dominant side was significantly higher than that of the non-dominant side among the VT practitioners ($P = 0.044$) (Table 2).

The grip-strength values of both dominant and non-dominant hands were higher in the VT group by 13.5% ($P = 0.034$) and 11.2% ($P = 0.026$), respectively, than in the control group (Table 2). Additionally, the dominant hand demonstrated significantly higher hand-grip strength than the non-dominant hand ($P = 0.010$) (Table 2). For the SOT-derived scores, between-group differences were found in the ES of conditions 1 ($P = 0.037$) and 6 ($P = 0.004$) and the composite ES ($P = 0.005$). No significant difference was shown in the ES of SOT conditions 2 to 5. For the outcome variables that showed nonsignificant between-group differences, the partial eta-squared values ranged from 0.084 to 0.107, indicating medium-to-large effect sizes (except for the ES of SOT condition 2) (Table 2).

Post hoc power analysis showed that the statistical powers for the comparisons of radial bone strength (SOS T-score) between the VT and control groups were 0.68 (dominant side) and 0.39 (non-dominant side). For the between-group comparisons of hand-grip strength, the statistical powers were 0.57 (dominant side) and 0.63 (non-dominant side). For the comparisons of SOT-derived ES between the two groups, statistical powers were low, ranging from 0.07 to 0.59 for SOT conditions 1 to 5, but high for SOT condition 6 (0.87) and for the composite ES (0.85). This may explain why the ES of SOT conditions 2 to 5 failed to show a significant between-group difference in the MANOVA analysis (Table 2).

4. Discussion

This is the first study to investigate bone strength in older VT practitioners. Our results show that the bone strength of the distal radius (dominant side) was significantly higher in the VT practitioners than among the control participants. This finding was anticipated because VT training, which includes wooden dummy training (Figure 1), sticking-hand drills (Figure 2), and sandbag workouts, involves many upper limb striking movements that load the bones in the forearms with repeated high peak forces and impacts [18]. According to Wolff's law of bone remodeling, the internal structure of bone is adapted to mechanical demands such that the trabecular patterns (i.e., orientation of trabeculae) coincide with stress trajectories. That is, if loading on a bone increases, the bone will remodel to become stronger to resist that particular type of load [30]. Previous studies have reported that athletes who engage in high-impact sports such as karate display higher bone mineral density in specific regions than sedentary controls [31]. We postulated that long-term regular high-impact VT training might improve radial bone strength, therefore minimizing the risk of distal radius fractures in elderly males [32].

Despite the positive finding on the dominant side, our results demonstrated no between-group difference in radial bone strength on the non-dominant side with a medium effect size of 0.088. Secondary analysis showed that radial bone strength on the non-dominant side was actually 66.7% lower than that of the dominant side. This may be because fewer striking movements are performed with the left arm during wooden dummy training [18]. In addition, VT practitioners might use their non-dominant arm less frequently than their dominant arm during dynamic sticking-hand exercise or even during daily activities [33]. Therefore, the mechanical stresses placed on the non-dominant radius were decreased, and the bone became weaker as a result [30].

Another encouraging finding of this study is that VT practitioners demonstrated higher hand-grip strength, especially on the dominant side, than the control participants. This may be attributed to the repeated practice of punching (e.g., vertical fist or "one-inch punch") and grasping (e.g., grappling-hand) techniques during VT training [18, 19]. Extrinsic and intrinsic hand muscles might have been strengthened through these kinds of gripping exercises.

Our present finding actually concurs with a previous study that showed a significant improvement in hand-grip strength after Tai Chi training. The authors proposed that contraction and relaxation of forearm muscles might increase the muscle tone and hand-grip strength [34]. Previous studies have also suggested that grip strength is independently associated with radial bone mineral density [35, 36]. Perhaps higher hand-grip strength and stronger forearm muscles contribute to the higher radial bone strength among the VT practitioners. Further study might fruitfully explore the relationships between grip strength, forearm bone mineral density, and bone mineral content among VT practitioners.

VT practitioners seem to have better standing balance control under various sensory conditions, as demonstrated by their higher ES (SOT conditions 1 and 6) and composite ES. Although there were no significant differences between groups in the ES of SOT conditions 3 to 5, the effect sizes were moderate to large (0.084–0.107), indicating that the insignificant results might simply be due to the decreased statistical power (0.37–0.50). We might be able to detect significant differences between the two groups if the sample size was increased to 752 participants per group. For the ES of SOT condition 2, the effect size was exceptionally small (0.005) together with a large P value ($P = 0.703$). We postulated that VT practitioners may not be superior to their sedentary counterparts when standing with eyes closed. Indeed, training with eyes closed is not common during VT practice [19]. VT practitioners are conditioned to maintain postural stability under normal (i.e., SOT condition 1), reduced, and conflicting sensory environments (SOT conditions 3 to 6) instead.

One possible reason for the better standing balance (i.e., less postural sway) in VT practitioners under normal sensory environment (i.e., SOT condition 1) may be the tremendous time they spent in practicing static balance control. VT practitioners practice the basic "Siu Nim Tao" form in the static "goat-gripping" stance during every training session because it is the foundation of all VT techniques [19]. Practitioners are required to maintain postural stability (i.e., minimize postural sway) during different upper limb movements, and this may have trained the static and anticipatory postural control systems of the practitioners [19, 37]. If this is so, then why did VT practitioners sway less than the control participants when standing under sensory-depriving and conflicting environments? Perhaps VT practitioners develop better visual (reflected by the ES of SOT condition 4) and vestibular (reflected by the ES of SOT condition 5) senses for postural control [27, 28] through the dynamic sticking-hand exercise [19]. Further study is needed to explore the mechanisms through which VT practice could improve postural control under various sensory environments.

Our present findings shed light on the use of VT exercise to prevent fall and fall-related fractures of the distal radius in male elders. However, it is not definitive whether participating in VT lessons would increase one's exposure to risk of falling and fracture. The advanced VT practitioners in our study started VT training at a relatively young age (average 35.2 years old). Therefore, it is advisable to start VT training early, preferably before the deterioration of balance ability [5] and before the onset of osteopenia [2]. For people who are receiving VT training, our findings hint that they could exercise both upper limbs in a more symmetrical manner so that their bilateral radii, forearm, and hand muscles might be strengthened.

This study has several limitations. First, the small sample size may have compromised the statistical power. This could explain some of our insignificant findings. Second, it was a cross-sectional study. No causal relationship between practicing VT and the aforementioned beneficial effects could be established. Third, our participants were exclusively in their fifties. They were not frail elders with high fall or fracture risks. Further studies could consider using a randomized controlled study design that includes a larger sample of older males. Moreover, it may be necessary to modify the traditional VT training to suit the weaker participants.

5. Conclusions

Male elder VT practitioners had higher radial bone strength, hand-grip strength, and better standing balance control than nonpractitioners. Our findings may inspire the development of VT exercise as an evidence-based medium for preventing fall and fall-related fractures in male seniors.

Conflict of Interests

The authors declare that they have no conflict of interests with respect to the authorship or publication of this paper. No funding was provided for its preparation.

Acknowledgments

The authors thank Mr. Alex Ngai, Mr. Sunny So, Mr. Fung Man, and Mr. So Yip for their advice on Ving Tsun martial art and the recruitment of participants.

References

[1] T. Masud and R. O. Morris, "Epidemiology of falls," *Age and Ageing*, vol. 30, no. 4, pp. 3–7, 2001.

[2] E. M. Haney and M. M. Bliziotes, "Male osteoporosis: new insights in an understudied disease," *Current Opinion in Rheumatology*, vol. 20, no. 4, pp. 423–428, 2008.

[3] R. S. Lindle, E. J. Metter, N. A. Lynch et al., "Age and gender comparisons of muscle strength in 654 women and men aged 20–93 yr," *Journal of Applied Physiology*, vol. 83, no. 5, pp. 1581–1587, 1997.

[4] B. K. S. Chan, L. M. Marshall, K. M. Winters, K. A. Faulkner, A. V. Schwartz, and E. S. Orwoll, "Incident fall risk and physical activity and physical performance among older men: the osteoporotic fractures in men study," *American Journal of Epidemiology*, vol. 165, no. 6, pp. 696–703, 2007.

[5] P. W. Overstall, A. N. Exton Smith, F. J. Imms, and A. L. Johnson, "Falls in the elderly related to postural imbalance," *British Medical Journal*, vol. 1, no. 6056, pp. 261–264, 1977.

[6] S. R. Lord, J. A. Ward, P. Williams, and K. J. Anstey, "An epidemiological study of falls in older community-dwelling women: the Randwick falls and fractures study," *Australian Journal of Public Health*, vol. 17, no. 3, pp. 240–245, 1993.

[7] J. S. W. Lee, T.-W. Auyeung, T. Kwok, E. M. C. Lau, P.-C. Leung, and J. Woo, "Associated factors and health impact of sarcopenia in older Chinese men and women: a cross-sectional study," *Gerontology*, vol. 53, no. 6, pp. 404–410, 2008.

[8] S. Khosla, S. Amin, and E. Orwoll, "Osteoporosis in men," *Endocrine Reviews*, vol. 29, no. 4, pp. 441–464, 2008.

[9] R. G. Crilly, L. Delaquerriere Richardson, and J. H. Roth, "Postural stability and Colles' fracture," *Age and Ageing*, vol. 16, no. 3, pp. 133–138, 1987.

[10] J. L. Kelsey, M. M. Prill, T. H. M. Keegan et al., "Reducing the risk for distal forearm fracture: preserve bone mass, slow down, and don't fall!," *Osteoporosis International*, vol. 16, no. 6, pp. 681–690, 2005.

[11] C. P. Iglesias, A. Manca, and D. J. Torgerson, "The health-related quality of life and cost implications of falls in elderly women," *Osteoporosis International*, vol. 20, no. 6, pp. 869–878, 2009.

[12] A. J. Campbell, M. C. Robertson, M. M. Gardner, R. N. Norton, M. W. Tilyard, and D. M. Buchner, "Randomised controlled trial of a general practice programme of home based exercise to prevent falls in elderly women," *British Medical Journal*, vol. 315, no. 7115, pp. 1065–1069, 1997.

[13] S. E. Sihvonen, S. Sipilä, and P. A. Era, "Changes in postural balance in Frail Elderly women during a 4-week visual feedback training: a randomized controlled trial," *Gerontology*, vol. 50, no. 2, pp. 87–95, 2004.

[14] J. O. Judge, C. Lindsey, M. Underwood, D. Winsemius, and E. A. Keshner, "Balance improvements in older women: effects of exercise training," *Physical Therapy*, vol. 73, no. 4, pp. 254–265, 1993.

[15] W. W. Tsang, V. S. Wong, S. N. Fu, and C. W. Hui-Chan, "Tai Chi improves standing balance control under reduced or conflicting sensory conditions," *Archives of Physical Medicine and Rehabilitation*, vol. 85, no. 1, pp. 129–137, 2004.

[16] L. J. Melton III, E. J. Atkinson, M. K. O'Connor, W. M. O'Fallon, and B. L. Riggs, "Bone density and fracture risk in men," *Journal of Bone and Mineral Research*, vol. 13, no. 12, pp. 1915–1923, 1998.

[17] T. A. Green, *Martial Arts of the World: An Encyclopedia*, ABC-CLIO, Goleta, Calif, USA, 2001.

[18] C. Yip, *116 Wing Tsun Dummy Techniques as Demonstrated by grandmaster Yip Man*, Leung's Publications, Hong Kong, China, 1981.

[19] D. Peterson, *Look Beyond the Pointing Finger—the Combat Philosophy of Wong Shun Leung*, Melbourne Chinese Martial Arts Club, Victoria, Australia, 2001.

[20] Z. Zadik, D. Price, and G. Diamond, "Pediatric reference curves for multi-site quantitative ultrasound and its modulators," *Osteoporosis International*, vol. 14, no. 10, pp. 857–862, 2003.

[21] BeamMed Ltd, *Sunlight Miniomni Bone Sonometer User Guide*, BeamMed, Petach-Tikva, Israel, 2010.

[22] D. Hans, A. M. Schott, and P. J. Meunier, "Ultrasonic assessment of bone: a review," *European Journal of Medicine*, vol. 2, no. 3, pp. 157–163, 1993.

[23] K. M. Knapp, G. M. Blake, T. D. Spector, and I. Fogelman, "Multisite quantitative ultrasound: precision, age- and menopause-related changes, fracture discrimination, and T-score equivalence with dual-energy X-ray absorptiometry," *Osteoporosis International*, vol. 12, no. 6, pp. 456–464, 2001.

[24] R. Barkmann, E. Kantorovich, C. Singal et al., "A new method for quantitative ultrasound measurements at multiple skeletal sites: first results of precision and fracture discrimination," *Journal of Clinical Densitometry*, vol. 3, no. 1, pp. 1–7, 2000.

[25] W. M. Drake, M. McClung, C. F. Njeh et al., "Multisite bone ultrasound measurement on North American female reference population," *Journal of Clinical Densitometry*, vol. 4, no. 3, pp. 239–248, 2001.

[26] A. Peolsson, R. Hedlund, and B. Oberg, "Intra- and inter-tester reliability and reference values for hand strength," *Journal of Rehabilitation Medicine*, vol. 33, no. 1, pp. 36–41, 2001.

[27] NeuroCom, *Balance Manager Systems—Instructions for Use*, NeuroCom International, Clackamas, Ore, USA, 2008.

[28] L. M. Nashner, "Computerized dynamic posturography," in *Handbook of Balance Function and Testing*, Mosby Year book, St. Louis, Mo, USA, 1997.

[29] L. G. Portney and M. P. Watkins, *Foundations of Clinical Research—Applications to Practice*, Pearson Education, Cranbury, NJ, USA, 2009.

[30] C. Ruff, B. Holt, and E. Trinkaus, "Who's afraid of the big bad Wolff?: "Wolff's law" and bone functional adaptation," *American Journal of Physical Anthropology*, vol. 129, no. 4, pp. 484–498, 2006.

[31] A. Andreoli, M. Monteleone, M. Van Loan, L. Promenzio, U. Tarantino, and A. De Lorenzo, "Effects of different sports on bone density and muscle mass in highly trained athletes," *Medicine and Science in Sports and Exercise*, vol. 33, no. 4, pp. 507–511, 2001.

[32] Y. Jiang, J. Zhao, C. Rosen, P. Geusens, and H. K. Genant, "Perspectives on bone mechanical properties and adaptive response to mechanical challenge," *Journal of Clinical Densitometry*, vol. 2, no. 4, pp. 423–433, 1999.

[33] L. B. Bagesteiro and R. L. Sainburg, "Handedness: dominant arm advantages in control of limb dynamics," *Journal of Neurophysiology*, vol. 88, no. 5, pp. 2408–2421, 2002.

[34] K.-M. Chen, J.-N. Lin, H.-S. Lin et al., "The effects of a Simplified Tai-Chi Exercise Program (STEP) on the physical health of older adults living in long-term care facilities: a single group design with multiple time points," *International Journal of Nursing Studies*, vol. 45, no. 4, pp. 501–507, 2008.

[35] M. Di Monaco, R. Di Monaco, M. Manca, and A. Cavanna, "Handgrip strength is an independent predictor of distal radius bone mineral density in postmenopausal women," *Clinical Rheumatology*, vol. 19, no. 6, pp. 473–476, 2000.

[36] S. Tsuji, N. Tsunoda, H. Yata, F. Katsukawa, S. Onishi, and H. Yamazaki, "Relation between grip strength and radial bone mineral density in young athletes," *Archives of Physical Medicine and Rehabilitation*, vol. 76, no. 3, pp. 234–238, 1995.

[37] A. Shumway-Cook and M. H. Woollacott, "Development of postural control," in *Motor Control Translating Research Into Clinical Practice*, A. Shumway-Cook and M. H. Woollacott, Eds., Lippincott Williams and Wilkins, Philadelphia, Pa, USA, 2007.

9

The Influence of Self-Efficacy on Mood States in People with Spinal Cord Injury

Ashley Craig,[1] Nirupama Wijesuriya,[1] and Yvonne Tran[1,2]

[1] *Rehabilitation Studies Unit, Sydney Medical School-Northern, The University of Sydney, P.O. Box 6, Ryde, Sydney, NSW 1680, Australia*
[2] *Key University Centre for Health Technologies, University of Technology, Broadway, Sydney, NSW 2007, Australia*

Correspondence should be addressed to Ashley Craig; a.craig@sydney.edu.au

Academic Editors: P. Czarnecki, J. D. Kingsley, J. J. Sosnoff, and M. Yu

Objective. Negative mood is prevalent in people with a neurological injury such as spinal cord injury (SCI). However, research is needed for determining those people with SCI who are vulnerable to negative mood states, as well as establishing the influence of self-efficacy, that is, expectations of their control over their lives. The objective of this research was to investigate the protective role that self-efficacy may play in adult people with SCI compared to able-bodied controls. *Methods*. Participants included 41 adults with SCI living in the community and 41 able-bodied controls similar in age, sex ratio, and education. All participants completed a psychological assessment regimen in a relaxed environment. Measures consisted of validated measures of self-efficacy and negative mood states. *Results*. The SCI group was found to have significantly elevated levels of depressive mood, anxiety, stress, and poor self-efficacy. SCI participants with low levels of self-efficacy were shown to have significantly elevated levels of depressive mood and anxiety in comparison to those SCI participants with high levels of self-efficacy and able-bodied controls. *Conclusions*. People with a neurological injury such as SCI are vulnerable to experiencing clinically elevated negative mood states if they have poor expectations of control over their lives. Implications for SCI rehabilitation are discussed.

1. Introduction

Spinal cord injury (SCI) is a chronic neurological disorder that involves the cord being severely bruised, lacerated, or severed during a traumatic injury or damaged as a result of disease. The risk of suffering an SCI is low; however, when it occurs it is usually very traumatic and debilitating with substantial negative impacts on quality of life (QOL) [1, 2]. Most injuries to the spinal cord in adults involve damage to the surrounding protective vertebral column, consisting of the cervical, thoracic, lumbar, sacral, and the coccygeal vertebrae. Neurological damage resulting from an SCI depends upon the degree to which the injury disturbs or intrudes into the spinal cord [1]. Extreme damage to the spinal cord leads to loss of sensation and paralysis of voluntary muscles, resulting in reduced mobility and independence in activities of daily living and impairment of social and vocational skills. Potential negative influences on respiratory, cardiovascular, urinary, gastrointestinal, and reproductive systems also occur [1]. Furthermore, chronic pain, chronic fatigue, and mental health dysfunction are common secondary conditions that contribute to decreased QOL [3–10]. Mental health dysfunction in the form of negative mood states such as depression is a risk for up to 40% of adults with SCI living in the community [7]. This high prevalence rate highlights the need for careful screening of SCI patients, especially as they come to the end of their inpatient rehabilitation and are about to be discharged into the community [5]. Arguably, if those at risk of depression can be offered early treatment, then adjustment to SCI would improve substantially.

Outcomes like restrictions in mobility, barriers to employment and social engagement, and a high dependence on caregivers will combine to challenge expectations of control (called self-efficacy) in people with SCI [7]. Among other goals, SCI rehabilitation should enhance feelings of self-management (or self-efficacy) by teaching skills that convince the person they can control and reduce the negative impacts of associated impairment, as well as lower social barriers by improving locomotor function and enhancing vocational capacity [2]. Self-efficacy and expectations of control [11] have been shown to be important factors influencing health in diverse areas including weight loss [12], improvement following stroke [13], and improvement in stuttering [14] and in SCI rehabilitation outcomes [15–18]. Self-efficacy has been defined as a person's belief or sense of confidence in his or her own ability to perform a particular task or behavior successfully in the future [11]. Horn and colleagues found significant associations between low self-efficacy and level of neurological impairment [16]. Craig and colleagues found an association between low self-efficacy in people with SCI with long-term risks of depressive mood and poor outcomes in rehabilitation [17, 18].

Controlled research investigating the association of self-efficacy with negative mood states like depressive mood and anxiety in adult people with SCI is scarce. Therefore, the major objective of this research was to investigate more carefully the association between negative mood states and self-efficacy in adult people with SCI and able-bodied controls. To achieve this goal, differences in negative mood states were compared with adult people with SCI with low versus high self-efficacy, as well as with able-bodied controls. It was hypothesized that higher levels of negative mood states would occur in people with SCI with low self-efficacy compared to people with high self-efficacy with or without SCI.

2. Materials and Methods

2.1. Study Participants. Participants included 41 adults with SCI living in the community and 41 able-bodied controls. The SCI participants were enrolled into the study from rehabilitation units as well as through advertising in disability newsletters. The controls were enrolled by advertising and were admitted into the study if they stated they were free of chronic physical or psychiatric disease at the time of assessment. The 41 controls were selected and matched to the SCI participants for sex and age (±5 years) on a case by case basis from a sample of around 100 able-bodied participants who, along with the SCI participants, were enrolled in a neuropsychophysiological study.

The mean age for the SCI group was 47.1 years (SD = 12; min = 21, max = 70) consisting of 39 males and 2 females. The mean age for the controls was 46.8 years (SD = 12; min = 21, max = 70) also consisting of 39 males and 2 females. The two females in each group were aged in their mid 50s to early 60s. The two females were left in the study as the statistical outcomes with the two removed did not change. Their inclusion increases the statistical power of the study. Twenty-seven SCI participants had paraplegia, 14 had tetraplegia, while 23 were assessed by a medical specialist to have an incomplete lesion with the remaining 18 having complete lesions. The mean time since the injury was 16.5 years (SD = 14). The majority (n = 23) sustained an SCI in a road accident, 9 by a fall, 6 in sporting injury, and 3 due to a medical condition. The SCI and control groups had similar years of education (15.9 years, SD = 2.0; 14 years, SD = 2.6, resp.). Most of the SCI participants (n = 24) were on medications, the main types taken being analgesics, antispasmodics, hypnotics, and antidepressants. Most (n = 32) of the SCI sample did not have a comorbid TBI.

Research ethics approval was received from the local institutional human research ethics committee, and written consent was obtained prior to participation in the study. Inclusion criteria for SCI participants consisted of (a) the presence of a chronic SCI, (b) age 20 or more and less than 75 years old at the time of interview, and (c) ability to speak and understand instructions in English. Inclusion criteria for the controls were the same for points (b) and (c). Exclusion criteria for the controls included the presence of a chronic neurological injury.

2.2. Psychological Measures. Psychological questionnaires were completed in a relaxed environment in either the participants' home or in a clinic. All participants completed the Depression Anxiety Stress Scales (DASS), a self-report questionnaire assessing anxiety, depressive mood, and stress [19]. High scores indicate elevated mood states. The DASS has acceptable reliability and discriminate validity [20]. They also completed the Lifestyle Appraisal Questionnaire (LAQ) which is a standardized two-part self-report Likert measure of cumulative health risks (LAQ1) and self-efficacy (LAQ2) [21]. Only LAQ2 data is presented in this paper. The LAQ2 measures a person's self-efficacy, specifically, their perceived ability to influence life challenges. High scores indicate low self-efficacy. The LAQ2 has acceptable test-retest reliability and internal reliability (Cronbach's coefficient alpha of 0.89), as well as acceptable construct validity and low social desirability [21].

2.3. Data Analysis. Differences between groups for the psychological measures were determined by first conducting MANOVA, followed by one-way ANOVA analyses to determine where differences occurred. The influence of self-efficacy on negative mood states was determined by dichotomizing the groups into low and high self-efficacy subgroups on the basis of the population mean LAQ2 score of 20 [21]. Scores lower than 20 indicate enhanced self-efficacy, while scores equal to or over 20 indicate poor self-efficacy [21]. The DASS depressive mood, anxiety, and stress scores were then calculated for the SCI and able-bodied participants who were then placed into low versus high self-efficacy subgroups. Those participants with self-efficacy scores less than 20 constituted the high self-efficacy subgroups, while scores equal to or above 20 constituted the low self-efficacy subgroups in the SCI and control groups. MANOVA was performed first to determine whether differences occurred between the three mood state measures for the four subgroups. This was followed by a series of factorial ANOVAs so as to determine whether interaction effects were significant for differences in negative mood states as a function of high versus low self-efficacy. Bonferroni protected t-tests were then used to determine where differences occurred. Eta-squared (η^2) values are provided for all analyses as an indication of the size of the difference between the two samples. An η^2 of around .03 is considered small, .13 is considered

TABLE 1: Negative mood states (DASS) and self-efficacy (LAQ2) scores for the SCI group ($n = 41$) and the able-bodied controls ($n = 41$). ANOVA statistics, probabilities of difference, and effect sizes (η^2) are shown.

Variable	SCI group mean (SD) 95% CI	Able-bodied controls mean (SD) 95% CI	F	η^2
Dep. mood	9.5 (11.1) 6.0–13.0	2.9 (3.6) 1.7–4.0	13.0**	0.14
Anxiety	5.3 (7.7) 2.9–7.8	2.6 (2.9) 1.7–3.6	4.2*	0.05
Stress	10.5 (8.7) 7.7–13.3	7.3 (4.8) 5.8–8.8	4.3*	0.05
LAQ2	19.8 (16.1) 14.7–24.9	14.1 (7.3) 11.7–16.4	4.2*	0.05

*$P < .05$, **$P < .01$.

TABLE 2: DASS depressive mood, anxiety, and stress domain scores across low versus high levels of self-efficacy.

DASS mood states	Low self-efficacy ≥20 on the LAQ2		High self-efficacy <20 on the LAQ2	
	SCI mean (SD)	Controls mean (SD)	SCI mean (SD)	Controls mean (SD)
Dep. mood	20.5 (10.9)	6.2 (4.5)	3.1 (3.9)	2.3 (3.1)
Anxiety	10.7 (10.5)	4.0 (1.8)	2.2 (2.5)	2.4 (3.0)
Stress	17.6 (9.1)	12.0 (4.8)	6.4 (5.3)	6.5 (4.4)

There were 15 in the low self-efficacy SCI subgroup and 26 in the high self-efficacy SCI subgroup. There were 6 in the low self-efficacy able-bodied control group and 35 in the high self-efficacy subgroup.

a medium difference, and over .2 is considered a large and substantial difference [22]. Post hoc statistical power of the test is also provided. All analyses were performed using Statistica Software (Version 9, StatSoft).

3. Results

Age, sex, and years of education were not found to influence significantly the level of mood states. Table 1 shows DASS domains depressive mood, anxiety, and stress scale scores, as well as LAQ2 self-efficacy scores for the two groups, including ANOVA results and effect sizes (η^2). The SCI group was found to be significantly different from the able-bodied control group for the three DASS mood state domains and for the LAQ2 self-efficacy measure: Wilks $\lambda = .85$, $F_{4,77} = 3.5$, $P < .05$, $\eta^2 = .16$, power = 85%. Table 1 also shows the ANOVA results for differences between groups for each individual domain. Inspection of Table 1 shows that the overall SCI group had significantly higher levels of depressive mood, anxiety, stress, and poorer self-efficacy when compared to the able bodied group.

3.1. The Impact of Self-Efficacy on Mood States. After dichotomizing into the self-efficacy subgroups, the mean LAQ2 scores for the high self-efficacy SCI and able-bodied subgroups were 10.2 (SD = 5.4; 95% CI: 8.0–12.4) and 11.9 (SD = 4.7; 95% CI: 10.3–13.5), respectively. The mean LAQ2 scores for the low self-efficacy SCI and able-bodied subgroups were 36.4 (SD = 14.9; 95% CI: 28.1–44.7) and 26.5 (SD = 6.8; 95% CI: 19.3–33.7), respectively. Table 2 shows DASS depressive mood, anxiety, and stress domain scores as a function of low versus high levels of self-efficacy for the SCI ($n = 15$ with low self-efficacy and $n = 26$ with high self-efficacy) and control groups ($n = 6$ with low self-efficacy and 35 with high self-efficacy). MANOVA indicated that significant effects occurred for group: $F_{3,76} = 8.3$, $P < .001$, $\eta^2 = .25$, power = 99%; for level of self-efficacy: $F_{3,76} = 16.5$, $P < .0001$, $\eta^2 = .39$, power = 99%; and for the interaction effect: $F_{3,76} = 6.8$, $P < .001$, $\eta^2 = .21$, power = 97%.

Factorial ANOVA results indicated that a significant interaction effect occurred for depressive mood as a function of low versus high self-efficacy across the two groups: $F_{1,78} = 18.8$, $P < .001$, $\eta^2 = .19$, power = 99%. Post hoc Bonferroni protected t-tests confirmed that the low self-efficacy SCI subgroup had significantly elevated depressive mood compared to the high self-efficacy SCI subgroup and the two able-bodied subgroups ($P < .01$). Factorial ANOVA indicated that a significant interaction effect also occurred for anxiety as a function of low versus high self-efficacy across the two groups: $F_{1,78} = 6.1$, $P < .01$, $\eta^2 = .07$, power = 68%. Post hoc Bonferroni protected t-tests confirmed that the low self-efficacy SCI subgroup had significantly elevated anxiety compared to the high self-efficacy SCI subgroup and the two able-bodied subgroups ($P < .05$). The interaction effect for stress was close to significance ($P < .07$). Figure 1 illustrates the interaction effects for self-efficacy on the depressive mood, anxiety, and Stress domains in the four subgroups.

4. Discussion

Unsurprisingly, the distress and upset associated with sustaining a severe neurological injury like SCI can be extreme. For instance, as stated previously, evidence suggests that up to 40% of adults with SCI will be at risk of developing a mental health disorder such as depression [7], about 56% will develop excessive levels of chronic fatigue [8, 9], and up to 70% will develop chronic pain [23]. Interestingly, based on DASS norms [19], Table 1 shows that the SCI group as a whole had a depressive mood score at the bottom of the mild depressive mood range. The SCI group anxiety score was in the normal range as was the stress score. This suggests that as a group, the participants with SCI are adjusting well enough. However, there is clearly a proportion of participants with SCI who are scoring at least into the moderate range

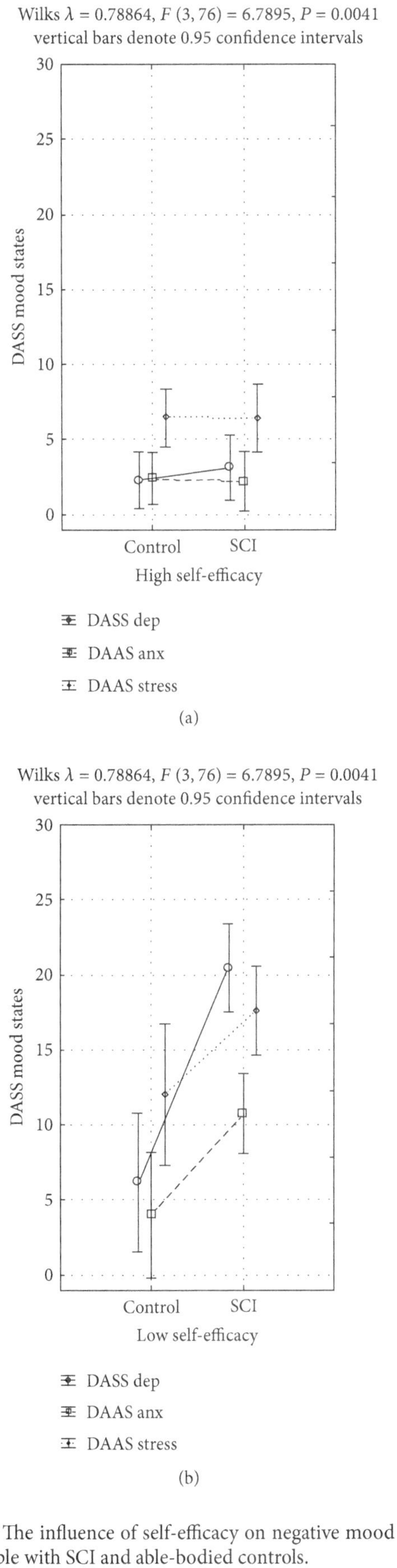

FIGURE 1: The influence of self-efficacy on negative mood states in adult people with SCI and able-bodied controls.

for depressive mood and anxiety, given the standard deviations scores shown in Table 1. Given the previously mentioned risk of chronic secondary conditions and consequent risks of poor adjustment when coping with the impairment and pain associated with SCI, rehabilitation strategies are needed that can protect people from the constant distress associated with SCI. The findings presented in this paper provide some direction in this regard, that is, the important role played by self-efficacy as a possible protective factor in people suffering an SCI.

Poor self-efficacy in adult people with SCI was found to be highly associated with elevated levels of depressive mood and anxiety. The low self-efficacy SCI subgroup had significantly elevated depressive mood and anxiety compared to SCI participants with high self-efficacy and to the able-bodied controls. Based on DASS norms [19], Table 2 shows that the low self-efficacy SCI subgroup had a Depressive mood score in the moderate to severe range, an Anxiety score in the moderate range, and Stress score in the mild range. Conversely, the high self-efficacy SCI subgroup had mood state scores in the normal DASS range [19], similar to the able-bodied group scores regardless of self-efficacy (though there was a trend for the low self-efficacy able-bodied subgroup to have higher levels of negative mood states than the high self-efficacy subgroup).

Self-efficacy has been established as a protective factor against negative mood in prior studies [24–27]. It has been suggested that it mediates between adverse life events and adjustment in people with SCI [7]. For example, Maciejewski and colleagues [27] showed that self-efficacy was a significant predictor of depressive symptom severity. They showed that having a higher level of self-efficacy resulted in fewer depressive mood symptoms in adults and that self-efficacy mediated around 40% of the effects of stressful life events on depressive mood. They concluded that maintaining a healthy self-efficacy, that is, a strong sense of control over one's life and environment, serves to protect a person from psychopathology, perhaps by ameliorating the negative effect of stressful life events [27]. Rutter [24] also argued that stressful life events may serve to precipitate psychopathology and that self-efficacy can act as a protective factor against the negative influence of stressful life events. Arnstein and colleagues showed that chronic pain was mediated by self-efficacy [26] and concluded that the belief in one's ability to cope with pain and disability protects against depression and anxiety. Middleton et al. [2] conducted research with over 100 adult persons with SCI living in the community and found that low self-efficacy was associated with substantially reduced QOL, above and beyond the effect of any physical impairment of the SCI. While the findings presented in this paper cannot conclude that self-efficacy plays a mediator role, the strong relationship found, coupled with prior research, does suggest that self-efficacy protects against the development of negative mood symptoms in people with SCI.

There are limitations in this study that require discussion. Participant numbers in the two groups were moderate, resulting in lowered statistical power [22], and dichotomizing the samples into self-efficacy subgroups would have lowered statistical power further. However, effect sizes for group differences were shown to be moderate to large, and post hoc power estimates confirmed that the statistical power in the study was robust, ensuring that the risk of a Type II error rate was low [22]. Furthermore, to clarify the mediator role of self-efficacy as a protective agent, research is now required that employs a longitudinal design in which participants are followed and measured over time, providing the necessary data to establish whether self-efficacy is indeed a mediator of stress or just a significant correlate.

5. Conclusions

Important clinical implications arise for improving the life of people with SCI. As argued before, problems like sadness related to their injury and impairment, chronic pain, and chronic fatigue have been reported by patients with SCI as a major source of distress and disablement [4, 7, 9] which can lead to social isolation, anxiety, depression, and reduced QOL [2, 5]. On the positive side, many people with SCI are coping satisfactorily, gaining employment, and socially integrating into their communities [28]. Therefore, clever assessment strategies are required during SCI rehabilitation that can detect in a reliable manner those who are at risk of maladaptive adjustment. Poor levels of self-efficacy may well be a primary risk factor for maladaptive adjustment. That is, those people with SCI who have no or little expectation of managing their lives and daily functions may well be those who are most at risk of depression, social withdrawal, pain, and so on. Validated self-efficacy measures are required to detect those at risk, and there are such measures available that could be used for this purpose [15, 21]. Furthermore, there is a crucial need for studies that evaluate the efficacy of psychological-based rehabilitation strategies that can improve and enhance the self-efficacy of patients with SCI when in hospital and when living in the community [18, 25]. This remains a challenge for future research in the area.

Acknowledgments

The authors acknowledge the support of the New South Wales Premier SCI Grant (RIPG4) and by a Grant from the Australian Research Council (LP0560590).

References

[1] M. F. Sommer, *Spinal Cord Injury. Functional Rehabilitation*, Prentice Hall, New Jersey, NJ, USA, 2001.

[2] J. Middleton, Y. Tran, and A. Craig, "Relationship between quality of life and self-efficacy in persons with spinal cord injuries," *Archives of Physical Medicine and Rehabilitation*, vol. 88, no. 12, pp. 1643–1648, 2007.

[3] J. Middleton and A. Craig, "Psychological challenges in treating persons with spinal cord injury," in *Psychological Dynamics Associated with Spinal Cord Injury Rehabilitation: New Directions and Best Evidence*, A. Craig and Y. Tran, Eds., Nova Science, New York, NY, USA, 2008.

[4] N. Westgren and R. Levi, "Quality of life and traumatic spinal cord injury," *Archives of Physical Medicine and Rehabilitation*, vol. 79, no. 11, pp. 1433–1439, 1998.

[5] C. H. Bombardier, J. S. Richards, J. S. Krause, D. Tulsky, and D. G. Tate, "Symptoms of major depression in people with spinal cord injury: implications for screening," *Archives of Physical Medicine and Rehabilitation*, vol. 85, no. 11, pp. 1749–1756, 2004.

[6] M. J. Haran, B. B. Lee, M. T. King, O. Marial, and M. R. Stockler, "Health status rated with the medical outcomes study 36-item short-form health survey after spinal cord injury," *Archives of Physical Medicine and Rehabilitation*, vol. 86, no. 12, pp. 2290–2295, 2005.

[7] A. Craig, Y. Tran, and J. Middleton, "Psychological morbidity and spinal cord injury: a systematic review," *Spinal Cord*, vol. 47, no. 2, pp. 108–114, 2009.

[8] N. Wijesuriya, Y. Tran, J. Middleton, and A. Craig, "The impact of fatigue on the health related quality of life in persons with spinal cord injury," *Archives Physical Medicine Rehabilitation*, vol. 93, pp. 319–324, 2012.

[9] A. Craig, Y. Tran, N. Wijesuriya, and J. Middleton, "Fatigue and tiredness in people with spinal cord injury," *Journal of Psychosomatic Research*, vol. 73, pp. 205–210, 2012.

[10] M. P. Jensen, M. J. Chodroff, and R. H. Dworkin, "The impact of neuropathic pain on health-related quality of life: review and implications," *Neurology*, vol. 68, no. 15, pp. 1178–1182, 2007.

[11] A. Bandura, "Self-efficacy: toward a unifying theory of behavioral change," *Psychological Review*, vol. 84, no. 2, pp. 191–215, 1977.

[12] P. D. Martin, G. R. Dutton, and P. J. Brantley, "Self-efficacy as a predictor of weight change in African-American women," *Obesity Research*, vol. 12, no. 4, pp. 646–651, 2004.

[13] G. Robinson-Smith, M. V. Johnston, and J. Allen, "Self-care self-efficacy, quality of life, and depression after stroke," *Archives of Physical Medicine and Rehabilitation*, vol. 81, no. 4, pp. 460–464, 2000.

[14] G. Andrews and A. Craig, "Prediction of outcome after treatment for stuttering," *British Journal of Psychiatry*, vol. 153, pp. 236–240, 1988.

[15] J. W. Middleton, R. L. Tate, and T. J. Geraghty, "Self-efficacy and spinal cord injury: psychometric properties of a new scale," *Rehabilitation Psychology*, vol. 48, no. 4, pp. 281–288, 2003.

[16] W. Horn, W. Yoels, D. Wallace, D. Macrina, and M. Wrigley, "Determinants of self-efficacy among persons with spinal cord injuries," *Disability and Rehabilitation*, vol. 20, no. 4, pp. 138–141, 1998.

[17] A. R. Craig, K. M. Hancock, and H. G. Dickson, "Spinal cord injury: a search for determinants of depression two years after the event," *British Journal of Clinical Psychology*, vol. 33, no. 2, pp. 221–230, 1994.

[18] A. R. Craig, K. Hancock, and E. Chang, "The influence of spinal cord injury on coping styles and self-perceptions two years after the injury," *Australian and New Zealand Journal of Psychiatry*, vol. 28, no. 2, pp. 307–312, 1994.

[19] S. H. Lovibond and P. F. Lovibond, *Manual for the Depression Anxiety Stress Scales*, Psychology Foundation, Sydney, Australia, 1995.

[20] J. D. Henry and J. R. Crawford, "The short-form version of the depression anxiety stress scales (DASS-21): construct validity and normative data in a large non-clinical sample," *British Journal of Clinical Psychology*, vol. 44, no. 2, pp. 227–239, 2005.

[21] A. Craig, K. Hancock, and M. Craig, "The lifestyle appraisal questionnaire: a comprehensive assessment of health and stress," *Psychology and Health*, vol. 11, no. 3, pp. 331–343, 1996.

[22] J. Cohen, *Statistical Power Analysis for the Behavioral Sciences*, LEA, New Jersey, NJ, USA, 1988.

[23] P. J. Siddall, J. M. McClelland, S. B. Rutkowski, and M. J. Cousins, "A longitudinal study of the prevalence and characteristics of pain in the first 5 years following spinal cord injury," *Pain*, vol. 103, no. 3, pp. 249–257, 2003.

[24] M. Rutter, "Resilience in the face of adversity: protective factors and resistance to psychiatric disorder," *British Journal of Psychiatry*, vol. 147, pp. 598–611, 1985.

[25] A. Craig, "Resilience in people with physical disabilities," in *The Oxford Handbook of Rehabilitation Psychology*, P. Kennedy, Ed., chapter 26, Oxford University Press, Oxford, UK, 2012.

[26] P. Arnstein, M. Caudill, C. L. Mandle, A. Norris, and R. Beasley, "Self efficacy as a mediator of the relationship between pain intensity, disability and depression in chronic pain patients," *Pain*, vol. 80, no. 3, pp. 483–491, 1999.

[27] P. K. Maciejewski, H. G. Prigerson, and C. M. Mazure, "Self-efficacy as a mediator between stressful life events and depressive symptoms. Differences based on history of prior depression," *British Journal of Psychiatry*, vol. 176, pp. 373–378, 2000.

[28] A. Craig, K. Hancock, and H. Dickson, "Improving the long-term adjustment of spinal cord injured persons," *Spinal Cord*, vol. 37, no. 5, pp. 345–350, 1999.

10

An Exploratory Study of the Elements of Successful Service Dog Partnerships in the Workplace

Margaret K. Glenn

West Virginia University, P.O. Box 6122, 502 Allen Hall, Morgantown, WV 26506, USA

Correspondence should be addressed to Margaret K. Glenn; margaret.glenn@mail.wvu.edu

Academic Editors: J. McDougall and C. Zwingmann

The use of service or assistance dogs has increased over the past three decades but is still considered by many to be an emerging concept for assisting people with disabilities to navigate a number of environments. This is predominately due to the minimal research that has been done on the effect and promising practices. One area, employment, has been completely overlooked in research related to service dogs. This research project undertook an exploratory study to gather data on the elements of service dog partnerships that have been successful in the workplace. A structured methodology using mixed methods was used to gather ideas from a diverse group of stakeholders, people with service dogs, trainers, vocational rehabilitation counselors, and other healthcare professionals, to form a common framework for addressing the issue in future research and development of interventions. The results identified 68 elements that respondents perceived and rated to be important or highly important to the phenomenon. They were categorized into six clusters: (1) dog preparation, (2) monitoring, (3) employee competence, (4) legal knowledge, (5) information and education, and (6) coworker preparation. The discussion identified key points that might support the development of successful employment outcomes for people working with service dogs.

1. Introduction

Service animals provide support for people with disabilities at a level we could not have foreseen just decades ago. They have expanded our understanding of the variety of tasks that can be done, different types of people with disabilities who can be served, and the effect of the animal on the lives of people with disabilities. Given this capacity, many people with significant disabilities are seeking entry into the workplace with their animals in an effort to allow themselves to benefit from the more normal rhythm of life afforded to others [1]. That is creating a challenge for employers and employees alike as they navigate the legal and social implications of animals in the workplace and work to understand the validity of the service [2].

The terminology used to label specific types of work dogs perform for people with disabilities has not even been standardized. At present, Assistance Dogs International (n.d.) defines three types of assistance dogs: (1) guide dogs for the blind and the visually impaired, (2) hearing dogs for the deaf and hard of hearing, and (3) service dogs for people with disabilities other than those related to vision or hearing [3]. The third category broadens into distinctions of trained dogs such as medical response, mobility assistance, psychiatric service, and seizure response. These dogs are trained to work with people who use power or manual wheelchairs, have balance issues, have various types of autism, need seizure alert or response, need to be alerted to other medical issues like low blood sugar, or have psychiatric disabilities.

The staff of the Job Accommodation Network, a service of the Office of Disability Employment Policy of the U.S. Department of Labor, field thousands of inquiries about workplace accommodations from employers every year, including questions about service animals. According to the staff, the calls include inquiries about more than the traditional guide dog, hearing, or mobility support animal. The majority is now focused on uncharted territory for employers, such as justifying an animal as a reasonable accommodation in the workplace for people with mental health disorders and hidden disabilities (personal communication, Hendricks).

There exist anecdotal stories of why employers may be concerned about having a dog in the workplace. These include issues around allergens, potential for disruptive behavior, employee phobias, and liability. A rising concern promoted in the media is the possible proliferation of people falsely identifying their dog as a service animal to go on public transportation, into businesses and restaurants [4]. One would expect employers to become skeptical as well, especially given the variety of emerging breeds of dogs and reasons people use them. The traditional perception that service animals were Golden Retrievers, Labradors, and German Shepherds are being challenged as Papillons, Great Danes, and a host of other dog breeds and mixed breeds are trained to serve. They are also serving people who experience extreme vertigo, migraines, epilepsy, diabetes, and other medical conditions that limit activities of daily living. The changes are occurring faster than in the past. For instance, guide dogs for people who are blind had an official start shortly after World War I but those for mobility limitations did not follow for another 40 years. Hearing, psychiatric service, autism, and medical alert dogs, among others, have been a much more recent occurrences. Now, people are even using other animals such as monkeys, horses, cats, and birds to provide service and support.

The Americans with Disabilities Act has provided guidance around legal rights and limits to the use of a service dog in the workplace and related environments, such as transportation, public access, and housing. Yet there is little research based information about what it means and requires for a service dog partnership to navigate these environments successfully.

Federal law defines service animal as, "any dog that is individually trained to do work or perform tasks for the benefit of an individual with a disability, including a physical, sensory, psychiatric, intellectual, or other mental disability. Other species of animals, whether wild or domestic, trained or untrained, are not service animals for the purposes of this definition. The work or tasks performed by a service animal must be directly related to the individual's disability" (DOJ, n.d.).

According to the Department of Justice (n.d.), "examples of work or tasks include, but are not limited to, assisting individuals who are blind or have low vision with navigation and other tasks, alerting individuals who are deaf or hard of hearing to the presence of people or sounds, providing nonviolent protection or rescue work, pulling a wheelchair, assisting an individual during a seizure, alerting individuals to the presence of allergens, retrieving items such as medicine or the telephone, providing physical support and assistance with balance and stability to individuals with mobility disabilities, and helping persons with psychiatric and neurological disabilities by preventing or interrupting impulsive or destructive behaviors. The crime deterrent effects of an animal's presence and the provision of emotional support, well-being, comfort, or companionship do not constitute work or tasks for the purposes of this definition." These tasks and their applicability to the workplace as a reasonable accommodation is a concern of larger proportions than just a decade ago.

The use of service animals can be considered a reasonable accommodation in employment settings by law as well as an opportunity for increased independence in educational and the general community environments. The key word in the former sentence is "can." The ADA requires that service animal use by a person with a disability be allowed public access, but Title I, the employment section of the ADA does not require employers to allow employees to bring their service animals to work. Instead, it is considered a form of reasonable accommodation. Although, on the other hand, Title I expands the options available to people who wish to use a service animal as they do not limit the definition to dogs.

Expanded use of service animals to support people with disabilities in community participation and employment needs promising practices that will inform policies and procedures and possibly regulation. Data-driven approaches are needed to navigate the expectations of defining reasonable accommodation in the workplace, a significantly underresearched phenomenon even in service dog use.

The goal of this paper is to provide a foundation for understanding the role of service dogs in the lives of people with disabilities and the practices that may allow for appropriate access and positive outcomes in the workplace. Dogs were chosen because they have a longer history than other animals in providing services for people with disabilities. A study was conducted with funding from the National Institute on Disability and Rehabilitation Research's Switzer Distinguished Rehabilitation Research Fellowship. The study undertook a mixed methods form of structural conceptualization to assess the complex issues from the perspective and needs of a diverse group of stakeholders and generated a graphic depiction of major concepts.

The primary research question that was posed for the study was "*What elements are present in the process of creating successful service dog partnerships in the workplace?*" In addition, there was an investigation of the relative importance of specific recommended elements to the overall process.

2. Method

2.1. Participants. Participants were recruited through listservs and membership lists of Assistance Dog International, International Association of Assistance Dog Partners, followers of the International Assistance Dog Week pages, and State vocational rehabilitation agencies in the Mid-Atlantic, southern and western regions. A snowball sampling approach was used to reach a larger group. In each contact made with individuals associated with these organizations, they were asked to forward the request to participation to others in their network that met the participation criteria.

Participation was limited to include only individuals who were experienced with the use of service dogs in the workplace either as handler, service dog trainer, vocational rehabilitation counselor, or health care professional. The population was constrained to experience with hearing dogs for the deaf and hard of hearing, service dogs that provide mobility and stability assistance, seizure alert or response, and other medical issues such as diabetic alert medical service dogs for people with disabilities other than those related to vision or hearing. Those whose experience focused on service dogs for people with low vision or blindness were excluded due to their differences in training as well as level of experience.

The seminal work of Trochim recommended 10 to 20 people as a suitable participant size in the concept mapping system (1989). For this study, this was applied to the subpopulations, seeking a minimum of 10 participants who had experience with mobility/stability and hearing assistance dogs and 10 who had experience with medical alert service dogs, to include psychiatric. This minimum was also applied to the roles of service dog user, trainer, vocational rehabilitation counselor, other healthcare professional, and employers.

Sixty-eight (68) individuals participated in the process. The largest group was service dog users (n = 38; 56%). Predominately, the experience was with dogs who provide mobility/stability assistance (n = 37; 54%). This is not surprising, as one would expect the number of handlers or users to outnumber the number of trainers and vocational rehabilitation counselors. There is a longer history of training mobility and stability dogs than medical alert dogs as well. Further information on the participant demographics is provided in Table 1.

Of the 68 participants, 64 completed the demographic questions, 24 participated in the brainstorming exercise, 10 sorted the elements once the brainstorming was completed, and 40 finished rating the overall importance of the elements in the overall process. Individuals may have participated in more than one activity.

TABLE 1: Demographic characteristics of participants with service dog experience (N = 68).

Participant Question	Option	Frequency	%
Primary role	Person who uses a service dog	38	55.88%
	Service dog trainer	11	16.18%
	Vocational rehabilitation counselor	12	17.65%
	Employer (to include human resources personnel, or supervisors)	0	0.00%
	Other health care professional	3	4.41%
	Did not respond	4	5.88%
		68	**100.00%**
Primary type of service dog in experience	Hearing assistance	8	11.76%
	Mobility/stability assistance	37	54.41%
	Psychiatric/psychological service	13	19.12%
	Seizure alert/response	1	1.47%
	Diabetic alert	2	2.94%
	Other medical response	3	4.41%
	Did not respond	4	5.88%
		68	**100.00%**
Experience with service dogs	1	21	30.88%
	2–5	27	39.71%
	6–10	3	4.41%
	11–20	6	8.82%
	More than 20	7	10.29%
	Did not respond	4	5.88%
		68	**100.00%**

Note. Experience is measured in number of service dog partnerships in the workplace the respondent has been part of, as a trainer, handler, vocational rehabilitation counselor, or healthcare professional.

2.2. Research Design. An integrative mixed methods research design geared toward exploratory research was used in this study [5–7], specifically concept mapping pattern matching. Trochim [8] provided the following definition of *concept mapping*: "a pictorial representation of the group's thinking which displays all of the ideas of the group relative to the topic at hand, shows how these ideas are related to each other, and optionally, shows which ideas are more relevant, or appropriate" (p. 2). This type of design is especially useful when no formal hypotheses important exist and allows for potential hypotheses to be generated from the findings. It is also a method that, when examined across a range of projects, has been shown to yield reliable results [9].

For this research, there was a need to establish a baseline understanding of what was occurring in successful service dog partnerships in the workplace from the perspective of those with experience. The structured methodology we used gathers ideas from a diverse group of stakeholders to form a common framework for addressing the issue while simultaneously creating potential hypotheses for future research. In the representation of the participants as a geography of thought, engaging different communities of interest, the methodology allows us to create a new quantitative framework out of a qualitative process [10].

The process started with preparation and selection of participants, to include gathering of quantitative data to provide a demographic portrait of the participant pool. Online, asynchronistic group processes allowed for generation of ideas through brainstorming. The statements are then synthesized and sorted into clusters according to commonality. The ideas are rated according to variables of interest, then analyzed with multivariate statistics such as multidimensional scaling and cluster analysis [11].

2.3. Data Collection. In the announcement sent to prospective participants, a link (url) was provided for a web-based survey with an open-ended question. They were first asked to respond to the demographic questions, self-identifying as meeting the participation criteria. Then they were asked to brainstorm responses to the focus prompt *What elements are important to a successful service dog partnership in the workplace?* Data was collected from 24 participants who submitted individually with anonymity. The brainstorming website was updated in real time so participants could see ideas as they were generated. Members of the research team then refined the statements to remove duplicate statements,

TABLE 2: Brainstormed elements of successful service dog partnerships in the workplace organized by clusters (N = 68).

Cluster	Id #	Statement	Bridging
(1) Dog preparation			**0.50**
	1	The dog is well behaved; controlled by vocal command.	0.33
	38	That the service dog has received training appropriate for the specific workplace.	0.47
	39	Maintenance of behavior and task completion is expected of the service dog team.	0.49
	41	The use of service dog program trainers to do annual maintenance checks and address problems as they occur.	0.70
		Count = 4, Std. Dev. = 0.13, Variance = 0.02, Min = 0.33, Max = 0.70, Median = 0.48.	
(2) Monitoring			**0.30**
	17	The person who is bringing the dog into the workplace must take responsibility for the dog's behavior and reinforce appropriate boundaries with colleagues.	0.31
	33	The employee provides proper physical maintenance of the animal, to include grooming, bathing, and feeding to minimize smells and shedding.	0.00
	36	That the employee assumes responsibility to balance the need to interact with the dog throughout the workplace, maintain appropriate work productivity, and minimize disruption of the worksite.	0.27
	43	The person with the service dog needs to be able to reinforce the dog's skills and use a "no excuse for bad behavior" policy.	0.27
	48	A willingness of both the dog and the employee to work together.	0.61
	58	The ability to cite examples of how a service dog benefits may benefit the employer, through reduction in stress among employees, public relations, and so forth.	0.33
	60	An understanding of the employee/applicant's knowledge of training and dog handling.	0.21
	61	The dog's ability to be invisibly present at work (not distracting or stressed).	0.52
	62	Employee/applicant ability to maintain training rules and regulations in order to maintain the dog's behavior around colleagues and others.	0.15
		Count = 9, Std. Dev. = 0.17, Variance = 0.03, Min = 0.00, Max = 0.61, Median = 0.61.	
(3) Employee competence			**0.18**
	3	An understanding by the service dog owner that permission to have a service dog in the workplace must be agreed upon by the employer prior to the dog entering the workplace.	0.23
	12	For those who are already working, having a discussion with the employer as part of the decision to obtain a service dog.	0.30
	25	That the employee or job applicant is able to articulate a well-founded argument for the use of a service dog in the workplace as a reasonable accommodation.	0.07
	26	The employee or job applicant is able to articulate the specific job related or supportive task(s) that will include the service dog.	0.07
	31	The employee or job applicant is able to outline specific needs of the animal in the workplace, including breaks for walks, water, food, and bathroom breaks.	0.18
	34	An understanding of the consequences if the employee does not maintain proper control or maintenance of the service dog.	0.22
	37	The job applicant with a service dog is prepared to address behavior of interviewers that reveals a lack of understanding of service dog etiquette, that is, petting the dog.	0.12
	40	If the dog has been owner trained, that the handler has written documentation of the training which may include obedience classes, special sessions with trainers, and reinforcement procedures.	0.16
	46	That the dog is identifiable through the use of a service dog vest, cape, or harness.	0.24
	56	A process for ensuring the dog handler can provide testing and certification or evidence of training which establishes the dog is a service dog.	0.27
	66	A procedure for addressing alternative accommodations\if the dog is not able to be present (e.g., during illness).	0.17

Table 2: Continued.

Cluster	Id #	Statement	Bridging
	68	That there is a procedure for verifying that the dog has had appropriate vaccinations and health maintenance.	0.15
		Count = 12, Std. Dev. = 0.07, Variance = 0.01, Min = 0.07, Max = 0.30, Median = 0.17.	
(4) Legal knowledge			**0.25**
	4	An informed understanding by employer and employee or applicant of the parameters, including limits, regarding the person with disabilities' legal rights, both state and federal, to the use of service dogs in the workplace.	0.21
	5	An understanding among employer, supervisor, and coworkers of practices that are legally deemed discriminatory.	0.18
	6	An informed understanding of the employer's legal responsibilities and rights related to the decisions associated with a service dog team in the workplace.	0.18
	7	An informed understanding of any related insurance and workers compensation implications and requirements of the employer.	0.33
	8	Clear communication between supervisor and employee regarding needs of both parties related to work performance standards.	0.16
	9	An established collaborative procedure for communication within the workplace among coworkers, service dog partner and any related customer interaction, and so forth, regarding issues, problems, and suggestions.	0.25
	13	A supportive procedure for allowing the employee to participate in an intensive 2 to 4 week training program with a new service dog.	0.24
	15	A procedure for establishing options in response to coworkers who are allergic to animals.	0.30
	16	A procedure for establishing areas within the workplace that a service dog cannot go.	0.31
	28	If the person will work in an office setting, workspace is provided that is close to a door or out of high traffic areas.	0.34
	35	The employer understands the need for and the process used to address misbehavior by the dog, to include having a private or quiet place to address the issue.	0.24
	54	Protocols for human resource departments in large companies or agencies to use when interviewing people with service dogs.	0.18
	55	A system for allowing "play breaks" for the service dog to exercise and "blow off" the energy they bottle up in the work environment.	0.42
	64	A system for notifying potential customers of the presence of a service dog in the place of business.	0.21
	65	Standard operating procedures in place to effectively distinguish between service dogs and pets to prevent other employees from attempting to bring nonservice dogs into work environment.	0.33
	67	Flexibility to allow the dog handler to have time to address any health problems that arise for the service dog (use of sick leave).	0.14
		Count = 16, Std. Dev. = 0.08, Variance = 0.01, Min = 0.14, Max = 0.42, Median = 0.31.	
(5) Information and education			**0.47**
	2	If the type of job may require the service dog to go into environments other than one workplace, the dog/handler team needs a means to educate in different professional settings.	0.67
	18	Training and information for employers on what it means to have a service dog in the workplace.	0.45
	22	A willingness on the part of employer to consider allowing a service dog at work and not immediately deny access on potentially unfounded concerns.	0.20
	27	A job analysis is done to determine the specific tasks associated with the position, identification of those tasks that need accommodation and where the dog will provide assistance.	0.54
	42	To have the service dog trainer initially assess the workplace and provide suggestions for problem areas.	1.00
	44	The knowledge that service dogs in the workplace break down barriers and facilitate positive social interactions and workplace relationships.	0.29

TABLE 2: Continued.

Cluster	Id #	Statement	Bridging
	45	An understanding of the fact that animals present in the workplace can ameliorate stress.	0.25
	47	An employer who understands that the service dog interaction is part of mitigating limitations associated with a disability, is a type of assistive device.	0.28
	49	The availability of educational materials about service dog teams in the workplace for potential employers and job seekers.	0.53
	50	The availability of educational workshops and information about use of service dogs in the workplace at workforce development conferences at the state and national levels.	0.59
	51	The involvement of vocational rehabilitation counselors and resources to assist both the business and individual in the modification or adaptation of the workplace.	0.39
	52	The involvement of vocational rehabilitation counselors to help with the negotiation or address any communication problems related to the use of the service dog.	0.40
	53	The awareness of the secondary benefits of having a service dog team in their corporation, which may include positive public relations.	0.41
	57	An understanding in the workplace that service dogs alert in a wide variety of ways, including sitting and staring, pawing, placing head on lap, leaning, nosing, and so forth.	0.47
	59	Dog enhances employee productivity; ensuring the dog does not distract employee from performing essential functions of the job.	0.65
	63	An understanding of what safety or health concerns for customers may exist if a dog is present at work (i.e., a service dog may not be appropriate in a kitchen).	0.33
		Count = 16, Std. Dev. = 0.19, Variance = 0.04, Min = 0.20, Max = 1.00, Median = 0.41.	
(6) Coworker preparation			**0.35**
	10	An employer demonstrating leadership through support of the service dog team by educating coworkers before the team enters the workplace, fielding concerns, complaints, and questions.	0.28
	11	The establishment and respecting of boundaries for the service dog, handler, coworkers, and customers.	0.38
	14	To engage workplace partners to feel a sense of ownership, pride, and support for the service dog team in a way that respects the team's autonomy and privacy.	0.43
	19	Orientation session for personnel to address the dog, breed and name, and the tasks the dog will perform.	0.59
	20	Orientation for personnel to address the roles and responsibilities of the handler in the care of the service dog.	0.52
	21	Orientation for personnel regarding the rules of service dog etiquette to include the fact that this is a service dog not a pet, speak to the person and not dog, and do not feed or pet animal without handler's permission.	0.52
	23	A tone set by the supervisor that values and appreciates what a service dog team brings to the employment setting, modeling for the entire workforce.	0.16
	24	The modeling of appropriate behavior and responses to the dog and person in the service dog team by the employer and supervisor(s).	0.35
	29	In the case of coworkers with allergies, air purifiers are provided and the work area is cleaned regularly to minimize problems related to having a dog in the workplace.	0.22
	30	In the case of coworkers or others who have a fear of dogs, a procedure for addressing ways to maximize their ability to avoid the dog.	0.18
	32	A work environment that is able to respond with flexibility to the needs of the animal.	0.21
		Count = 11, Std. Dev. = 0.14, Variance = 0.02, Min = 0.1, Max = 0.59, Median = 0.52.	

Note. The bridging value, ranging from 0 to 1, provides information on how often a statement was sorted with others that are close to it or disparate on the map. Lower bridging values indicate closer relationships while higher means there is less of a relationship between the statements in the cluster. It correlates with the average rating. Abbreviations used in the table include: Std, Dev. is standard deviation; Min. is minimum rating on a 0-1 scale; Max. is maximum rating on 0-1 scale; Median is median rating on a 0-1 scale.

clarify the language, and ensure that only one idea is represented in each.

A second call for participation was made of those who participated in the brainstorming part of the project. In order to ensure that the demographic groups were represented, a secondary call was made to the group that represented people with disabilities who use service animals and trainers. Ten participants individually sorted the elements into clusters or categories of common or similar elements. They were asked to create conceptual "piles" online and drag the elements into piles according to "how they seem to go together." Forty participants then ranked each element within those categories on a Likert scale of 1 to 5 in response to the question *How important do you think this item is in the OVERALL process?* (1—not important to 5—essential).

2.4. Data Analysis. Once the ideas were generated and sorted, the participants' work was aggregated to create a concept map using a nonmetric multidimensional scaling procedure. It arranges points representing the elements along orthogonal axes reflecting the distance between any two points, reflecting the frequency the items were sorted together. Conceptually, a small area suggests that the statements reflect a similar, probably well-defined underlying concept. Hierarchical cluster analysis was then used to draw boundaries around groups of ideas, turning them into conceptual clusters. The procedure provides a spatial representation of potentially unknown relationships among the elements and other variables [12].

The ratings regarding the participants' perceptions of the importance of each element were average for each element and each cluster of elements. The research team was then tasked to interpret the rating maps that were chosen to most effectively present the results. They overlay the rating of importance data onto the cluster map to show which cluster of ideas was most important to the participants (see Figure 1).

All data were collected and analyzed using Concept Systems Global MAX software. This software allows stakeholders to brainstorm, sort, and provide rating input via the Internet or offline. It includes online analysis tools, creating point and cluster rating and bridging maps, pattern matches, and go zones. It is also able to perform analysis for significance.

3. Results

The brainstorming process produced 68 elements considered relevant to a successful service dog partnership (see Table 2). This was well over the required minimum of 30 to 40 statements to ensure a valid concept mapping analysis. The elements were then organized into six clusters, reflecting the following content (1) dog preparation, (2) monitoring, (3) employee competence, (4) legal knowledge, (5) information and education, and (6) coworker preparation. (see Figure 1). This model provided the maximum number of interpretable clusters without losing between-group distinctions.

The 68 items were rated according to relative importance of an element in the overall perspective regarding what may constitute a successful service dog partnership in the workplace. For each participant, cluster scores were computed using the sum of all ratings for items within a particular cluster. Table 3 illustrates the descriptive statistics by cluster of the relative importance of each item in the overall process of creating a successful service dog partnership in the workplace as rated by participants.

Noting that higher means represent a higher perceived importance rating, clusters are shown in decreasing order of perceived importance. The items comprising monitoring

TABLE 3: Importance ratings by cluster ($N = 40$).

Cluster	Count	Min	Max	Mean	Std Dev.
Monitoring	9	0.00	0.61	4.38	0.17
Dog preparation	4	0.33	0.70	4.15	0.13
Coworker preparation	11	0.16	0.59	3.97	0.14
Legal knowledge	16	0.14	0.42	3.94	0.08
Information and education	16	0.20	1.00	3.84	0.19
Employee competence	12	0.07	0.30	3.85	0.07

Note. The count is the number of elements in the cluster. Abbreviations used in the table include: Std Dev. is Standard Deviation; Min. is minimum bridging values of ratings on 0-1 scale; Max. is maximum bridging values of ratings on 0-1 scale. The bridging value, ranging from 0 to 1, provides information on how often a statement was sorted with others that are close to it or disparate on the map. Median is median rating of level of importance on a 1–5 scale.

received overall the highest rating of importance (mean = 4.38), while information and education, received the lowest rating of importance (mean = 3.84).

4. Discussion

This project sought stakeholder input to understand the elements that may exist in service dog partnerships that have been successful in the workplace. The participants, including service dog handlers and trainers, vocational rehabilitation counselors, and other healthcare professionals, generated a list of 68 items, all of which were then rated as important or highly important to the process, showing an internal consistency of the items. A limitation of the study was the researcher's inability to engage employers in responding to the survey items. The length of the exercise, and possibly perceived liability in responding to questions, may have prevented their involvement.

The strength of the project was its use of a methodology that allowed for community-based participatory research. Concept mapping pattern matching employs various strategies to reduce researcher bias. First, the elements are generated by the study participants. Then, the sorting of the elements into meaningful categories is done by the participants which eliminates the interpretation by researchers that is inherent in a traditional qualitative process. The statistical analysis of the participant-determined sortings eliminated the need for specifying attributes to the sorting of the elements [10].

The researcher sought to establish working hypotheses on the subject of service dog use in the workplace for researchers and others seeking to design or evaluate effective employment programs. This exercise was to identify key elements that support a partnership and were not intended as a mandatory checklist. The project did not have the resources to investigate the elements in a wide participant population in the workplace, with accompanying instruments to measure validity of the findings. It is exploratory in nature.

One possible use of this data by the person who has the service dog is to develop a strategy to address any potential employer questions, spoken or unspoken. While

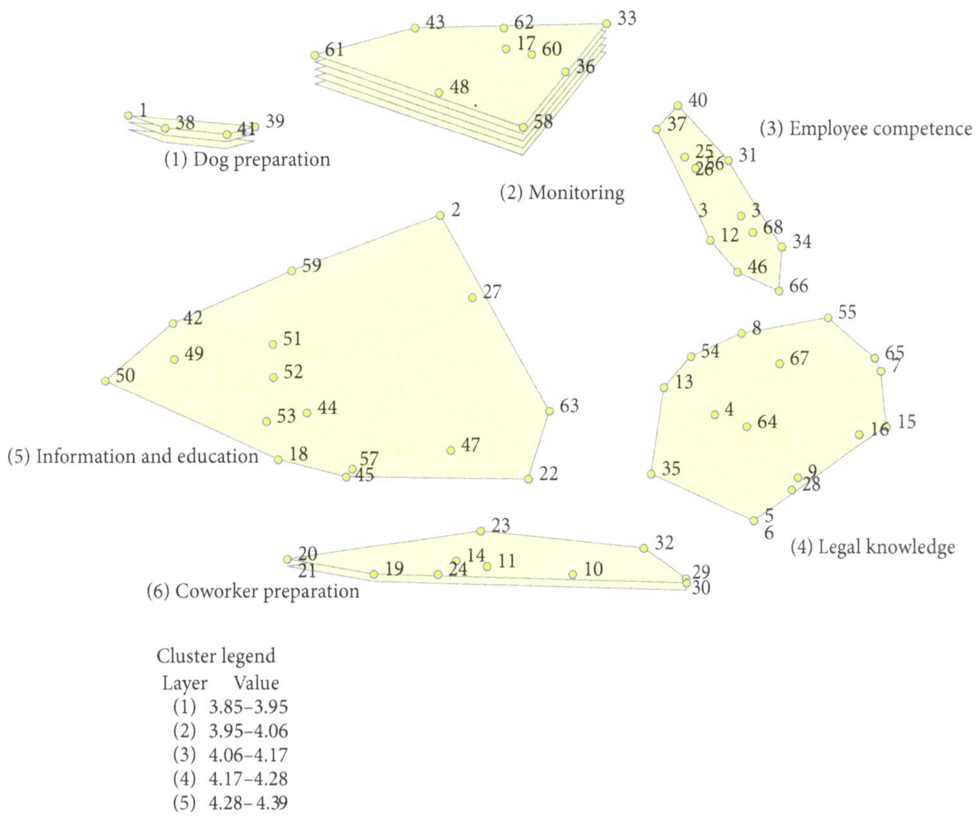

FIGURE 1: Visual depiction of the cluster rating map. The named clusters are comprised of the elements of successful service dog partnerships in the workplace. Each point number ($N = 68$) corresponds with elements listed on Table 2. The cluster legend provides the level of importance range of each cluster established by participants. Layers provide visual perspective of levels of importance.

employers were not represented in the group, the participants represented individuals who had experience negotiating with employers on behalf of people who require reasonable accommodations, as well as people who have successfully navigated with work world with their four-legged support system. Although it should be noted that the participants self-reported demographic information and were given the option to do so anonymously. So, the researcher was unable to verify the authenticity of the demographic information in all cases.

The service dog handler has control of a number of the items listed in this project, most importantly those in the monitoring category. There was overwhelming consistency among participants that this area is of high importance to a person obtaining and maintaining employment with a service dog. Addressing these with an employer would be of benefit during discussions regarding the request for a reasonable accommodation. The items focused on the responsibility of the individual with the service dog for behavior, care, and hygiene of the dog in the workplace.

It also supports the practice of many programs to require ongoing assessments of the maintenance of the partnership's skills and behaviors. Even people who have undertaken alternative training preparation for their dogs can, at a minimum, show successful completion of Public Access tests under the guidance of a trainer. An example of such a test has been made available, within an accompanying warning, by Assistance Dogs International on their website at http://www.assistancedogsinternational.org/standards/public-access-test/. If this is not available, there might be a benefit to identifying key informants who could provide more informal feedback of their observation of the dog's behavior and ability to perform tasks. This may be family members or a local dog trainer. Again, the intent of this recommendation is the importance of ensuring maintenance levels and not creating a restrictive requirement.

The participants rated the need for information and education as the category of least importance, although they considered it important. At this point, we must discuss problems within the brainstorming process that reflected a true need for dissemination of information to all the stakeholder groups. One survey respondent noted that, even within this group of experienced individuals, there was a lack of consistency in interpretation of the Americans with Disabilities Act with regard to service dogs and employment. Specifically, there was confusion regarding Title 1.

According to the Civil Rights Division of the U.S. Department of Justice, "Title I of the Americans with Disabilities Act of 1990 prohibits private employers, State and local governments, employment agencies and labor unions from discriminating against qualified individuals with disabilities in job application procedures, hiring, firing, advancement, compensation, job training, and other terms, conditions, and privileges of employment [13]. The ADA covers employers with 15 or more employees, including State and local governments. It also applies to employment agencies and to labor organizations." http://www.ada.gov/ada_title_I.htm. The confusion appears to stem from the differences between Titles I, II, and III of the Act with regard to requiring entities to comply with requests for access with a service dog. Allowing a service dog to accompany an employee on the job, under the guidelines of Title I, is held to the expectations of "reasonable accommodation." An employer may refuse to comply if the situation will create undue hardship.

Employers also have the right to ask for documentation of the need for the accommodation, within reason (EEOC, [14]). They can also ask if the service dog is trained but the documentation may come from a variety of sources, beyond healthcare professionals [15]. And the tasks may not be work specific but there could be needs associated with a medical condition.

Misunderstanding of these regulations can create missed opportunities for the person with a disability to forge a successful employment outcome. In order to make a strong argument for access, one needs the correct framework. More information can be found on the *ADA 2010 Revised Requirements Specific to Service Animals* as published by the Civil Rights Division of the U.S. Department of Justice. http://www.ada.gov/service_animals_2010.htm. The Job Accommodation Network provides guidelines specific to the workplace as part of the Accommodation and Compliance Series, at http://askjan.org/media/servanim.html.

5. Conclusion

The number of items ($N = 68$) generated in this exercise indicates the complexity of navigating the world of work with a service dog. Yet, as the items or elements of a successful service dog partnership were clustered into six categories, there are indicators that members of the stakeholder groups, trainers, vocational rehabilitation counselors, and employers, can play a part in making it happen for and with the person with a disability. Trainers are involved in (1) dog preparation and (2), while vocational rehabilitation counselors and employers would be mostly addressing (3) employee competence, (4) legal knowledge, (5) information and education, and (6) coworker preparation.

The most important element as rated by the participants was in the area of monitoring which meant that ongoing work would be done to ensure achievement of acceptable task completion and behavior of the service dog team and monitoring to prevent any problems. Once the service dog team is trained and comfortable with their respective roles, employers and vocational rehabilitation counselors can help establish a supportive work environment with the person working with the dog using the listed elements as a guide. In all, the service dog partnership is successful when all operate with guidelines that provide recommendations for all concerned.

Future research would be of great benefit as we seek to create data-driven responses to the questions that arise from new opportunities for people with disabilities to achieve independence and work. The benefits appear to be many and outweigh any potential barriers, with the right mix of information and innovation on the part of employers and employees alike.

Acknowledgement

This study was funded under Grant no. H133F120031 from the National Institute on Disability and Rehabilitation Research (NIDRR), the U.S. Department of Education's Office of Special Education and Rehabilitative Services (OSERS). However, these contents do not necessarily represent the policy of the U.S. Department of Education, and no endorsement by the Federal government should be assumed.

References

[1] D. H. Rintala, R. Matamoros, and L. L. Seitz, "Effects of assistance dogs on persons with mobility or hearing impairments: a pilot study," *Journal of Rehabilitation Research and Development*, vol. 45, no. 4, pp. 489–504, 2008.

[2] E. Eames, "Reasonable accommodation and assistance dogs in the workplace," CPER No. 189, 2008, http://www.iaadp.org/work_access6.html.

[3] Assistance Dogs International (n.d.), "Types of assistance dogs," 2013, http://www.assistancedogsinternational.org/about-us/types-of-assistance-dogs/.

[4] J. Hay, "Fake service dogs anger owners of trained pets," The Press Democrat, 2013, http://www.pressdemocrat.com/article/20130807/articles/130809625#page=1.

[5] V. J. Caracelli and J. C. Greene, "Data analysis strategies for mixed-method evaluation designs," *Educational Evaluation and Policy Analysis*, vol. 15, pp. 195–207, 1993.

[6] W. Trochim, "Concept mapping: soft science or hard art?" in *A Special Issue of Evaluation and Program Planning*, W. Trochim, Ed., vol. 12, pp. 87–110, 1989.

[7] W. Trochim and R. Linton, "Conceptualization for evaluation and planning," *Evaluation and Program Planning*, vol. 9, pp. 289–308, 1986.

[8] W. M. K. Trochim, "Concept mapping. Soft science or hard art?" *Evaluation and Program Planning*, vol. 12, no. 1, pp. 87–110, 1989.

[9] W. Trochim, "The reliability of concept mapping. Working document for paper presented at the Annual Conference of the American Evaluation Association, Dallas, Texas," 1993, http://www.socialresearchmethods.net/research/Reliable/reliable.htm.

[10] D. Truscott, B. L. Paulson, and R. D. Everall, "Studying participants' experiences using concept mapping," *The Alberta Journal of Educational Research*, vol. 45, no. 3, pp. 320–323, 1999.

[11] K. M. Jackson and W. M. K. Trochim, "Concept mapping as an alternative approach for the analysis of open-ended survey responses," *Organizational Research Methods*, vol. 5, no. 4, pp. 307–336, 2002.

[12] L. F. Fitzgerald and L. J. Hubert, "Multidimensional scaling: some possibilities for counseling psychology," *Journal of Counseling Psychology*, vol. 34, no. 4, pp. 469–480, 1987.

[13] "Civil Rights Division of the U.S. Department of Justice. (n.d.). Information and technical assistance on the Americans with Disabilities Act," 2013, http://www.ada.gov/ada_title_I.htm.

[14] Equal Employment Opportunity Commission (EEOC), "EEOC enforcement guidance: reasonable accommodation and undue hardship under the Americans with Disabilities ActEEOC Notice Number 915.002," 2013, http://www.eeoc.gov/policy/docs/accommodation.html.

[15] L. C. Bastiste, "Accommodation and compliance series: service animals in the workplace, Job Accommodation Network Accommodation Ideas," 2013, http://askjan.org/media/servanim.html.

11

Clinical Features of Bell's Palsy in Children and Outcomes of Physical Therapy: A Retrospective Study

Duygu Cubukcu,[1] Unsal Yilmaz,[2] Hakan Alkan,[3] Ferda Metinkisi,[1] and Muazzez Ozcan[4]

[1] *Department of Physical Medicine and Rehabilitation, Dr. Behcet Uz Children's Diseases Training and Research Hospital, Sezer Dogan Street No. 11, Konak, 35210 Izmir, Turkey*
[2] *Department of Pediatric Neurology, Dr. Behcet Uz Children's Diseases Training and Research Hospital, Sezer Dogan Street No. 11, Konak, 35210 Izmir, Turkey*
[3] *Department of Physical Medicine and Rehabilitation, Pamukkale University Faculty of Medicine, Kınıklı 20070, Denizli, Turkey*
[4] *Department of Otorhinolaryngology, Dr. Behcet Uz Children's Diseases Training and Research Hospital, Sezer Dogan Street No. 11, Konak, 35210 Izmir, Turkey*

Correspondence should be addressed to Hakan Alkan; alkangsc@yahoo.com

Academic Editors: S. Eyigor and E. E. Hansson

The aim of this study was to describe clinical features of Bell's palsy (BP) in children and outcomes of physical therapy interventions. Medical records of 186 patients with diagnosis of BP were reviewed. The severity of facial nerve dysfunction was graded according to House Brackmann Facial Nerve Grading Scale (HB FGS). After one month, patients who had HB FGS grade three or more were included in a physical therapy programme consisting of superficial heat, massage, exercises, and electrical stimulation. Among 186 children with BP, 167 children had a severity of HB FGS grade three or more and 19 had the incomplete type at the time of the diagnosis. After one month follow-up, 144 patients fully recovered, 35 patients recovered partially, while 7 patients had no recovery. Patients who had not fully recovered one month after onset of paralysis were included in the physical therapy programme. There was statistically significant difference between pretreatment and posttreatment HB FGS scores in patients who had not fully recovered one month after onset of paralysis. We concluded that the prognosis of BP in children seems to be good with higher recovery rate and physical therapy programme might be an effective method to facilitate recovery in patients with poor prognosis.

1. Introduction

The most common type of facial paralysis in children is Bell's palsy (BP), which is defined as an acute, idiopathic, unilateral paralysis of the facial nerve without any associated disorders. Known congenital, genetic, and acquired causes of facial nerve paralysis need to be ruled out before the diagnosis of BP is made [1]. It has an incidence rate of 18.8 cases per 100.000 in children younger than 18 years old [2]. BP is an important cause of disability in some pediatric patients with major facial dysfunction and reduced quality of life [3].

Facial functions are multidimensional, serving emotional, social, and physical aspects of a person's health. Incomplete recovery from facial nerve damage has significant social and psychological consequences. The prognosis of BP in pediatric population is generally good with a high rate of recovery. In spite of high complete recovery rate, some patients with BP do not achieve even satisfactory recovery. Moreover children with complete facial palsy and absence of recovery within 3 weeks may suffer poor outcomes as frequently as adults [4, 5]. In contrast with adults, the natural course of BP in children is not well documented and there are still many unresolved issues regarding the treatment and prognosis. Even though the treatment and prognosis of BP differ among children and adults, there are only a few studies focused on children [6–10]. Furthermore to our knowledge, there is no study in the literature which evaluates the outcomes of physical therapy interventions solely in children with BP.

Knowledge on the course of disease and clinical features of BP in children largely depends on the studies of BP among adults. Little is known regarding the clinical features and outcomes of physical therapy programme among children with BP. In this study, we aimed to investigate clinical features of BP as well as the outcomes of physical therapy programme in pediatric patients who had not fully recovered one month after onset of paralysis.

2. Patients and Methods

Medical records of patients younger than 18 years old, attending one of the Physical Medicine and Rehabilitation outpatient clinics at Dr. Behçet Uz Children's Diseases Training and Research Hospital between January 2007 and December 2012, were retrospectively reviewed and children who had the diagnosis of BP were identified. Children with facial paralysis due to central causes were excluded. The study protocol was approved by local ethics committee.

Each child had been examined by a pediatric neurologist, an otolaryngologist, an ophthalmologist, and a physiatrist during initial evaluation as it is a routine in Dr. Behçet Uz Children's Diseases Training and Research Hospital. All patients were referred to Physical Medicine and Rehabilitation outpatient clinic by pediatric neurologist. Each child was assessed by pediatric neurologist as well as a physiatrist with a standardized work-up and follow-up. Following a thorough history, a detailed physical and neurologic examination were performed. Moreover, selected laboratory testing such as serological viral markers for various viruses, including human immunodeficiency, Epstein-Barr, hepatitis B, and herpes simplex virus and also serologic test to rule out Lyme disease were obtained based on the suspected diagnosis. All patients in whom secondary facial nerve palsy is suspected a diagnostic work-up for the presence or absence of possible causes had been promptly initiated.

Detailed information including demographic characteristics, time of presentation in regard to the season of the year, medical history, family history and outcome were collected. The diagnosis of BP had been made when no obvious cause was identified by medical history, physical examination, or radiologic studies.

The severity of facial nerve dysfunction and the recovery rate after treatment were evaluated according to House-Brackmann Facial Nerve Grading Scale (HB FGS), an easily administered, widely used clinical system for grading recovery from facial nerve paralysis caused by damaged to lower motor neurons [11]. On this scale, grade I represents normal face function while grade VI refers to total paralysis; II mean slight weakness (mild dysfunction); III moderate dysfunction; IV moderate to severe; V represents severe dysfunction. In IV and V grades patient can not close the eye and could only barely move the mouth at V [11].

In patients with BP, when HB FGS was grade three or more, oral prednisolone therapy was initiated with a dose of 2 mg/kg up to 60 mg daily for 5 days followed by 5 days taper. When a viral infection is suspected, antiviral medication was initiated. In addition, a home based exercise programme consisting of training the facial muscles following a standardized protocol were initiated in all patients at the time of the diagnosis. A standard exercise handout for home programmes was given to each subject on the initial consultation with the physiatrist. Exercises were chosen to include different muscle groups supplied by each branch of the facial nerve repeated 10 times a day. Exercises were performed for both sides of the face by using a mirror to promote symmetry and feedback. The exercises included in the home programme were shown to the patient on the initial treatment.

Recovery was defined as the achievement of HB FGS grade one or two. All children with BP were followed up until complete recovery. Recovery was assessed with follow-up visits once a week during the first month and subsequently every month until satisfactory recovery.

Patients who had HB FGS grade more than two within one month after onset of paralysis, were included in the physical therapy programme. The physical therapy programme consisted of infrared application, massage to the face musculature, electrical stimulation, and exercise. Local superficial heat therapy by the application of infrared was performed for 15 min/session for the facial muscles prior to electrical stimulation (ES), massage or exercises. Massage was applied for 10 minutes to both sides of the face. ES was aplied to the facial muscles which have no active motion or muscle strength lower than three out of five. For stimulating muscles which is completely denervated, interrupted galvanic stimulation of 100 ms rectangular pulses may be given at rate of 1 pulse/s for 30–100 contraction/session. During each session, ES should be stopped once muscle fatigue occurs. ES was stopped as soon as the active motion of muscle seen. Exercises carried out on consultation with the physiotherapist were based on current trends of the facial retraining rehabilitation programme. This physical therapy programme was applied once daily for 5 days a week in patients who had HB FGS grade more than two. Median number of physical therapy sessions were 10 (range 5–32).

3. Statistical Analysis

All statistical analyses were performed using the SPSS version 17.0 for Windows software program (SPSS Inc., Chicago, IL, USA). Kolmogorov-Smirnov test was used to assess whether continuous variables were normally distributed or not. Descriptive statistics were used for the demographic characteristics. For continuous variables, the significance of the differences was analyzed using Student's t-test for normally distributed variables while categorical variables were analyzed with a chi-square test. Wilcoxon Singed Rank test was used to analyze the difference between the pretreatment and postreatment HB FGS. In all analyses, P values < 0.05 were considered statistically significant.

Table 1: Demographic characteristics and clinical features in patients with Bell's palsy.

	Patients (n = 186)
Gender, n (%)	
Male	79 (42.5%)
Female	107 (57.5%)
Age (years) (mean ± SD)	9.56 ± 3.45
Affected side, n (%)	
Right	97 (52.2%)
Left	89 (47.8%)
Season, n (%)	
Winter	42 (22.6%)
Spring	47 (25.3%)
Summer	30 (16.1%)
Autumn	67 (36%)
Severity, n (%)	
Mild	19 (10.2%)
Severe	167 (89.8%)
Recurrence, n (%)	
No	174 (93.5%)
Yes	12 (6.5%)
Family history, n (%)	
No	177 (95.2%)
Yes	9 (4.8%)
HB FGS, n (%)	
Grade II	19 (10.2%)
Grade III	31 (16.7%)
Grade IV	44 (23.7%)
Grade V	77 (41.4%)
Grade VI	15 (8.0%)
After first month, n (%)	
Full recovery	144 (77.4%)
Partial recovery	35 (18.8%)
No recovery	7 (3.8%)
After rehabilitation, n (%)	
Full recovery	35 (83.3%)
Partial recovery	7 (16.7%)
No recovery	—

HB FGS: House Brackmann Facial Nerve Grading scale.

Table 2: Demographic and clinical features of Bell's palsy patients according to severity of disease.

	Mild (n = 19)	Severe (n = 167)	P value
Gender, n (%)			0.51
Male	11 (57.9%)	68 (40.7%)	
Female	8 (42.1%)	99 (59.3%)	
Age (years) (mean ± SD)	8.84 ± 2.69	9.64 ± 3.52	0.21
Season, n (%)			0.22
Winter	1 (5.3%)	41 (24.6%)	
Spring	5 (26.3%)	42 (25.1%)	
Summer	5 (26.3%)	25 (15.0%)	
Autumn	8 (42.1%)	59 (35.3%)	
Affected side, n (%)			0.66
Right	9 (47.4%)	88 (52.7%)	
Left	10 (52.6%)	79 (47.3%)	
Recurrence, n (%)			0.23
No	19 (100%)	155 (92.8%)	
Yes	0 (0%)	12 (7.2%)	
After first month, n (%)			0.004*
Full recovery	19 (100%)	104 (62.3%)	
Partial recovery	0 (0%)	56 (33.5%)	
No recovery	0 (0%)	7 (4.2%)	

*Statistically significant difference.

4. Results

A total of 186 patients with BP reviewed of whom 79 were male and 107 were female, with a mean age of 9.56 ± 3.45 years ranging from 0 to 18 years. The majority of patients were seen in the autumn (67) and spring (47), respectively. The smallest number of the patients were seen on summer. There were 97 right and 89 left facial palsies. Out of 186 patients 9 (4.8%) had a positive family history of BP and 12 (6.5%) children had recurrent facial nerve palsy (Table 1).

Also, we could not demonstrate a significant difference on demographic and clinical features of BP patients with mild or severe disease ($P > 0.05$). On the other hand children with mild BP had significantly higher full recovery rate than children with severe BP ($P < 0.05$) (Table 2).

Among 186 children with BP, 167 (89.8%) children had a severity of HB FGS grade three or more and 19 (10.2%) had the incomplete type at the time of the diagnosis. After one month follow-up, 144 (77.4%) patients fully recovered, 35 (18.8%) patients recovered partially while 7 patients (3.8%) had no recovery.

A total of 42 patients who had not fully recovered one month after onset of paralysis, were included in the physical therapy programme. After the physical therapy programme at a mean 10 sessions totally; 35 (83.3%) patients out of 42 were fully recovered while 7 (16.7%) had partial recovery. There was a statistically significant difference between pretreatment and posttreatment HB FGS scores ($P < 0.001$) (Table 3). Finally at the end of one year follow-up, all patients except three were fully recovered. Moreover sequela such as contracture and synkinesis were not shown in children with BP.

5. Discussion

In this study, we describe a retrospective analysis designed specifically to determine the clinical features of BP and outcomes of physical therapy programme in pediatric patients with BP. Our results demonstrated that the majority of patients were diagnosed in spring and also had a complete BP. However the prognosis of BP was good with higher recovery

TABLE 3: Outcome of physical therapy programme in children with Bell's palsy who had no full recovery within one month after onset of paralysis.

	Before rehabilitation ($n = 42$)	After rehabilitation ($n = 42$)	P value
According to HB FGS, n (%)			<0.001
Full recovery	0 (0%)	35 (83.3%)	
Partial recovery	35 (83.3%)	7 (16.7%)	
No recovery	7 (16.7%)	0 (0%)	
HB FGS			
Median (minimum–maximum)	4 (3–6)	2 (1–4)	<0.001

HB FGS: House Brackmann Facial Nerve Grading scale.

rate. On the other hand physical therapy programme seems to be an effective method to facilitate recovery in patients with poor prognosis.

It is important that we have a clear understanding about the clinical features of BP. In a recent retrospective study which 51 cases (60.7%) were classified as BP, it was demonstrated that the number of girls and boys were equal with 42 patients of each gender and the mean age was 9.6 years. Also the facial palsy affected the right side in 40 patients (47.6%), the left side in 43 cases (51.2%) and in one patient (1.2%) it appeared bilaterally [6]. In another retrospective study it was reported that the male to female ratio was 0.9 in children with BP as well as the ratio of the affected side was left/right 1/0.8 also the mean age was 6 years 7 months and the peak age distribution was under 3 years [7]. The mean age in the pediatric population lies between 5 and 11 years with no significant difference between female and male patients [7, 12, 13]. Comparable to these studies, we found no difference concerning the gender or the affected side of the face.

Reports of children with recurrent BP is uncommon. Recurrent BP was found in only two children (4.3%) out of 47 children with BP in a Thai study [9]. In another study, 3 (10.3%) out of 29 children with BP admitted during 1995–2003 had recurrent facial nerve palsy [7]. We showed an incidence of 6.5% of 186 pediatric patients had recurrent BP, which was similar to these studies. On the other hand exposure to cold may trigger the BP. However, it is not clear that cold has a significant independent effect on risk of disease. Although seasonal variations in BP rates were observed, they were usually lower in summer. Cambell and Brundage [14] demonstrated that incidence rates for BP during colder months of the year were consistently higher than incidence rates during warmer months of the year.

Prognosis of BP in pediatric population were rarely studied. In a recent retrospective study it was reported that 75 patients (89.3%) recovered completely among 84 children with peripheral facial palsy of whom 51 cases (60.7%) were classified as BP [6]. In the Copenhagen facial nerve study which evaluated the natural history of 463 children with peripheral facial nerve palsy over a 25-year period, full recovery was achieved by 90% of these children [15]. In another retrospective study, the recovery rate within 3 weeks for children with BP was 68.8% whereas the complete recovery rate was high, 31 episodes (96.9%) had complete recovery within 32 episodes of BP in 29 children at the end of the 7 months from onset [7]. A recent study Jenke et al. reported a 97% spontaneous complete recovery of their patients, even though only 3.7% had been treated with corticosteroids [8]. In spite of high complete recovery rate, children with complete facial palsy and absence of recovery within 3 weeks can be indicators of poor prognosis in patients with BP (4). In accordance with these findings we also found that complete recovery was achieved by 77.4% children with BP and partial recovery was 18.8% while 3.8% achieved no recovery after the first month. We also demonstrated that out of remaining 42 patients who had not fully recovered after the first month 35 (83.3%) patients got full recovery while 7 (16.7%) had partial recovery after the physical therapy programme. Moreover, at the end of one year we observed that all except three patients had full recovery. In contrast to these, in a recent study [16] it was concluded that facial nerve palsy in children is not as benign as it was previously supposed. Surprisingly this study found that 21% of the participants had persistent mild to moderate dysfunction.

The prognosis of BP is primarily related to the severity of the initial dysfunction. We can say that clinically incomplete lesions tends to recover. Patients with incomplete facial nerve palsy have a better prognosis compared with those who have complete paralysis [15, 17]. This is in accordance with results of our study which demonstrated children with mild BP had significantly higher full recovery rate than children with severe BP.

It is still controversial whether children with BP should be given any medical treatment or applied physical therapy programme. Main goals of treatment are to expedite recovery without any sequela such as contracture and synkinesis [4]. Evaluation of any therapy for BP is difficult due to the high rates of spontaneous and complete recovery. The main question is whether results would be better if some treatment were given [18]. Most studies include only adults or a mixed population. Although a systematic review showed a higher recovery rate with corticosteroid and antiviral treatments, these data mostly refer to adults and trials including children are sparse [19]. Unüvar et al. described a quicker recovery, but no better outcome of facial palsy in children when treated with corticosteroids [20]. Currently, there is no sufficient evidence showing any clear benefit in the use of steroids or antiviral agents in the treatment of acute peripheral facial palsy in children [6]. However, in the present study when a patient had HB FGS grade three or more, steroid was initiated with a dose of 2 mg/kg up to 60 mg daily and whenever a viral infection is suspected antiviral medication was also initiated. Since all of the patients had received treatment, we could not make any conclusions on its effect on the natural outcome of the disease.

BP is commonly treated with various rehabilitation strategies and therapeutic modalities. There are many questions about their efficacy and effectiveness. Exercise is the most commonly used method for the rehabilitation of BP. Thermal methods, electrotherapy, massage and biofeedback are other forms that could be used for rehabilitation [18, 21]. The Cochrane Systematic Review [21] concludes that high-quality evidence to support significant benefit or harm from any physical therapy for idiopathic facial paralysis is lacking. There is, however, low-quality evidence that facial exercises can help improve facial function, mainly for people with moderate paralysis and chronic cases, and that facial exercise reduces sequelae in acute cases [21]. The possibility that facial exercise reduces time to recover and sequelae needs confirming with good quality randomised controlled trials. Physical therapy agents are often used in the treatment of idiopathic facial paralysis in adults, but the effectiveness is not known exactly. It is still unclear whether rehabilitation affects the natural course of BP. To our knowledge this is the first study that found physical therapy programme to be an effective method to facilitate recovery in children with BP who had not fully recovered within one month after onset of paralysis.

Major limitations of this study are its retrospective design rather than longitudinal follow up, relatively small number of patients who were included in the physical therapy programme, unequal number of physical therapy sessions and due to the lack of control group, difficulty in determining the outcome of treatment. Since this is a retrospective study, we were not able to assess the separate contribution of all possible confounders that have been associated with severity and also outcome of BP, which reduced the statistical power of our study. Despite these limitations, to our knowledge this is the first study focusing on the effect of comprehensive physical therapy programme in children with BP who had partial recovery after one month. Further longitudinal, prospective studies are warranted to evaluate the efficacy of physical therapy interventions in children with BP who had poor prognosis.

6. Conclusions

Prognosis of BP seems to be good with higher recovery rate in children with BP and physical therapy programme might be an effective method to facilitate recovery in patients who had not fully recovered within one month after onset of paralysis.

Conflict of Interests

The authors declare that there is no conflicts of interests.

References

[1] M. Lorch and S. J. Teach, "Facial nerve palsy: etiology and approach to diagnosis and treatment," *Pediatric Emergency Care*, vol. 26, no. 10, pp. 763–769, 2010.

[2] A. Rowhani-Rahbar, R. Baxter, B. Rasgon et al., "Epidemiologic and clinical features of Bell's palsy among children in Northern California," *Neuroepidemiology*, vol. 38, no. 4, pp. 252–258, 2012.

[3] J. Shargorodsky, H. W. Lin, and Q. Gopen, "Facial nerve palsy in the pediatric population," *Clinical Pediatrics*, vol. 49, no. 5, pp. 411–417, 2010.

[4] N. J. Holland and G. M. Weiner, "Recent developments in Bell's palsy," *The British Medical Journal*, vol. 329, no. 465, pp. 553–557, 2004.

[5] J. Holland, "Bell's palsy," *Clinical Evidence*, vol. 2008, article 1204, 2008.

[6] F. Drack and M. Weissert, "Outcome of peripheral facial palsy in children—a catamnestic study," *European Journal of Paediatric Neurology*, vol. 17, no. 2, pp. 185–191, 2013.

[7] W. X. Chen and V. Wong, "Prognosis of Bell's palsy in children—analysis of 29 cases," *Brain and Development*, vol. 27, no. 7, pp. 504–508, 2005.

[8] A. C. Jenke, L. M. Stoek, M. Zilbauer, S. Wirth, and P. Borusiak, "Facial palsy: etiology, outcome and management in children," *European Journal of Paediatric Neurology*, vol. 15, no. 3, pp. 209–213, 2011.

[9] K. Dhiravibulya, "Outcome of Bell's palsy in children," *Journal of the Medical Association of Thailand*, vol. 85, pp. 334–339, 2002.

[10] C. H. Wang, Y. C. Chang, H. M. Shih, C. Y. Chen, and J. C. Chen, "Facial palsy in children: emergency department management and outcome," *Pediatric Emergency Care*, vol. 26, no. 2, pp. 121–125, 2010.

[11] J. W. House and D. E. Brackmann, "Facial nerve grading system," *Otolaryngology—Head and Neck Surgery*, vol. 93, no. 2, pp. 146–147, 1985.

[12] H. J. Christen, F. Hanefeld, H. Eiffert, and R. Thomssen, "Epidemiology and clinical manifestations of Lyme borreliosis in childhood. A prospective multicentre study with special regard to neuroborreliosis," *Acta Paediatrica*, vol. 386, pp. 1–75, 1993.

[13] M. Peltomaa, H. Saxen, I. Seppälä, M. Viljanen, and I. Pyykkö, "Paediatric facial paralysis caused by Lyme borreliosis: a prospective and retrospective analysis," *Scandinavian Journal of Infectious Diseases*, vol. 30, no. 3, pp. 269–275, 1998.

[14] K. E. Campbell and J. F. Brundage, "Effects of climate, latitude, and season on the incidence of Bell's palsy in the US Armed Forces, October 1997 to September 1999," *The American Journal of Epidemiology*, vol. 156, no. 1, pp. 32–39, 2002.

[15] E. Peitersen, "Bell's palsy: the spontaneous course of 2,500 peripheral facial nerve palsies of different etiologies," *Acta Oto-Laryngologica*, no. 549, pp. 4–30, 2002.

[16] A. Biebl, E. Lechner, K. Hroncek et al., "Facial nerve paralysis in children: is it as benign as supposed?" *Pediatric Neurology*, vol. 49, no. 3, pp. 178–181, 2013.

[17] K. K. Adour, F. M. Byl, R. L. Hilsinger Jr., Z. M. Kahn, and M. I. Sheldon, "The true nature of Bell's palsy: analysis of 1,000 consecutive patients," *Laryngoscope*, vol. 88, no. 5, pp. 787–801, 1978.

[18] T. S. Shafshak, "The treatment of facial palsy from the point of view of physical and rehabilitation medicine," *Europa Medicophysica*, vol. 42, no. 1, pp. 41–47, 2006.

[19] G. M. Thaera, K. E. Wellik, D. M. Barrs, E. D. D. Dunckley, D. M. Wingerchuk, and B. M. Demaerschalk, "Are corticosteroid and antiviral treatments effective for bell palsy? A critically appraised topic," *Neurologist*, vol. 16, no. 2, pp. 138–140, 2010.

[20] E. Unüvar, F. Oğuz, M. Sidal, and A. Kiliç, "Corticosteroid treatment of childhood Bell's palsy," *Pediatric Neurology*, vol. 21, no. 5, pp. 814–816, 1999.

[21] L. J. Teixeira, B. G. Soares, V. P. Vieira, and G. F. Prado, "Physical therapy for Bell's palsy (idiopathic facial paralysis)," *Cochrane Database of Systematic Reviews*, no. 16, Article ID CD006283, 2008.

12

First-Year Outcomes after Stroke Rehabilitation: A Multicenter Study in Thailand

Vilai Kuptniratsaikul,[1] Apichana Kovindha,[2] Krisna Piravej,[3] and Piyapat Dajpratham[1]

[1] *Rehabilitation Medicine Department, Faculty of Medicine Siriraj Hospital, Mahidol University, 2 Prannok, Bangkok 10700, Thailand*
[2] *Rehabilitation Medicine Department, Faculty of Medicine, Chiang Mai University, Chiang Mai 50200, Thailand*
[3] *Rehabilitation Medicine Department, Faculty of Medicine, Chulalongkorn University, Bangkok 10330, Thailand*

Correspondence should be addressed to Vilai Kuptniratsaikul; sivkp@mahidol.ac.th

Academic Editors: K. Hashimoto, J. D. Kingsley, K. Masani, M. Syczewska, and M. Yu

Stroke affects the long-term quality of life and the well-being of patients and families. Stroke patients gain benefits from rehabilitation. Authors reported 1-year outcomes of stroke rehabilitation in 327 patients registered to the Thai Stroke Rehabilitation Registry. The outcomes included death rate, readmission rate, functional ability score (Barthel Index, BI), and factors affecting BI score. Of 327 patients, 214 (65.4%) had adequate follow-up data for analysis. The average age was 62.1 ± 12.5 years, and 57.9% were male. The mortality rate was 2.5% and the readmission rate was 11.2%. The number of the patients who could function independently increased from 5.5% at discharge to 22.9% and 25.5% at month 6 and month 12, respectively. The change in functional ability level of 214 patients included improvement (51.5%), deterioration (12.8%), and equivocal (35.7%). The low functional score at month 12 was significantly correlated with longer length of stay (LOS), longer onset to admission interval, and higher depression score at month-12. In conclusion, approximately half of the patients had an improvement in the disability level for at least one grade at 1-year follow-up. The low functional score by the end of the first year is associated with longer LOS during the first admission, delay in rehabilitation program, and psychological depression.

1. Introduction

Stroke is one of the leading causes of mortality [1]. It is the most common cause of physical and mental disability in the elderly worldwide, particularly East Asian populations [2]. It affects the long-term quality of life and well-being for both the patients themselves and their families. Stroke patients need medical rehabilitation to enable optimal functions that will overcome the patient's disability. A Canadian guideline in 2008 recommended that all stroke patients should receive rehabilitation therapy as soon as their medical conditions were stable [3]. Rehabilitation for stroke patients has been shown to improve functional ability of stroke survivors and to decrease burden of their families and society [4].

The outcomes of stroke and rehabilitation vary among patients. Teasell et al. revealed, the evidence-based stroke rehabilitation care which is more efficient in functional gain, had fewer complications, had lower mortality rate, and had lower need for institutionalization [5]. The median length of survival among ischemic stroke patients independent in daily living was longer than that of those who are dependent (9.7 years (95% CI 8.9 to 10.6) versus 6.0 years (95% CI 5.7 to 6.4), resp.) [6]. The result from rehabilitation affects not only longer survival period but also the quality of life of stroke patients for functional independence [6–8].

Thai Stroke Rehabilitation Registry (TSRR) was the first multicentre and hospital-based registry in Thailand. It was founded in 2008 by a group of rehabilitation medicine specialists of six university hospitals and three rehabilitation centres [9]. The patients in TSRR received conventional rehabilitation program including range of motion (ROM) exercise for the paralyzed limb to prevent contracture, strengthening exercise for the sound limb to strengthen muscles, balancing training, and ambulation training if possible. In addition, activities to improve hand functions and self-care training were also rehabilitated. They were discharged from hospitals when they reached the rehabilitation goals or when their Barthel Index (BI) scores were stable for 2 consecutive weeks. In 2009, we reported the immediate outcomes of the patients at the time of discharge from rehabilitation wards [10]. In this study, we presented the outcomes of stroke patients in TSRR at the first year after discharge from rehabilitation ward and its correlated factors in order to find the long-term effect of receiving intensive rehabilitation.

2. Materials and Methods

The present prospective study was conducted on a cohort of stroke patients in TSRR project which was a multicenter registry established in 2008 [9]. The study was conducted in accordance with the ethical principles stated in the most recent version of the Declaration of Helsinki. The study protocol was approved by the Institutional Review Board of 9 tertiary hospitals.

The outcomes of the rehabilitation inpatient period of 327 patients in TSRR were reported in our previous study [10]. After discharge from rehabilitation ward, the patients were followed up at month 6 and month 12. All patients or their representatives signed an informed consent to release the information for the present study. The inclusion criteria of this study were all subjects from TSRR who could be followed up. The patients whose follow-up data were not available due to any reasons, for example, unable to contact, living in rural areas, or being unable to come to the hospitals, were excluded from the study.

Demographic data including age, sex, type of stroke, bowel/bladder problems, and associated medical diseases of the patients were recorded using a structured record form. The assessment of all outcomes was performed at the hospital setting at month 6 and month 12. At each follow-up visit or appointment, the patients were interviewed or evaluated for the continuing home programs, types of vocations, sources of income, readmission rate, and mortality rate. The patients who were able to come to the hospital were evaluated for self-care and mobility functions using the BI (score 0–20; the higher score means the better functions) [11]. The BI represents severity of disability and is categorized into 5 scales according to the scores. Those were very severely disabled (score 0–4), severely disabled (score 5–9), moderately disabled (score 10–14), mildly disabled (score 15–19), and independent (score 20) [12].

In addition, factors associating with the change of BI between 1-year follow-up and discharge periods were also explored. Those factors were sex, age, previous stroke, length of stay (LOS), type of stroke, having medical diseases, onset to admission interval, perceptual dysfunctions, having bowel/bladder dysfunctions, having complications during admission from previous study (TSRR), and anxiety and depression scores at month 12. The anxiety and depression scores were evaluated using the Thai version of the Hospital Anxiety and Depression scale (HADS) [13]. It is composed of 14 items of 2 dimensions of anxiety and depression. The score ranges from 0 to 21 for each dimension. Patients who had a score ≥11 of each part were considered as having clinical anxiety or depression.

TABLE 1: Characteristics of 214 stroke patients.

Demographic data	Mean ± SD or *n* (%)
Age (yrs)	62.1 ± 12.5 (range 21–93)
Sex: male	124 (57.9)
Marital status: married	151 (70.6)
Urban residence	132 (61.7)
Type of stroke: infarction	155 (72.4)
Current cigarette smoking	34 (15.9)
Current alcohol drinking	63 (29.4)
Presence of dysphagia	33 (15.4)
Presence of bowel/bladder problems	65 (30.4)
Associated medical diseases:	
(i) Hypertension	162 (75.7)
(ii) Dyslipidemia	118 (55.1)
(iii) Diabetes Mellitus	62 (29.0)
(iv) Cardiac diseases	40 (18.7)
(v) Previous stroke/TIA	32 (15.0)
(vi) Others (carotid stenosis, diabetic retinopathy, hypothyroid, parkinsonism, seizure, spinal stenosis)	41 (19.2)

TIA: transient ischemic attack.

3. Statistical Analysis

Data was collected at baseline (discharge period of TSRR project), month 6, and month 12 and was presented in mean and standard deviation (SD), or number (n) and percent (%). Kolmogorov-Smirnov test was used to examine the normality of data distribution. The functional ability levels of each visit were compared using Chi-square. Unpaired t-test was used to survey the factors associating with the change of BI score. The factors with a P value less than 0.2 were entered into multiple linear regression analysis because there were chances that those might be confounders in a multiple linear regression even though they were not significant in univariate analysis [14].

4. Results

Among 327 patients registered in TSRR during October 2008 to September 2009, only 214 patients (65.4%) could be followed up for at least one-year duration. During the study period, 8 cases (2.5%) died, 3 cases (0.9%) withdrew, and 102 cases (31.2%) were lost to follow up. Causes of death included myocardial infarction (2 cases), chronic renal failure (2 cases), hypoglycemic shock (1 case), brain edema (1 case), and unknown causes (2 cases). Concerning drop-out analysis, the 214 studied cases and the 102 lost-to-follow-up cases were not different in age, sex, and types of stroke (data not shown).

Demographic data of the 214 patients were presented in Table 1. The average age was 62.1 ± 12.5 years old and 57.9% were male. Most patients were married (70.6%) and lived in urban areas (61.7%). The majority (72.4%) of the patients

TABLE 2: Continuing treatment programs after discharge and places of treatments of stroke patients at 1-year after discharge (N = 202).

Treatment programs	N (%)	Places of treatments[#]		
		Hospital	Home	Others
ROM exercise[@]	179 (88.6)	21 (11.7)	164 (91.6)	6 (3.4)
Balancing training	144 (71.3)	20 (13.9)	130 (90.3)	4 (2.8)
Herbal spa	12 (5.9)	2 (16.7)	6 (50.0)	5 (41.7)
Thai traditional massage	88 (43.6)	7 (8.0)	57 (64.8)	26 (29.5)
Acupuncture	23 (11.4)	19 (82.6)	0 (0.0)	4 (17.4)

[#] Patients may receive treatments in more than one place.
[@] ROM: range of motion exercise.

TABLE 3: Severity of disability of stroke patients at various periods.

Severity of disability	Discharge N = 327	Month 6 N = 175	Month 12 N = 196	P value
Very severely disabled (BI = 0–4)	21 (6.4%)	8 (4.6%)	6 (3.1%)	
Severely disabled (BI = 5–9)	54 (16.5%)	16 (9.1%)	21 (10.7%)	
Moderately disabled (BI = 10–14)	97 (29.7%)	41 (23.4%)	35 (17.9%)	<0.001
Mildly disabled (BI = 15–19)	137 (41.9%)	70 (40.0%)	84 (42.8%)	
Independent (BI = 20)	18 (5.5%)	40 (22.9%)	50 (25.5%)	

Data are the number of patients (percentage) and are compared using Chi-square tests.
BI: Barthel Index.

had ischemic stroke. The most common associated medical diseases were hypertension (75.7%), followed by dyslipidemia (55.1%), diabetes mellitus (29.0%), cardiac diseases (18.7%), and previous stroke (15.0%). At the end of one year, 15.9% were still smoking, 29.4% were drinking alcohol, 15.4% had dysphagia, and 30.4% had bowel/bladder problems.

Readmission occurred in 24 patients (readmission rate = 11.2%), 19 cases of single and 5 of double readmission. As the causes of readmission in some patients were more than 1, the total number of events was 29 including recurrent stroke (6 events), urinary tract infection (7 events), gastrointestinal bleeding (3 events), convulsion (3 events), heart failure (2 events), lung infection (2 events), bradycardia (2 events), severe knee pain from osteoarthritis (2 events), warfarin overdose (1 event), and hydrocephalus (1 event).

Concerning the continuing programs after discharge from hospital, almost all of the continuing programs, except acupuncture, were home-based rather than institutional-based programs. The top three programs that patients still performed at home were ROM exercise (88.6%), balance training (71.3%), and Thai traditional massage (TTM, 43.6%) (Table 2). Only 28 cases (13.1%) could continue working on their own jobs. Nearly half of them could work full time. The main sources of income came from their relatives (54.5%), their own pensions (29.1%), or their spouses' pensions (10.3%).

Table 3 presents the number (percentage) of patients classified according to the severity of disability level at discharge, month 6 and month 12. The number of the patients who were moderately to severely and very severely disabled decreased while number of the patients who could function independently increased from 5.5% at discharge to 22.9% and 25.5% at month 6 and month 12 respectively. Table 4 shows the association between the severity of disability levels at discharge and at month 12. Approximately half (101 from 196, 51.5%) of the patients had improvement of the disability level for at least 1 grade, 25 patients (12.8%) got deterioration whereas 70 (35.7%) had no change in disability level.

Table 5 demonstrates the factors associated with the change in BI score between 1-year follow up and discharge periods. Only 196 from 214 patients have completed data on BI. After using multiple linear regression analysis, LOS ≥ 1 month, onset to admission interval ≥3 months, and depression score at month 12 of ≥11 were independent factors associating with poor functional score at 1-year follow up period.

5. Discussion

Our result showed that the functional outcome (BI) at month 6 and month 12 increased significantly compared to the score at discharge. It may be because most patients continued rehabilitation program at home after discharge. Vibo et al. reported disability level using the BI score of stroke patients at month 12 and found that 31% of patients were mildly to moderately disabled (BI score = 10–19), 54% were very severely disabled (BI score = 0–4), and 15% were independent (BI score = 20) [15]. Compared with our results, only 3.1% were very severely disabled, 60.7% were mildly to moderately disabled, and 25.5% could function independently. However, Vibo's data and ours could not directly be compared because the patients in Vibo's study were in acute stage while ours were in a rehabilitation phase. In contrast, our subjects were more stable and able to receive rehabilitation program in an inpatient ward. Therefore, our patients seemed to have better outcomes than Vibo's study.

There are pieces evidence concerning various predictors for the recovery of functional ability during the first year after stroke. Those significant predictors are age and baseline

TABLE 4: The association between severity of disability at discharge and month 12 ($N = 196$).

Severity of disability at discharge	Severity of disability at month 12: Very severely disabled (BI = 0–4)	Severely disabled (BI = 5–9)	Moderately disabled (BI = 10–14)	Mildly disabled (BI = 15–19)	Independent (BI = 20)	P-value
Very severely disabled (BI = 0–4)	2	4	2	0	0	
Severely disabled (BI = 5–9)	3	7	7	11	1	<0.001
Moderately disabled (BI = 10–14)	1	7	17	32	12	
Mildly disabled (BI = 15–19)	0	3	9	39	32	
Independent (BI = 20)	0	0	0	2	5	

Data are number of the patients and are compared using McNemar Chi-square test.
BI: Barthel Index.

disability [15–18]. The study of Khan et al. reported that older age was one of the independent predictors of poor functional outcome with adjusted OR of 2.1 [19]. In our study, the independent factors associated with the improvement in functional score included LOS, onset to admission interval, and depression score. In contrast to previous studies, we did not find the association between the functional score and age. This might be due to the fact that our subjects were younger than others. Moreover, our subjects had high functional score at the time of discharge and nearly half of them were classified as mildly disabled and independent groups. The relatively young patients would have faster recovery resulting in shorter LOS as shown in our data.

Most of our subjects performed continuing home programs, that is, ROM exercise, and balancing and ambulation training after discharge. Consequently, the percentage of mildly disabled to independent groups was higher (68.3%) compared to that of moderately to severely and very severely disabled ones (31.7%) at 1-year follow up. The rehabilitation outcomes depend on patients' continuing program as reported by Legg et al. [8]. The authors stated that community stroke rehabilitation could reduce the incidence of functional deterioration and maintain or improve activities of daily living (ADL). Van Peppen et al. found strong evidence that task-oriented exercise training could restore balance and gait, and strengthen the lower paretic limb, when applied intensively and early after stroke onset [20]. In addition, stroke survivors got benefit from participation in physical activity and exercise training [21]. All of these pieces of evidences may support the benefits of rehabilitation program for stroke patients. In contrast, Aziz et al. performed the Cochrane review in 2008 to investigate the effect of the long-term therapy-based rehabilitation interventions in functional ability for stroke patients. They found that there was inconclusive evidence on whether therapy-based rehabilitation intervention one year after stroke can affect the proportion of participants who had deteriorated or were dependent in personal activities of daily living. This may due to quality of trial included [22].

Concerning the complementary and alternative medicine (CAM), the most preferable CAM used on our patients was TTM followed by acupuncture. The TTM is popular among Thai people because it provides sense of comfort from muscle relaxation effect. Moreover, TTM is easy to access as this service is available all over our country. Some believe that massage can improve neurological recovery. Apart from massage, acupuncture is also one of the most popular CAMs among Thai people. Some physicians prefer to use acupuncture in addition to the conventional programs for decreasing pain and muscle spasm [23]. It is carried out for 2-3 cycles of treatment with each of 10–12 sessions. In 2007, a meta-analysis by Shiflett revealed that acupuncture was an effective adjunctive treatment for facilitating stroke recovery [24].

The limitation of this study was the only 65.4% of stroke patients could be followed up for at least one year. As nearly 40% of our subjects lived in rural areas, the shortage in patients' transportation facility might be the major obstacle to follow-up the patients at the hospitals. However, the first year mortality rate of 2.5% in our population was much lower than that in other studies whose mortality rates varied from 14 to 44% [15–17, 25]. This could be due to a possibility that younger subjects or those with TIA were recruited. There are plenty of evidence showing that the mortality rate increases with age of the patients [16, 17, 26]. Musicco et al. found that the mortality rate in stroke patients increased 2-fold for the 74-years-old patients compared with the 65-years-old parients and the rate increased to 5-fold in the group of patients older than 75-years-old compared with those younger than 65 years old [27]. Liu et al. reported that advanced age was one of the independent predictors for the first year mortality rate (hazard ratio, HR = 5.65, 95% CI = 4.54–8.23) [25]. Our subjects were of a younger age group compared to those in other studies. However, the mortality rate in our study may be underestimated due to the large number of patients (31.2%) who were lost to follow up. It is possible that some patients may have died in the year following stroke. Therefore, this should be interpreted with caution that our results only represent data of stroke patients who could be followed up. These patients might have better physical condition and higher economical status, and as a result they would have better outcomes than the lost-to-follow-up subjects.

TABLE 5: Factors associated with the change in Barthel Index (BI) scores#.

Variables		Univariate analysis		Multiple linear regression		
		Change in BI score#				
	n	Mean ± SD	*P*	*b*	SE (*b*)	*P*
Sex						
Female (1)	83	1.90 ± 3.81	0.486	—		
Male (0)	113	2.32 ± 4.32				
Age (yr)						
≥60 (1)	117	2.11 ± 4.21	0.896	—		
<60 (0)	79	2.19 ± 3.97				
Previous stroke						
Yes (1)	28	1.57 ± 5.10	0.428	—		
No (0)	168	2.24 ± 3.92				
LOS						
≥1 month (1)	74	1.05 ± 4.20	0.004	−1.292	0.587	0.029*
<1 month (0)	122	2.80 ± 3.91				
Type of stroke						
Infarction (1)	142	2.06 ± 4.18	0.633	—		
Hemorrhage (0)	54	2.37 ± 3.93				
Medical diseases						
Yes (1)	128	1.95 ± 4.06	0.357	—		
No (0)	68	2.52 ± 4.18				
OAI						
≥3 mo (1)	40	0.23 ± 3.61	0.001	−1.737	0.717	0.016*
<3 mo (0)	156	2.64 ± 4.09				
Perceptual dysfunction						
Presence (1)	118	2.02 ± 3.94	0.599	—		
Absence (0)	78	2.33 ± 4.37				
Bowel / bladder problem						
Yes (1)	63	2.35 ± 4.53	0.629	—		
No (0)	133	2.05 ± 3.90				
Complication at admission						
Yes (1)	92	1.75 ± 4.41	0.208	—		
No (0)	104	2.49 ± 3.80				
Anxiety score at month-12						
≥11 (1)	19	0.74 ± 4.37	0.067	−0.036	1.083	0.974
<11 (0)	165	2.48 ± 3.84				
Depression score at month-12						
≥11 (1)	37	0.87 ± 4.11	0.009	−1.684	0.813	0.040*
<11 (0)	146	2.72 ± 3.75				

#Change in BI: BI score at 1-year FU-BI score at DC.
LOS: length of stay, OAI: onset to admission interval means time between stroke and being transferred from acute care to a rehabilitation unit.
*Statistical significance.

6. Conclusions

Approximately half of the patients had an improvement in the disability level for at least one grade at 1-year follow-up compared to those of at discharge. The low functional score by the end of the first year is associated with longer LOS during the first admission, delay in rehabilitation program, and psychological depression.

Conflict of Interests

The authors declare that they have no conflict of interests.

Acknowledgments

Authors would like to thank the Thai Stroke Rehabilitation Registry Group for their contribution as site coordinators for data collection. This study was supported by the National Research Council of Thailand, the Clinical Research Collaboration Network, and the Royal College of Physiatrists of Thailand, on behalf of the Thai Stroke Rehabilitation Registry Group.

References

[1] F. Levi, L. Chatenoud, P. Bertuccio, F. Lucchini, E. Negri, and C. L. Vecchia, "Mortality from cardiovascular and cerebrovascular diseases in Europe and other areas of the world: an update," *European Journal of Cardiovascular Prevention and Rehabilitation*, vol. 16, no. 3, pp. 333–350, 2009.

[2] J. S. Jeng and P. K. Yip, "Epidemiology of cerebrovascular disease in the elderly in East Asia," *Geriatrics & Gerontology International*, vol. 4, pp. S198–S201, 2004.

[3] P. Lindsay, M. Bayley, A. McDonald, I. D. Graham, G. Warner, and S. Phillips, "Toward a more effective approach to stroke: Canadian best practice recommendations for stroke care," *Canadian Medical Association Journal*, vol. 178, no. 11, pp. 1418–1425, 2008.

[4] S. M. Samuelsson, M. Mähönen, D. Hassaf, J. Isaksen, and G. Berg, "Short-term functional outcome of hospitalised first-ever strokes in Finnmark, Norway in 1998-1999. Results from the Finnmark Stroke Register," *International Journal of Circumpolar Health*, vol. 60, no. 2, pp. 235–244, 2001.

[5] R. W. Teasell, N. C. Foley, K. L. Salter, and J. W. Jutai, "A blueprint for transforming stroke rehabilitation care in Canada: the case for change," *Archives of Physical Medicine and Rehabilitation*, vol. 89, no. 3, pp. 575–578, 2008.

[6] K. B. Slot, E. Berge, P. Dorman, S. Lewis, M. Dennis, and P. Sandercock, "Impact of functional status at six months on long term survival in patients with ischaemic stroke: prospective cohort studies," *British Medical Journal*, vol. 336, no. 7640, pp. 376–379, 2008.

[7] P. Chaiyawat, K. Kulkantrakorn, and P. Sritipsukho, "Effectiveness of home rehabilitation for ischemic stroke," *Neurology International*, vol. 1, no. 1, pp. 36–40, 2009.

[8] L. Legg, P. Langhorne, A. E. Drummond, J. R. Gladman, P. A. Logan, and M. F. Walker, "Rehabilitation therapy services for stroke patients living at home: systematic review of randomised trials," *Lancet*, vol. 363, no. 9406, pp. 352–356, 2004.

[9] V. Kuptniratsaikul, A. Kovindha, P. Massakulpan et al., "An epidemiologic study of the Thai Stroke Rehabilitation Registry (TSRR): a multi-center study," *Journal of the Medical Association of Thailand*, vol. 91, no. 2, pp. 225–233, 2008.

[10] V. Kuptniratsaikul, A. Kovindha, P. Dajpratham, and K. Piravej, "Main outcomes of stroke rehabilitation: a multi-centre study in Thailand," *Journal of Rehabilitation Medicine*, vol. 41, no. 1, pp. 54–58, 2009.

[11] F. I. Mahoney and D. W. Barthel, "Functional evaluation: the Barthel Index," *Maryland State Medical Journal*, vol. 14, pp. 61–65, 1965.

[12] D. T. Wade and R. L. Hewer, "Functional abilities after stroke: measurement, natural history and prognosis," *Journal of Neurology Neurosurgery and Psychiatry*, vol. 50, no. 2, pp. 177–182, 1987.

[13] T. Nilchaikovit, M. Lotrakul, and U. Phisansuthideth, "Development of Thai version of Hospital anxiety and depression scale in cancer patients," *Journal of The Psychiatric Association of Thailand*, vol. 41, pp. 18–30, 1996.

[14] D. W. Hosmer and S. Lemeshow, *Applied Logistic Regression*, John Wiley, New York, Ny, USA, 1989.

[15] R. Vibo, J. Kõrv, and M. Roose, "One-year outcome after first-ever stroke according to stroke subtype, severity, risk factors and pre-stroke treatment. A population-based study from Tartu, Estonia," *European Journal of Neurology*, vol. 14, no. 4, pp. 435–439, 2007.

[16] K. N. Vemmos, M. L. Bots, P. K. Tsibouris et al., "Prognosis of stroke in the south of Greece: 1 year mortality, functional outcome and its determinants: the Arcadia Stroke Registry," *Journal of Neurology Neurosurgery and Psychiatry*, vol. 69, no. 5, pp. 595–600, 2000.

[17] P. Appelros, I. Nydevik, and M. Viitanen, "Poor outcome after first-ever stroke: predictors for death, dependency, and recurrent stroke within the first year," *Stroke*, vol. 34, no. 1, pp. 122–126, 2003.

[18] G. J. Hankey, K. Jamrozik, R. J. Broadhurst, S. Forbes, and C. S. Anderson, "Long-term disability after first-ever stroke and related prognostic factors in the Perth Community Stroke Study, 1989-1990," *Stroke*, vol. 33, no. 4, pp. 1034–1040, 2002.

[19] M. Khan, B. Ahmed, M. Ahmed et al., "Functional, cognitive and psychological outcomes, and recurrent vascular events in Pakistani stroke survivors: a cross sectional study," *BMC Research Notes*, vol. 5, article 89, 2012.

[20] R. P. S. Van Peppen, G. Kwakkel, S. Wood-Dauphinee, H. J. M. Hendriks, P. J. Van der Wees, and J. Dekker, "The impact of physical therapy on functional outcomes after stroke: what's the evidence?" *Clinical Rehabilitation*, vol. 18, no. 8, pp. 833–862, 2004.

[21] P. D. Thompson, D. Buchner, I. L. Piña et al., "Exercise and physical activity in the prevention and treatment of atherosclerotic cardiovascular disease: a statement from the council on clinical cardiology (subcommittee on exercise, rehabilitation, and prevention) and the council on nutrition, physical activity, and metabolism (subcommittee on physical activity)," *Circulation*, vol. 107, no. 24, pp. 3109–3116, 2003.

[22] N. A. Aziz, J. Leonardi-Bee, M. Phillips, J. R. Gladman, L. Legg, and M. F. Walker, "Therapy-based rehabilitation services for patients living at home more than one year after stroke," *Cochrane Database of Systematic Reviews*, no. 2, Article ID CD005952, 2008.

[23] J.-G. Zhao, C.-H. Cao, C.-Z. Liu et al., "Effect of acupuncture treatment on spastic states of stroke patients," *Journal of the Neurological Sciences*, vol. 276, no. 1-2, pp. 143–147, 2009.

[24] S. C. Shiflett, "Does acupuncture work for stroke rehabilitation: what do recent clinical trials really show?" *Topics in Stroke Rehabilitation*, vol. 14, no. 4, pp. 40–58, 2007.

[25] X. Liu, G. Xu, W. Wu, R. Zhang, Q. Yin, and W. Zhu, "Subtypes and one-year survival of first-ever stroke in Chinese patients: the Nanjing Stroke Registry," *Cerebrovascular Diseases*, vol. 22, no. 2-3, pp. 130–136, 2006.

[26] M. V. Shah, "Rehabilitation of the older adult with stroke," *Clinics in Geriatric Medicine*, vol. 22, no. 2, pp. 469–489, 2006.

[27] M. Musicco, L. Emberti, G. Nappi, and C. Caltagirone, "Early and long-term outcome of rehabilitation in stroke patients: the role of patient characteristics, time of initiation, and duration of interventions," *Archives of Physical Medicine and Rehabilitation*, vol. 84, no. 4, pp. 551–558, 2003.

13

Assessing the Discriminative Ability and Internal Consistency of the School Outcomes Measure

Sandra H. Arnold,[1] Thubi H. A. Kolobe,[1] David M. Thompson,[2] and Lindsay Boeckman[2]

[1] *Department of Rehabilitation Sciences, College of Allied Health, University of Oklahoma Health Sciences Center, 1200 N Stonewall Avenue, P.O. Box 26901, Oklahoma City, OK 73126-0901, USA*
[2] *Department of Biostatistics and Epidemiology, University of Oklahoma Health Sciences Center, 801 N.E. 13th Street, P.O. Box 26901, Oklahoma City, OK 73126-0901, USA*

Correspondence should be addressed to Sandra H. Arnold; sandra-arnold@ouhsc.edu

Academic Editors: M. P. Galea, H. Houdijk, and H. Unalan

The School Outcomes Measure (SOM) measures the outcomes of students who receive school-based occupational and physical therapies in the USA. This study examined the SOM's discriminative ability and internal consistency. Descriptive data from a previous study of 73 students, classified by gross motor function classification (GMFCS) level of disability, was computed to determine the frequency of use of the SOM items and differences in subscale scores by students with various ages and levels of disability. There were no differences in mean subscale scores based on age; however students with less severe disabilities (GMFCS I–III) had higher mean scores in all subscales except expresses learning all students and behavior. Cronbach's alpha coefficient was used to examine the internal consistency of items of the SOM. The correlations between many of the items within the subscales were high (.87–.99). Lower alpha coefficients were noted when the SOM was applied to students in GMFCS Levels II and III on two subscales when compared to GMFCS Levels I, IV, and V. On the basis of this evaluation, we revised the SOM to prepare it for a national field testing to measure its construct validity.

1. Introduction

Both individual and program outcomes measurement are important for determining effectiveness of student interventions and to provide occupational therapists and physical therapists, who work in the school setting, with information to make decisions about treatment approaches and program planning.Individual tools measure outcomes of individual students over time [1]. Program outcome measures compare outcomes over time in groups of students at local, state, or national levels. Used in multivariable models, program outcome measures can also identify variables with which various outcomes are associated, such as service delivery models, types of intervention, child characteristics (e.g., age, sex, and diagnosis), and service intensity [2]. Although school-based occupational therapists and physical therapists in the USA are expected to measure the effectiveness of their interventions with the students they serve [3–5], no tool currently exists that measures either individual or program outcomes of students with disabilities who receive school-based occupational therapy or physical therapy services. Nor does a minimal data set exist for school-based therapists to identify variables of service delivery, type and intensity of intervention, and student and therapist characteristics that may be associated with student outcomes.

The School Outcomes Measure (SOM) is a program outcome measure of occupational therapy and physical therapy services provided to students with disabilities in school settings [6]. The SOM, a minimal data set, gathers information about a large number of students on an ongoing basis, using the fewest number of items. The tool takes about 10 minutes to administer when a therapist is familiar with the student and requires no manipulatives or supplies other than the test form. The SOM includes 30 functional ability items that cover seven areas (subscales) of a student's ability to fulfill roles and complete tasks in school: self-care; mobility; assuming a student's role (for preschool/elementary school students and secondary students); expressing learning (for all students and those unable to use speech as primary means of communication); and behavior. These seven areas are addressed by school-based therapists and are based on the conceptual model described by Bundy [7] and her colleagues. McEwen et al. [6] further describe the constructs underlying these subscales.

Occupational therapists and physical therapists rate, through direct or by report, each of the 30 functional ability items on a 6-point scale according to the amount of assistance (from 1 = total assistance to 6 = independent) a student requires for each activity. The SOM also collects data on student and therapist demographics, pertinent information on the student's Individual Education Program (IEP) (e.g., disability category, educational placement, and frequency of therapy), therapy activities used (e.g., activities of daily living, assistive technology, and therapeutic interventions), and services provided, which are variables likely to be associated with student outcomes.

Research supports content validity and interrater reliability of the SOM [6]. Arnold and McEwen [8] further established item test-retest reliability of the SOM and indicated that the tool was responsive to change in students with mild/moderate functional limitations but less sensitive to change in students with severe disabilities.

However, research has not investigated if the SOM can discriminate students' performance in school based on the student's age or level of disability. Additionally, studies using the SOM have thus far used its total raw score without validating its subscales. Because the seven subscales assess diverse and sometimes unrelated tasks and activities, the use of a total raw score is questionable.

This study represents an important step in validating the SOM by assessing its discriminative ability and examining the internal consistency of its subscales. According to Portney and Watkins [9], items within each subscale should be internally consistent; that is, they should reflect "the extent to which items measure various aspects of the same characteristic and nothing else" (page 71). Evidence of internal consistency would allow the use and interpretation of the subscales scores and enhance therapists' confidence that the items within each subscale of the SOM measure the aspects of the same function (subscale).

The purpose of this study was to assess whether the mean scores on the SOM subscales differed based on student age or severity of disability and to determine the internal consistency of the functional ability items in each subscale of the SOM. In addition, we identified the frequency of use of the items and scoring criteria by students within various age groups and levels of disabilities to further refine the tool. The findings will be used in a national field test of the measure's construct validity.

2. Methods

2.1. Participants. Participants, all from the USA, were 73 students with disabilities (student participants) and 32 school-based occupational therapists and physical therapists (therapist participants) who completed the SOM for the students, from a previous study [8]. The University of Oklahoma Health Sciences Center Institutional Review Board (IRB) approved the study. The sample of students included 49 boys and 24 girls between the ages of 3 and 20 years. Tables 1, 2, and 3 present student characteristics, primary diagnosis, and primary individuals with disabilities education act (IDEA) disability categories, respectively.

The therapists, 14 occupational therapists and 18 physical therapists, provided services through IEPs for school-aged children who received special education and related services in eight local school districts. They reported their experience in providing school-based services as follows: (a) 1-2 years of experience $n = 2$ (6.3%), (b) >2–5 years of experience $n = 5$ (15.6%), and (c) 5+ years of experience $n = 25$ (78.1%). The length of time they have worked with the student participants ranged from less than 1 year $n = 16$ (21.9%) to more than 8 years $n = 1$ (1.4%), with the majority reporting 1–3 years $n = 38$ (52.1%).

2.2. Procedures. Following a 2-hour training, provided by the first author, in classifying student disability using the Gross Motor Function Classification System (GMFCS) [10], therapist participants classified the students on their caseloads into two groups: students with mild-to-moderate functional limitations (GMFCS Levels I, II, or III) and students with severe functional limitations (GMFCS Levels IV or V). Mild/moderate and severe functional limitations were classified to initially collect response to change data [8]. Although the GMFCS criteria for classification are validated only for children with cerebral palsy, it was employed in this study because no other system exists that classifies children's gross motor function. Therapists were asked to choose, using a table of random numbers, one student from their caseload with moderate functional limitations and one student with severe functional limitations. However, one of the therapists chose only one student from the overall caseload, and three therapists selected four students for a total of 39 students with mild-to-moderate functional limitations (disability) and 34 students with severe functional limitations (disability) ($N = 73$). Therapists completed the SOM three times during one school year for each of the randomly selected student participants. This study reports item-specific response frequencies and calculates internal consistency using responses from the first administration of the SOM.

2.3. Data Analysis. We used SAS v9.2 [11] to analyze the data. We tabulated the frequency of the student and therapist demographics, pertinent student IEP information, therapy activities used, and services provided, and the mean and SD for each item's SOM scores for groups defined by age (3–5 years, 6–11 years, 12–15 years, and >16 years), and level of disability (I, II, III, IV, and V). We used the ANOVA and t-tests to determine whether the mean scores on each subscale differed based on age and severity of disability, respectively.

The Cronbach's alpha statistic was calculated to determine the internal consistency of the items within each of the SOM's seven subscales. Cronbach's alpha, the most commonly used statistical measure of internal consistency, expresses the

TABLE 1: Student participant characteristics ($N = 73$) (number (%)).

	Total ($N = 73$)	Mild/moderate disability ($n = 39$)	Severe disability ($n = 34$)
Sex			
Male	49 (67.1)	28 (71.7)	21 (61.7)
Female	24 (32.8)	11 (28.2)	13 (38.2)
Age			
3–5 years	29 (39.7)	19 (48.7)	10 (29.4)
6–11 years	30 (41.1)	18 (46.1)	12 (35.2)
12–18 years	10 (13.7)	2 (05.1)	8 (23.5)
19-20 years	4 (05.4)	0 (0.0)	4 (11.7)
Ethnicity			
White	54 (73.9)	29 (74.3)	25 (73.5)
African American	15 (20.5)	8 (20.5)	7 (20.5)
Asian	1 (01.3)	1 (02.5)	0 (0.0)
Hispanic	1 (01.3)	0 (0.0)	1 (02.9)
Native American	1 (01.3)	0 (0.0)	1 (02.9)
Pacific Islander	0 (0.0)	0 (0.0)	0 (0.0)
Other: East Indian	1 (01.3)	1 (02.5)	0 (0.0)
Gross motor function classification level (GMFCS)			
Level I	27 (36.9)	27 (69.2)	0 (0.0)
Level II	9 (12.3)	9 (23.0)	0 (0.0)
Level III	3 (04.1)	3 (07.6)	0 (0.0)
Level IV	19 (26.0)	0 (0.0)	19 (55.8)
Level V	15 (20.5)	0 (0.0)	15 (44.1)

average correlation among a set of ordinally scaled items [9]. Alpha values range from 0.00 to 1.00, with values approaching 0.90 are considered to represent high consistency [9]. We also compared values for standard Cronbach's alpha, on items within each subscale between groups defined by students' age and level of disability. Raw Cronbach's alphas were calculated when the standard deviation of any variable was 0, and there were at least four responses. We did not compute Cronbach's alpha for observations of 3 or fewer.

3. Results and Discussion

3.1. Results: Discriminative Analysis. As expected there were very little differences between the mean scores based on age (see Table 4). For all subscales, age did not have a statistically significant effect ($P > .05$). However, in all disability levels, students in disability Level I, II, and III had higher mean scores compared to students in Levels IV and V in all subscale areas except expressing learning all students ($t = -1.016$; $P = 0.3$) and behavior ($t = 1.41$; $P = 0.2$) (see Table 5). Because there were just three students classified at Level III, we further analyzed the differences between Level I and II with Levels III, IV, and V (see Table 5). Similarly, Level I and II had higher mean scores compared to students in Level III, IV, and V in all subscales except Expressing Learning All Students ($t = -0.56$; $P = 0.6$) and Behavior ($t = 1.21$; $P = 0.2$).

3.2. Results: Internal Consistency. Table 6 presents Cronbach's alpha results for all students' ratings on the SOM and shows that the values for each subscale ranged from .87 to .99. The subscales demonstrated the same high internal consistency across age and level of disabilities with a few exceptions. Tables 7 and 8 present the values for age and level of disability, respectively. The alpha values for students aged 3–5 years ranged .65–.98; .89–.99 for ages 6–11; .91–.99 for ages 12–15; and .94–1.00 for ages 15 and above. The alpha values for students across the GMFCS levels were mixed. Values for students in Level 1 were consistently high (.91–.99) but ranged from −.28 to 1.00 for the scores of students in Levels II to V. The negative correlations, although not statistically significant, were between handwriting and computer and between copying and computer ($R = -0.48$ ($P = 0.3$) and $R = -0.047$ ($P = 0.9$) resp.). As student's score increased in computer, the score decreased in handwriting or copying. The alpha values for the self-care and mobility subscales were relatively lower for those in disability Level III (.56 and .67 resp.,) and the Expresses Learning All Students and Behavior subscales were low for Level II (−.28 and .41 resp.,). Because not all therapist participants answered each item in each subscale and because several therapist participants scored the same rating on at least one of the items, both the raw and standard Cronbach's alphas were analyzed (see Table 8).

TABLE 2: Primary diagnosis of student participants (N = 73) (number (%)).

	Total (N = 73)	Mild/moderate disability (n = 39)	Severe disability (n = 34)
Cerebral palsy	22 (30.1)	4 (10.2)	18 (52.9)
Developmental delay	8 (10.9)	6 (15.3)	2 (05.8)
Autism spectrum disorder	6 (08.2)	6 (15.3)	0 (0.0)
Down syndrome	5 (06.8)	4 (10.2)	1 (02.9)
Traumatic brain injury	3 (04.1)	3 (07.7)	0 (0.0)
Brain tumor	2 (02.7)	1 (02.5)	1 (02.9)
Hydrocephalus	2 (02.7)	0 (0.0)	2 (05.8)
Anoxia	1 (01.3)	1 (02.5)	0 (0.0)
ADHD	1 (01.3)	1 (02.5)	0 (0.0)
CVA	1 (01.3)	1 (02.5)	0 (0.0)
DiGeorge syndrome	1 (01.3)	1 (02.5)	0 (0.0)
Failure to thrive	1 (01.3)	0 (0.0)	1 (02.9)
Fetal alcohol syndrome	1 (01.3)	1 (02.5)	0 (0.0)
Lawrence-Moon	1 (01.3)	1 (02.5)	0 (0.0)
Learning disability	1 (01.3)	1 (02.5)	0 (0.0)
Muscular dystrophy	1 (01.3)	0 (0.0)	1 (02.9)
Mental retardation/cerebral palsy	1 (01.3)	0 (0.0)	1 (02.9)
Shaken baby syndrome	1 (01.3)	0 (0.0)	1 (02.9)
Rhett syndrome	1 (01.3)	0 (0.0)	1 (02.9)
Spina bifida	1 (01.3)	0 (0.0)	1 (02.9)
Sturge-Weber syndrome	1 (01.3)	1 (02.5)	0 (0.0)
Not identified	11 (15.0)	7 (17.9)	4 (11.7)

TABLE 3: Student participant primary IDEA disability category for eligibility for special education and related services (N = 73) (number (%)).

	Total (N = 73)	Mild/moderate disability (n = 39)	Severe disability (n = 34)
Multiple disabilities	26 (35.6)	5 (12.0)	21 (61.7)
Developmental delay	23 (31.1)	12 (30.6)	11 (32.5)
Traumatic brain injury	5 (06.5)	4 (10.6)	1 (02.4)
Specific learning disability	4 (05.8)	4 (10.6)	0 (0.0)
Speech or language impairment	4 (05.8)	4 (10.6)	0 (0.0)
Autism	3 (04.1)	3 (07.0)	0 (0.0)
Mental retardation	3 (04.1)	3 (07.0)	0 (0.0)
Other health impairment	3 (04.1)	3 (07.0)	0 (0.0)
Orthopedic impairment	2 (02.4)	1 (02.6)	1 (02.4)
Deafness	0 (0.0)	0 (0.0)	0 (0.0)
Deaf-blindness	0 (0.0)	0 (0.0)	0 (0.0)
Emotional disturbance	0 (0.0)	0 (0.0)	0 (0.0)
Hearing impaired	0 (0.0)	0 (0.0)	0 (0.0)
Visually impaired (blindness)	0 (0.0)	0 (0.0)	0 (0.0)

3.3. Results: Frequency of Responses. The frequency data showed that all the levels of the scaling criteria for the SOM ability items were used. The exceptions were responses related to types of activities and techniques used. *Therapy Activities Used* included a rating scale of "never," "rarely," "sometimes," "frequently," and "always" for each activity item. Analysis of these frequency counts showed that for some items, "frequently" and "always" were not selected (e.g., craniosacral therapy). Items that frequently scored "never" or "rarely" included casting/splinting, wheelchair training,

TABLE 4: Differences in subscale sum scores by age.

Source (age group)	DF	Type III SS	Mean square	F value	Pr > F
Self-care	3	356.8042219	118.9347406	2.72	0.0510
Mobility	3	1608.065248	536.021749	2.41	0.0773
Assuming students role—preschool/elementary	1	57.30158730	57.30158730	0.18	0.6799
Assuming student's role—secondary	1	120.3333333	120.3333333	0.27	0.6547
Expressing learning—unable to use speech	3	72.67478632	24.22492877	1.55	0.2198
Expresses learning—all students	3	137.3929737	45.7976579	2.58	0.0727
Behavior	3	245.9142424	81.9714141	2.46	0.0708

TABLE 5: Differences in sum scores by GMFCS Levels I–III versus IV-V and I-II versus III–V.

Subscale	Estimate	Standard error	t value	Pr > $\|t\|$
GMFCS Levels I–III versus IV-V				
Self-care	9.9473684	1.1218986	8.87	<.0001
Mobility	27.447500	1.9138478	14.34	<.0001
Assuming a student's role—preschool/elementary	25.428571	6.2482650	4.07	0.0016
Assuming a student's role—secondary	*	*	*	*
Expresses learning—unable to use speech	4.8333333	1.1893368	4.06	0.0003
Expresses learning—all students	−1.7777777	1.7642292	−1.01	0.3214
Behavior	2.0661696	1.4673178	1.41	0.1639
GMFCS Levels I-II versus III–V				
Self-care	9.6166666	1.1574110	8.31	<.0001
Mobility	26.757389	2.0214822	13.24	<.0001
Assuming a student's role—preschool/elementary	25.428571	6.2482650	4.07	0.0016
Assuming a student's role—secondary	*	*	*	*
Expresses learning—unable to use speech	5.4076923	1.2115481	4.46	<.0001
Expresses learning—all students	−1.0260869	1.7276662	−0.59	0.5569
Behavior	1.7757352	1.4628238	1.21	0.2292

*N/A as no secondary students in Levels I–III.

TABLE 6: Cronbach's alphas for all items in subscales.

Subscale	Cronbach's alpha
Self-care	0.9546
Mobility	0.9721
Assuming a student's role—preschool/elementary school	0.9897
Assuming a student's role—secondary school	0.9994
Expressing learning—students unable to use speech	0.9289
Expressing learning—all students	0.8769
Behavior	0.9380

craniosacral therapy, deep pressure brushing, and myofascial release. Eighty-six percent of students of age 12 years and older, were classified as having a severe disability (Level IV and V) and thus completed few subscale items related to preschool/elementary. Alternately, those classified with mild/moderate disabilities (Levels I, II, and III) completed few items in the subscale for secondary school students.

3.4. Discussion. The purpose of this study was to further refine the SOM by assessing whether the mean scores on the SOM subscales differed based on student age or severity of disability, and by determining the internal consistency of the functional ability items in each subscale of the SOM. In addition, we identified the frequency of use of the items and scoring criteria by students within various age groups and levels of disabilities.

As a minimum data set, the SOM was expected to discriminate amongst student's performance in the school setting based on level of disability. Our findings reveal differences in the mean SOM scores of the self-care, mobility, and assuming a student's role subscales, among students in Level I or II compared to Levels IV and V but not between Level I and II or Level IV and V. Although Level III was initially classified with Levels 1 & II, as Mild/Moderate, because there were only three students in this classification we reanalyzed the Level III data with Level IV and V data. These findings show that the SOM can discriminate among three rather than five levels of the GMFCS. One explanation may be related to the relatively few number of items in the SOM. In addition, the items of the SOM do not include the GMFCS level distinctions of need for hand-held mobility devices, wheeled mobility, or quality of movement [12]. For

TABLE 7: Standardized Cronbach's alphas for age.

Subscale	Mean Cronbach's alpha by age group			
	3–5 years old	6–11 years old	12–15 years old	Greater than 16 years old
Self-care	0.9153	0.9700	0.9154	0.9459
Mobility	0.9585	0.9780	0.9533	0.9731
Assuming a student's role—preschool/elementary school students	0.9810	0.9942	·	·
Assuming a student's role—secondary school students	·	·	·	0.9994
Expressing learning—students unable to use speech	0.8018	0.9556	·	·
Expressing learning—all students	0.6545	0.8932	·	1.0000
Behavior	0.8985	0.9513	0.9950	0.9439

(·) signifies 3 or fewer observations; therefore, Cronbach's alpha is not computed.

TABLE 8: Standardized and (raw) Cronbach's alphas for level of disability.

Subscale	Mean Cronbach's alpha by level of disability				
	I	II	III	IV	V
Self-care	0.9173	0.8531	0.5612	0.9190	0.8813
Mobility	0.9188	0.8093	0.6783	0.8482	(0.6070)
Assuming a student's role—preschool/elementary school students	0.9925	·	·	·	·
Assuming a student's role—secondary school students	·	·	·	1.0000	·
Expressing learning—students unable to use speech	0.9515	1.0000	·	(0.0259)	(0.6116)
Expressing learning—all students	0.9063	−0.2871	·	0.8455	·
Behavior	0.9322	0.4155	0.9883	0.9547	0.7889

(·) signifies 3 or fewer observations; therefore, Cronbach's alpha is not computed.

example, distinctions between children in Levels IV and V include children having limitations in head and trunk control, requiring extensive assistive technology, and learning how to operate a powered wheelchair [12]. These specific attributes are not included within the SOM's minimal data set items. Similarly, distinctions between Levels I and II include difficulty with balance and devices/support needed for travel [12]. The SOM items do not measure quality of movement or need for devices. Thus, sensitivity or responsiveness to change may be limited if the goal of the SOM was to differentiate between the five levels of GMFCS.

On the other hand, we did not observe differences in the three subscales based on age. These findings were not unexpected given that the items in the SOM target functional rather than developmental skills. The findings support the SOM as a contextual or setting a specific tool rather than a developmental assessment scale. Similarly, the Express Learning All Students and Behavior subscales did not discriminate among students based on age or severity of disability. However, further analysis of frequency data showed that the percentages of students who exhibited independence in behavior and learning were similar in all levels except those in Level V. This group needed more support in these two areas. This suggests that the level of disability does not distinguish student's learning and behavior or the inability of the SOM to discriminate.

Outcome measures require psychometric testing to be considered reliable and valid for the population they discern. In particular, internal consistency examines if items in a tool reflect the characteristics or subscales being measured. This research further examined the extent to which the items in each of the SOM's seven subscales were related. The results indicated that the items within the subscales of the SOM were homogeneous; that is, the items within each subscale correlated with each other, and the subscales correlated with the total scale.

Disagreement exists in the literature regarding the importance of Cronbach's alpha on establishing unidimensionality of a scale. In particular is the notion of redundancy among items leading to higher values of alpha and thus not truly guaranteeing internal consistency [13, 14]. Opponents of Cronbach's alpha as a measure of consistency base their argument on the literature from scales that measure social behavior in which evaluated behaviors could overlap. This important consideration may not apply to the SOM. First, because it is a minimal data set, efforts have been made to include a limited number of items in the SOM to capture a wide variety of areas or tasks. Second, the items are context based and assess the student's role and ability to function in the school setting and as such involves all the domains of development. As a result, a student may do well in some but not other domains regardless of age or level of disability. An example is the Behavior and mobility subscales in which the mean scores for the students in all five levels of the GMFCS were similar for the former but not for the latter.

Nunnally [15] and Nunnally and Berstein [16] consider an alpha coefficient of .70 to represent "high consistency" in the early stages of tool development. The high alpha values observed in this study suggest that the SOM's subscales have strong internal consistency. Although the coefficients were high, the results also suggest that some of the subscales may be more or less consistent depending on the severity of a student's disability or the assumed role expected of a student in the classroom. It should be pointed out that although Table 6 gives seven subscales, not every subscale would be appropriate for rating all students due to age and level of functioning; only five subscales would be appropriate for any given student.

Low alpha values were observed in the self-care and mobility subscales for students in the Level III category. This finding was unexpected. Previous findings from the literature on performance of children in Level III suggest that children in this category are not any more heterogeneous than the other groups. This group was underrepresented in the sample (3 students); therefore, the differences observed in our findings were more pronounced than might have been observed in a larger sample. The items in the self-care subscale such as eating, hygiene, and grooming or in the mobility subscale such as bus transfers, doors, and classroom mobility, as well as items in assuming students roles, such as obtaining classroom materials or getting teacher's attention, should not function differently for students who are in level I, II, or III [17]. The literature also suggests that where alphas are calculated for a very small number of observations (fewer than five), the alphas may not represent the subscale's performance in the larger population. Therefore, until additional studies are conducted that include a larger sample of students in Level III, these findings should be interpreted with caution.

Despite the high internal consistency of the subscales observed in the study, the inconsistency of the number of items for each subscale and the high number of subscales is a concern. For example, the mobility subscale contains eight items, and expresses learning for students unable to use speech contains only one item. An initial concern is that few items within a subscale threaten the sensitivity of scale [18]. That is, the SOM, may not be able to identify the number of students who can express learning without speech who actually can express learning, thus threatening the SOM's ability to identify positive results.

An analysis of frequency data revealed that despite the diversity of the students in terms of age and level of disability, some items were not frequently used. *Therapy activity* items such as casting/splinting, craniosacral therapy, and deep pressure brushing and subscale items such as opening and closing of lockers, going off campus for lunch, and assessing vending machines may be infrequently used in the school setting, and therefore they are not necessary items in a minimal data set. Items with frequencies of lower than 50% were eliminated from the SOM minimal data set.

In addition to removing items rarely used from the minimal data set, we expanded certain items in the functional ability subscales to distinguish specific tasks within an item. For example, in the original self-care subscale, item "eating" was expanded into two items: "eating 1" related to eating and drinking 75% of meal or snack without spilling and "eating 2" related to using a spoon and/or fork during a snack or meal. And we added two additional items in student demographics and therapy activities, respectively: state where student resides, to collect national data, and positive behavior support, as was an "other" item frequently listed.

Finally, we changed the *therapy activities used* rating from a Likert scale to a numerical scale that accumulates percentage scores that add up to 100%. That is, each item receives a score between 0 and 100% so that the total of all items equals 100%. This change allows every item or choice to receive a value or response, including zero. All of the revisions resulted in a reduced scale that included 25 therapist, student, therapy items, and 42 student functional ability items.

The changes made to the SOM further enhance its ability to become a quick and an easy to use minimal data set for occupational therapists and physical therapists in the school setting. In addition, the continued psychometric testing establishes the SOM as a reliable and valid tool. These steps are important in developing a user friendly, valid outcome measure for practicing therapists to collect outcomes on the students they serve.

3.5. Suggestions for Further Research. Additional psychometric research is recommended to evaluate the use of the SOM as a minimal data set for measuring outcomes of students who receive occupational therapy and physical therapy services in school settings. The benefit of having a scale with good internal consistency lies in the interpretation of the score. Based on the present findings, occupational therapists and physical therapists interpret an increase in the subscale scores as an improvement in the construct measured by the subscale. However, internal consistency does not provide information about whether or not there is overlap between items in the subscales. The current seven SOM subscales were theoretically derived and determined a priori. To evaluate the validity of the subscales, it requires more advanced statistics such as factor analysis or principal component analysis [9, 19]. Additionally, Rasch model analysis can be used to create a continuous scale that will place individual SOM items along a continuum from most difficult to least difficult [20]. The importance of developing an interval scale will allow therapists to clearly report change and the magnitude of such change, when change in student's abilities actually change. Then, subsequent studies can be performed to determine the minimally clinical important difference. These analyses will require a larger sample size than that which was available in the present study.

4. Conclusion

The SOM is intended to address the need for a program measure or outcomes management system to measure the outcomes of students receiving occupational therapy and physical therapy in school settings and meet the IDEA mandate for accountability for outcomes of students with disabilities across the USA. Reliability and validity estimates are necessary to establish the SOM as a valid outcomes measure.

To assess whether the mean scores on the SOM subscales differed based on student age or severity of disability, the results of the study demonstrated that there was no difference in mean subscale scores based on student age; however, students with less severe disabilities had higher mean scores in all subscales except expresses learning all students and behavior. In determining the internal consistency of the functional ability items in each subscale of the SOM, the study results supported internal consistency of the SOM's seven subscales, with the exception of low Cronbach's alpha for students in Levels II and III. In methodological research, correlation among all items should be determined prior to evaluation item analysis [19]. In addition, we identified frequency of use of the items and scoring criteria by students within various age groups and levels of disabilities to further refine the tool.

Therefore, the next steps in the development of the SOM are the validation studies that focus on sensitivity of each item, responsiveness of the various subscales, item difficulty [20], and the use of various scores as units of analysis. Such a process would require a large number of subjects and/or a national validation study.

Because, to date, no outcome measure exists that collects data on school-aged children, occupational therapists and physical therapists do not have a valid tool to measure change in the students they serve. A valid and reliable tool, such as the SOM, that can be used by all school-based occupational therapists and physical therapists with students of all ages and severity of disabilities will enable service providers to confidently measure the change in student ability. In addition, as a program outcome measure, the data collected from many therapists will provide national data to begin to evaluate student outcomes over time and identify variables such as type of intervention or intensity of service delivery that are associated with either positive or negative student outcomes.

Conflict of Interests

The authors declares that there is no conflict of interests.

Acknowledgment

This research was supported by funding from a grant from the Presbyterian Health Foundation.

References

[1] E. A. Dobrzykowski, *Essential Readings in Rehabilitation Outcomes Measurement: Application, Methodology, and Technology*, Aspen, Gaithersburg, Md, USA, 1998.

[2] W. T. F. Goossen, P. J. M. M. Epping, T. Feuth, T. W. N. Dassen, A. Hasman, and W. J. A. Van Den Heuvel, "A comparison of nursing minimal data sets," *Journal of the American Medical Informatics Association*, vol. 5, no. 2, pp. 152–163, 1998.

[3] American Occupational Therapy Association, "Occupational therapy practice framework: domain and process," *American Journal of Occupational Therapy*, vol. 56, pp. 609–639, 2002.

[4] American Physical Therapy Association, *Guide to Physical Therapist Practice*, American Physical Therapy Association, Alexandria, VA, USA, 2nd edition, 2001.

[5] "Individuals with Disabilities Education Improvement Act of 2004, 20 U.S.C. § 1400".

[6] I. R. McEwen, S. H. Arnold, L. H. Hansen, and D. Johnson, "Interrater reliability and content validity of a minimal data set to measure outcomes of students receiving school-based occupational therapy and physical therapy," *Physical and Occupational Therapy in Pediatrics*, vol. 23, no. 2, pp. 77–95, 2003.

[7] A. C. Bundy, Ed., *Making a Difference: OTs and PTs in Public Schools: A Conceptual Model of Practice for School System Therapists*, University of Illinois at Chicago, Chicago, Ill, USA, 1991.

[8] S. H. Arnold and I. R. McEwen, "Item test-retest reliability and responsiveness of the School Outcomes Measure (SOM)," *Physical and Occupational Therapy in Pediatrics*, vol. 28, no. 1, pp. 59–77, 2008.

[9] L. G. Portney and M. P. Watkins, *Foundations of Clinical Research: Application to Practice*, Prentice-Hall, Upper Saddle River, NJ, USA, 3rd edition, 2009.

[10] R. Palisano, P. Rosenbaum, S. Walter, D. Russell, E. Wood, and B. Galuppi, "Development and reliability of a system to classify gross motor function in children with cerebral palsy," *Developmental Medicine and Child Neurology*, vol. 39, no. 4, pp. 214–223, 1997.

[11] S. A. S. Institute Inc, "SAS/STAT user's guide Version 8," 1999, http://books.google.com/books?id=y7gDP_ELM3gC&pg=PA1306&lpg=PA1306&dq=SAS/STAT+user%E2%80%99s+guide,+tests+and+measures+of+agreement&source=bl&ots=GI5wusNAHB&sig=LG1jnLMwdFis2IRdZ5rAW7zDh98&hl=en&ei=2z13SoLfDo2QMcSbjbEM&sa=X&oi=book_result&ct=result&resnum=1#v=onepage&q=&f=false.

[12] R. Palisano, P. Rosenbaum, D. Bartlett, and M. Livingston, *Gross Motor Function Classification System Expanded and Revised (GMFCS -E & R)*, CanChild Center for Childhood Disability Research, McMaster University, 2007.

[13] G. J. Boyle, "Does item homogeneity indicate internal consistency or item redundancy in psychometric scales?" *Personality and Individual Differences*, vol. 12, no. 3, pp. 291–294, 1991.

[14] D. L. Streiner, "Starting at the beginning: an introduction to coefficient alpha and internal consistency," *Journal of Personality Assessment*, vol. 80, no. 1, pp. 99–103, 2003.

[15] J. C. Nunnally, *Psychometric Theory*, McGraw-Hill, New York, NY, USA, 2nd edition, 1978.

[16] J. C. Nunnally and I. H. Berstein, *Psychometric Theory*, McGraw-Hill, New York, NY, USA, 3rd edition, 1994.

[17] D. Oeffinger, G. Gorton, A. Bagley et al., "Outcome assessments in children with cerebral palsy, Part I: descriptive characteristics of GMFCS Levels I to III," *Developmental Medicine and Child Neurology*, vol. 49, no. 3, pp. 172–180, 2007.

[18] D. L. Streiner and G. R. Norman, *Health Measurement Scales: A Practical Guide to their Development and Use*, Oxford University Press, New York, NY, USA, 2nd edition, 2000.

[19] M. A. Pett, N. R. Lackey, and J. J. Sullivan, *Making Sense of Factor Analysis: The Use of Factor Analysis for Instrument Development in Health Care Research*, Sage, Thousand Oaks, Calif, USA, 2003.

[20] T. G. Bond and C. M. Fox, *Applying the Rasch Model: Fundamental Measurement in the Human Sciences*, Lawrence Erlbaum Associates, Mahwah, NJ, USA, 2001.

14

Psychometric Evaluation of the Perceived Stress Scale in Multiple Sclerosis

Salene M. Wu[1] **and Dagmar Amtmann**[2]

[1] *Group Health Research Institute, 1730 Minor Avenue, Seattle, WA 98101, USA*
[2] *Department of Rehabilitation Medicine, University of Washington, P.O. Box 354237, Seattle, WA 98195-4237, USA*

Correspondence should be addressed to Salene M. Wu; wu.582@osu.edu

Academic Editors: B. Murphy and C. Zwingmann

Multiple sclerosis (MS) is a progressive disease characterized by neurological symptoms and sometimes heightened levels of distress. The Perceived Stress Scale (PSS) is often used in MS samples to measure stress but has not been validated in this population. Participants (n = 446) completed the PSS as well as measure of depression, anxiety, and mental and physical health. Factor analyses indicated that the general factor of a bifactor model accounted for a large amount of the variance in the 14-item and 10-item versions of the PSS. The 4-item PSS had two factors, the Stress subscale and the Coping subscale, but a one-factor model also fits the data well. Total scores and both subscales had sufficient reliability and validity for all versions of the PSS, although a few items of the 14-item PSS had low item-total correlations. This study supports the use of the total score of the PSS in MS but also suggests that the 10-item PSS had better psychometric properties than the 14-item PSS.

1. Introduction

Multiple sclerosis (MS) is a neurological disease characterized by numbness, weakness, fatigue, vision problems, and spasticity and is often progressive [1]. People with MS often experience depression and anxiety, with as many as 50% of people with MS experiencing depression in their lifetime [2]. A common trigger of depression is stress [3], which can be defined objectively as stressful life events such as divorce or subjectively as perceptions of stress including perceptions that events are uncontrollable and unpredictable. One of the most common measures of subjective experiences of stress is the Perceived Stress Scale [4]. However, despite its use to measure perceived stress in MS [5, 6], this scale has not been psychometrically validated in this population.

The Perceived Stress Scale (PSS) measures the level to which a respondent considers his or her life stressful and was designed to assess how unpredictable and controllable a person appraises his or her life [4]. The original version had 14 items, seven negatively stated and seven positively stated. Two short forms are available, one with 10 items (six negatively stated and four positively stated items) and the other with four items (two negatively stated and two positively stated) [7]. The PSS is related to health behaviors such as smoking [8] as well as depression and anxiety [9]. Other measures of stress also are related to the PSS, supporting validity [10]. The 14-item and 10-item versions showed adequate internal consistency although the 4-item version had marginal reliability, such as a Cronbach's alpha of .67 [8, 10]. Cohen et al. specifically posited that perceived stress will be sensitive to daily hassles and other frequent changes, so test-retest reliability is not expected to be high [4]. The 14-item version showed test-retest reliability of .85 after two days but .55 after six weeks [4] and a .73 test-retest reliability after two weeks [9], consistent with this prediction. The 10-item PSS had a test-retest reliability of .86 using a 7-day interval [11], .77 using a two-week interval [9], and .53 to .61 using a 12-month interval [12].

In Cohen's original validation study, factor analyses of the 14-item and 10-item forms showed that two-factor model was the best model for the data while a one-factor model was a better fit for the 4-item version [7]. Cohen advised that for purposes of measuring stress, the distinction between the two factors was irrelevant. However, subsequent studies have consistently shown a two-factor structure for all three versions of the PSS [8, 10]. This two factor structure has been shown for the 10-item PSS in cancer patients [12], Turkish university students [13], and university teachers in Brazil [11]. One way of reconciling the use of the total PSS score and the two factor structure was the suggestion of a second order factor that influences the two factors [11, 12]. The first factor contains negatively stated items (unable to control important things and so forth) and has been termed "Stress" [12], "Negative stress" [11], and "Perceived Helplessness" [13]. The second factor contains positively stated items (things were going your way and so forth) and has been termed "Counter-stress" [12], "Positive stress" [11], and "Perceived Self-efficacy" [13]. Examination of the item content shows the first factor measures perceptions of uncontrollability, unpredictability, and inability to cope. The second factor items measure perceived success in coping. For the purposes of this study, the first factor will be referred to as "Stress" and the second factor as "Coping."

One way to examine the contribution of the general factor and the two subdomains to the summary score is the bifactor model. The bifactor model consists of a general factor and all items load on this factor [14]. Additional "group" factors are included and only certain items load on each group factor. See Figure 1. The bifactor model can be used to determine whether a measure is sufficiently unidimensional to support using a total score while still accounting for the inevitable multidimensionality of psychological measures [15]. The bifactor model also directly addresses and tests unidimensionality, unlike the second order model that has previously been used with the PSS. As no study has used the bifactor model to quantify the contribution of the potential factors to the PSS overall score, we examined the bifactor model for the PSS. In addition to the general factor, the bifactor model included group factors for the Stress and Coping factors shown in previous studies.

The current study examined the psychometric properties of the PSS in a sample of people with multiple sclerosis (MS) as this scale has not been validated in this rehabilitation population. Unidimensionality is an assumption of any scale that uses a total score, like the PSS, and we investigated whether the total score was supported and examined the contribution of the two factors previously described. To do so, we used a confirmatory factor analytic approach to investigate different factor structures for the three forms of the PSS. For all PSS versions, we compared one factor and two factor models. We also fit bifactor models and examined the amount of variance accounted for by the general and group factors for the 14-item and 10-item PSS. A bifactor model could not be fitted to the 4-item version due to the limited degrees of freedom. In addition to assessing reliability and floor and ceiling effects, we assessed validity by correlating the total PSS and two subscales with measures of depression, anxiety, and health. As stress is substantially related to depression and anxiety, we hypothesized that the PSS total score and both subscale scores would be more strongly associated with the mental health measures than with the physical health measures.

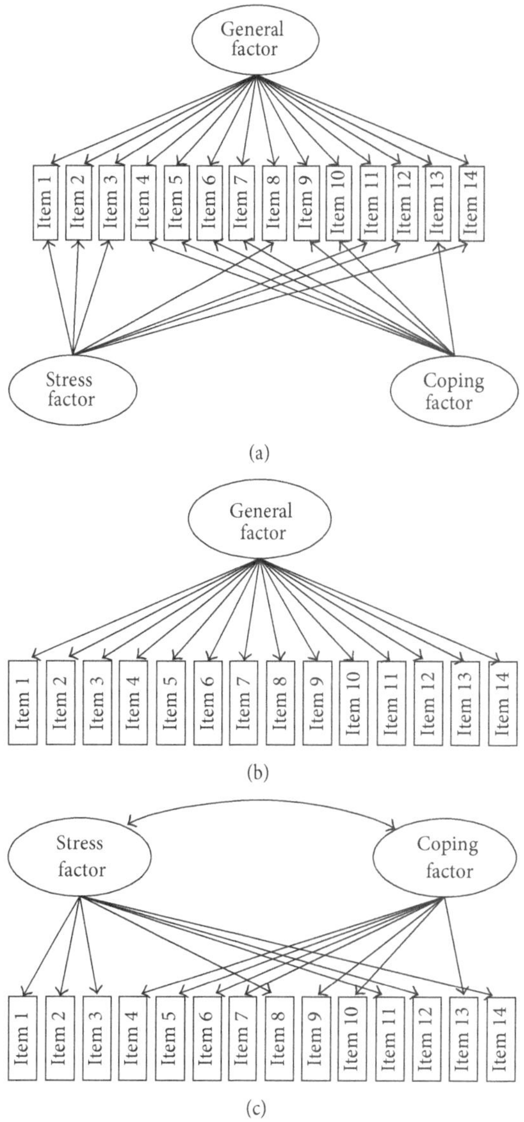

FIGURE 1: Simplified diagram of the bifactor model (a), one factor model (b), and two factor model (c) for the 14-item Perceived Stress Scale (PSS). The general and group (stress and coping) factors are not correlated in the bifactor model. The general factor has loadings on all items. The bifactor, one factor, and two factor models for the 10-item PSS were constructed in a similar way except items 4, 5, 12, and 13 which are not in the 10-item form.

2. Methods

2.1. Participants and Procedures. This study was approved by the University of Washington institutional review board before participants were recruited and informed consent was provided by participants before participation. Participants with self-reported MS were recruited for a longitudinal survey on symptoms and quality of life in multiple sclerosis through the greater northwest chapter of the National Multiple Sclerosis Society. The first survey was completed by 1,271 people with MS and 562 participants were randomly selected to participate in the longitudinal survey. Data for this study were collected between November 2008 and July 2009 at the

20-month followup (n = 446). A paper survey was mailed to participants and mailed back to study offices. In the event of missing data, study personnel called participants to obtain the missing data. Data were double entered and cleaned.

2.2. Measures

2.2.1. Perceived Stress Scale. The Perceived Stress Scale (PSS) was developed to measure how controllable and unpredictable people viewed their lives, an important component of the experience of stress. The original version had 14 items asking participants to rate their stress over the past month [4], with seven items negatively stated and seven items positively stated. For this study we refer to the subscale representing the negatively stated items as "Stress" and to the subscale representing the positively stated items as "Coping." Two short forms were also developed [7]. The first short form has 10 items, six negatively stated and four positively stated. The second short form has four items, two negatively stated and two positively stated. The response set ranges from 0 (never) to 4 (very often) and positively stated items are reverse coded before items are summed with higher scores indicating more perceived stress. Scores for the 14-item form range from 0 to 56, for the 10-item form range from 0 to 40, and from 0 to 16 for the 4-item form. Norms from a United States probability sample were 19.62, 13.02, and 4.49 for the 14-item, 10-item, and 4-item versions [7].

2.2.2. Patient Health Questionnaire-9. The Patient Health Questionnaire-9 (PHQ9) contains nine items corresponding to criteria symptoms for Major Depressive Disorder [16, 17]. Respondents are asked to rate their symptoms over the previous two weeks. The response options range from 0 (not at all) to 3 (nearly every day) and items are summed to create total scores. Higher scores indicate more depressive symptoms. The PHQ9 has been found to be reliable and valid in numerous medical populations [18].

2.2.3. Patient Health Questionnaire Anxiety. The Patient Health Questionnaire Anxiety [16] contains seven items measuring worry and other symptoms of anxiety. Response options range from 0 (not at all) to 2 (more than half the days) and respondents rate their symptoms over the past four weeks. Item responses are summed and then divided by the number of items to derive total scores in which higher scores indicate more anxiety.

2.2.4. Short Form 8. The short form 8 (SF8) is an abbreviated version of the SF36 questionnaire [19]. It contains eight items corresponding to the SF36 domains (general health, physical functioning, pain, social functioning, role limitations due to physical health, role limitations due to emotional health, vitality, and mental health) and scores are transformed onto a t-score metric with a mean of 50. Higher scores indicated better functioning. For this study, the overall physical health and overall mental health scales were used. The SF8 has shown good reliability and validity [19].

2.3. Analyses

2.3.1. Factor Structure. Factor structure was analyzed using categorical confirmatory factor analysis in Lisrel 8.8. Polychoric correlations were used as the data for these analyses and a diagonally weighted least squares estimator was used. Confirmatory factor analyses were run on each version of the PSS (PSS14, PSS10, and PSS4). For the PSS14 and PSS10, bifactor, one and two factor models were fit. For the PSS4, one and two factor models were fit to the data. The one factor analyses had all items load on a single factor while the two factor analyses had all negatively stated items load on the first factor, labeled Stress, and all positively stated items load on the second factor, labeled Coping. The bifactor model had a general factor on which all items were loaded. Both bifactor models also had two group factors, Stress (negatively worded items) and Coping (positively worded items).

Fit was evaluated using the chi-square tests for perfect and close fit, root mean square error of approximation (RMSEA), expected cross validation index (ECVI), comparative fit index (CFI), the standardized root mean residual (SRMR), and Akaike Information Criterion (AIC). The following criteria were used to assess goodness of fit: nonsignificance on tests of perfect and close fit, RMSEA $< .08$ but preferably $<.05$, CFI $>$ .96. ECVI and SRMR are used to compare models with lower levels indicating better fitting models so absolute values were not used for these measures. Lower levels of the AIC indicate a better fitting model and a difference of 10 was considered important [15].

2.3.2. Floor and Ceiling Effects. To examine floor and ceiling effects, we calculated the percentage of participants reporting the lowest scores (0 for all versions) and the highest possible scores (56, 40, and 16 for the PSS14, PSS10, and PSS4, resp.). We used the recommendations of Terwee et al. [20] to determine whether a floor or ceiling effect was present. Essentially, in any sample of 50 or more participants, having 15% or more of participants scoring at the lowest or highest score indicated a floor or ceiling effect.

2.3.3. Reliability and Validity. Reliability and validity analyses were conducted using SPSS. Cronbach's alpha was calculated for the total scores as well as for each of the two subscales. Item-total correlations (the correlation of an item with total of the remaining items) were also calculated to examine reliability in addition to the coefficient alpha. Ideally, item-total correlations are over .40 [21]. Convergent validity was assessed by correlating the PSS total and subscale scores with the PHQ9, PHQ-anxiety, and SF8 scores. The PSS scores were predicted to be strongly positively associated with depression and anxiety (PHQ9, PHQ-Anxiety) and strongly negatively associated with the mental health score (SF8-Mental Health score) and, while still moderately correlated with physical health (SF8-Physical Health score), the PSS scores would have lower correlations with physical health compared to mental health.

TABLE 1: Demographics, disease variables, and descriptive statistics.

Variable	*N* (%) or mean (SD)
Age	53.26 (10.94)
Gender (female)	368 (82.5%)
Race/ethnicity	
Caucasian	408 (91.5%)
African American	8 (1.8%)
Native American	14 (3.1%)
Asian	4 (0.9%)
Hispanic	13 (2.9%)
Married or in long-term relationship	306 (68.6%)
Income > $55,000	242 (54.3%)
Employed	163 (36.5%)
MS Type	
Relapsing remitting	254 (57.0%)
Other	183 (41.1%)
Time since MS diagnosis	12.59 (10.02)
Perceived Stress Scale	
PSS14 Total	21.35 (9.78)
PSS14 Stress	12.50 (5.52)
PSS14 Coping	8.85 (5.24)
PSS10 Total	14.90 (8.00)
PSS10 Stress	9.48 (5.23)
PSS10 Coping	5.42 (3.38)
PSS4 Total	5.59 (3.52)
PSS4 Stress	3.01 (2.06)
PSS4 Coping	2.58 (1.75)
Patient Health Questionnaire-9	6.66 (8.90)
PHQ-Anxiety	.09 (.29)
SF8	
Physical health	40.91 (10.51)
Mental health	47.10 (9.69)

3. Results

Participant demographics and disease-related variables are displayed in Table 1. The average participant was middle aged, female, Caucasian, and in a long-term relationship and was not currently employed. The majority had relapsing remitting MS and was more than 10 years post-MS diagnosis. The PHQ9 mean score of 6.66 indicated mild depression.

3.1. Factor Analyses. Results of the confirmatory factor analyses supported a bifactor structure for the 14-item and 10-item PSS forms. Factor loadings are reported in Table 2 and fit indices are reported in Table 3. For the PSS14, all items had acceptable factor loadings in the one factor model except for item 12. However, fit indices indicated that the one factor model did not have an optimal fit to the PSS14 data (RMSEA greater than .08, CFI < .96, both perfect and close fit tests were significant). The two factor model of the PSS14 had acceptable factor loadings and most fit indices indicated sufficient fit (RMSEA < .08, CFI > .96) although both tests of perfect and close fit were significant. When examining the bifactor model for the PSS14, the factor loadings on the general factor were all over .40 except for item 12 and some loadings on the group factors (Stress and Coping) which were low. The general factor in the bifactor model accounted for 45% of the total variance while the Stress factor accounted for 9% and the Coping factor accounted for 6%. The general factor accounted for 74% of the variance explained by the model and the group factors together accounted for 26%. The ratio of the total variance explained by the general and the group factors is consistent with what Reise and Haviland [22] suggested as supportive of sufficient unidimensionality.

For the one factor CFA model of the PSS10, the factor loadings were acceptable although, similar to the PSS14, several fit indices were not ideal (tests of perfect and close fit were significant, RMSEA > .08). The two factor structure of the PSS10 had adequate factor loadings and sufficient fit indices and the test of close fit was not significant (P = .350). The bifactor model of the PSS10 had some low factor loadings on the Stress and Coping factors but this was not as low as the PSS14. The general factor in the bifactor model accounted for 52% of the variance while the Stress factor accounted for 9% and the Coping factor accounted for 4% of the total variance. The general factor accounted for 80% of the explained variance and the group factors accounted for the remaining 20%. Similar to the PSS14, this is supportive of a general factor.

Factor loadings were acceptable for one and two CFA models of the PSS4. While fit indices for the PSS4 indicated that the two factor model fit the data better than the one factor model (lower RMSEA, RMSR, ECVI, and AIC), the one factor model still fits the data acceptably (RMSEA < .08, CFI > .96, test of close fit was nonsignificant). Results indicated that while the two factor model would be preferred, the one factor model was still tenable for the PSS4.

3.2. Floor and Ceiling Effects. The PSS was found to have negligible floor or ceiling effects. Only 2 (0.4%) responded "never" to all 14 questions on the PSS14, 5 (1.1%) were at the floor for the PSS10, and 32 (7.2%) endorsed the lowest category for PSS4. The ceiling effects were also low and ranged from 0 for PSS14 to 0.2 for PSS4. The breakdown of the responses at the floor and ceiling for the total score and subscales is listed in Table 4. More participants reported the lowest score than the highest score. For all the scales the proportion of responses at the floor and ceiling was far below the 15% threshold. Two subscales of the PSS4 had a higher number of participants reporting the lowest scores (12.3% and 12.6%) but they did not quite reach the threshold for a floor effect.

3.3. Reliability and Validity. Cronbach's alpha ranged from .73 for the PSS4-Stress to .91 for the PSS14-Total (see Table 4) and indicated adequate internal consistency for all versions and subscales. The Cronbach's alpha over .90 suggested likely redundancy in the full version (PSS14). Ranges for item-total correlations are also reported in Table 4. Some item-total correlations were below .40 for the PSS14 total score (2 of 14 correlations) and the PSS14 Stress subscale (1 of

Table 2: Factor analysis results: factor loadings.

Item	PSS-14						PSS-10						PSS-4		
	1F	2F-Stress	2F-Coping	Bifactor-general	Bifactor-Stress	Bifactor-Coping	1F	2F-Stress	2F-Coping	Bifactor-general	Bifactor-Stress	Bifactor-Coping	1F	2F-Stress	2F-Coping
PSS #1	.66	.70		.54	.53		.68	.71		.57	.55				
PSS #2	.82	.88		.77	.33		.83	.87		.81	.25		.81	.84	
PSS #3	.74	.78		.60	.61		.76	.79		.66	.52				
PSS #4	.49		.52	.41		.66									
PSS #5	.76		.79	.71		.55									
PSS #6	.84		.87	.83		.29	.81		.85	.81		.24	.83		.84
PSS #7	.83		.86	.86		.08	.83		.86	.79		.34	.84		.85
PSS #8	.67	.71		.63	.29		.68	.70		.67	.17				
PSS #9	.77		.79	.76		.20	.75		.78	.73		.26			
PSS #10	.86		.89	.88		.09	.85		.89	.81		.41			
PSS #11	.62	.66		.54	.40		.64	.67		.57	.38				
PSS #12	.15	.17		.05	.37										
PSS #13	.63		.65	.67		−.03									
PSS #14	.78	.83		.71	.40		.78	.82		.75	.30		.75	.76	

1F: one factor model, 2F: two factor model, PSS: Perceived Stress Scale.

TABLE 3: Factor analysis results: model fit indices.

	PSS-14			PSS-10			PSS-4	
	One factor	Two factor	Bifactor	One factor	Two factor	Bifactor	One factor	Two factor
Perfect Fit	$\chi^2 = 1124.54$, $P < .001$	$\chi^2 = 442.98$, $P < .001$	$\chi^2 = 181.28$, $P < .001$	$\chi^2 = 561.95$, $P < .001$	$\chi^2 = 156.23$, $P < .001$	$\chi^2 = 87.83$, $P < .001$	$\chi^2 = 11.18$, $P = .004$	$\chi^2 = .53$, $P = .470$
Close fit	$P < .001$	$P = .014$	$P = .99$	$P < .001$	$P = .350$	$P = .760$	$P = .430$	$P = .780$
RMSEA	.110	.064	.031	.120	.053	.041	.046	<.01
CFI	.95	.99	1.00	.97	.99	1.00	1.00	1.00
RMSR	.078	.057	.030	.063	.036	.022	.018	.004
ECVI	1.31	.61	.39	.66	.27	.23	.045	.043
AIC	584.57	270.92	173.58	293.73	118.54	103.41	19.89	18.23

RMSEA: root mean square error of approximation, CFI: comparative fit index, RMSR: root mean squared residual, ECVI: expected cross validation index, AIC: akaike information criterion.

Table 4: Floor effects and ceiling effects, reliability coefficients, and item-total correlations. Floor effects refer to the percentage of participants who reported the lowest possible score. Ceiling effects refer to the percentage of participants who reported the highest possible score. For floor and ceiling effects, more than 15% of the sample reporting the lowest or highest score is indicative of a floor or ceiling effect. Cronbach's alphas are ideally above .70 and item-total correlations should be above .40.

Scale	Floor effect % (*N*)	Ceiling effect % (*N*)	Cronbach's alpha	Item-total correlations range
PSS14-Total	0.4% (2)	0.0% (0)	.91	.126 to .758
PSS14-Stress	0.7% (3)	0.4% (2)	.84	.208 to .727
PSS14-Coping	4.9% (22)	0.0% (0)	.88	.488 to .770
PSS10-Total	1.1% (5)	0.0% (0)	.91	.588 to .771
PSS10-Stress	2.5% (11)	0.4% (2)	.87	.589 to .724
PSS10-Coping	7.2% (32)	0.0% (0)	.88	.688 to .785
PSS4-Total	7.2% (32)	0.2% (1)	.84	.643 to .706
PSS4-Stress	12.3% (55)	2.9% (13)	.73	.577
PSS4-Coping	12.6% (56)	0.9% (4)	.78	.639

PSS: Perceived Stress Scale.

Table 5: Convergent validity: correlations of PSS with PHQ9, PHQ-Anxiety, and SF8.

	PHQ9	PHQ-anxiety	SF8-physical	SF8-mental health
PSS14-Total	.371	.416	−.310	−.701
PSS14-Stress	.324	.461	−.246	−.654
PSS14-Coping	.351	.291	−.320	−.620
PSS10-Total	.378	.431	−.317	−.714
PSS10-Stress	.340	.460	−.268	−.672
PSS10-Coping	.369	.307	−.335	−.651
PSS4-Total	.368	.376	−.349	−.686
PSS4-Stress	.331	.413	−.328	−.633
PSS4-Coping	.351	.271	−.316	−.636

All correlations are significant at the $P < .001$ level. PSS: Perceived Stress Scale, PHQ: Patient Health Questionnaire, and SF: short form.

7 correlations) but all correlations for the PSS14 Coping subscale were over .40. Items on the PSS14 total scale with the lowest correlations were items 4 and 12. For the PSS10 and PSS4 total score and Stress and Coping subscales, all item-total correlations were above .40.

As indicated in Table 5, all PSS total scores (PSS14, PSS10, and PSS4) and PSS subscale scores were statistically significantly related to the PHQ9, PHQ-Anxiety, SF8-Physical Health scale, and SF8-Mental Health scale, indicating convergent validity. All associations were of the expected magnitude and in the hypothesized direction. The PSS scores showed a stronger relationship to the SF8-Mental Health scale (r's ranged from −.620 to −.714) compared to the SF8-Physical Health scale (r's ranged from −.246 to −.349), consistent with predictions.

4. Discussion

The present study evaluated the psychometric properties of the Perceived Stress Scale (PSS) in a sample of people living with MS. The analyses provided evidence for sufficient unidimensionality of all forms of PSS and supported the use of the summary score. Reliability and convergent validity was acceptable for the 10-item and 4-item PSS forms as well as for the subscales on those forms. Cronbach's alpha suggested redundancy of items for the 14-item PSS and some of the item-total correlations were low indicating that some items with low item-to-total correlations could be eliminated. These items, numbers 4 and 12, are also not included in the 10-item and 4-item PSS. The total scores and both subscales were related to measures of mental health and physical functioning.

The results of this study support previous evaluations of the PSS in healthy populations [7] and medical populations [12]. From one of the original validation studies, means for the 14-item, 10-item, and 4-item PSS total scores were 19.62, 13.02, and 4.49, respectively, in a healthy population [7]. These means for a healthy population were slightly lower than the means in this study suggesting that people living with MS report on average higher levels of stress compared to the healthy people. For women with cancer, means for the 10-item PSS were reported as 17.55 at initial cancer diagnosis, 14.13 one year later, and 14.04 two years later [12]. The mean of the 10-item PSS in this study was comparable to levels reported one and two years after diagnosis. In a sample of stroke patients, a mean on the 10-item PSS was reported at 12.27 right after hospital discharge and 10.47 at 12 months later, both lower than the present study [23]. Overall, people with MS reported levels of stress higher than those with other medical illnesses.

Previous studies have reported a two factor structure as opposed to a one factor structure [8, 10–13]. This study suggested that while there are separate Stress and Coping factors, a bifactor model suggested that the total scores of the PSS14 and PSS10 are driven by one underlying dimension: perceived stress. While the two factor model fits the 4-item PSS best, the one factor model still had acceptable fit indicating that a total score would still be tenable for the 4-item version. Unlike previous studies, sufficient reliability was shown for all forms of the PSS including the 4-item version suggesting that, at least for MS populations, the 4-item PSS is acceptable. This indicates that the total PSS scores are still acceptable to use. The shorter versions of the PSS or the subscales may be an appropriate choice for certain purposes, like epidemiological studies or patient screening and monitoring. The 4-item PSS may be particularly useful for research studies not primarily focused on stress and coping but for studies that may use stress and coping for secondary analyses. Ultimately these results suggest that the total score of the PSS is usable as the measure is sufficiently unidimensional. In addition, the PSS-10 appears to have better internal consistency than the PSS-14 and less participant burden due to fewer items and may be a better choice for MS researchers or clinicians.

The contributions of this study should be considered within the limitations. The sample in the study was a convenience sample and was not representative of people living with MS in the US. In addition, the diagnosis and the type of MS were self-reported. Also, as the full 14-item PSS was only administered at one time point in this study, we were unable to assess test-retest reliability. Regardless of the limitations, this study supports the use of the PSS in people with MS.

Conflict of Interests

The authors declare that there is no conflict of interests regarding the publication of this paper.

Acknowledgments

The authors would like to thank the study participants and the research staff who helped with this project. Dr. Wu is supported by a fellowship from the National Institute of Aging (T32 AG027677).

References

[1] National Multiple Sclerosis Society, "MS Prevalence," 2002, http://www.nationalmssociety.org/about-the-society/ms-prevalence/index.aspx.

[2] A. Feinstein, "Multiple sclerosis and depression," *Multiple Sclerosis*, vol. 17, no. 11, pp. 1276–1281, 2011.

[3] S. M. Monroe, G. M. Slavich, L. D. Torres, and I. H. Gotlib, "Major life events and major chronic difficulties are differentially associated with history of major depressive episodes," *Journal of Abnormal Psychology*, vol. 116, no. 1, pp. 116–124, 2007.

[4] S. Cohen, T. Kamarck, and R. Mermelstein, "A global measure of perceived stress," *Journal of Health and Social Behavior*, vol. 24, no. 4, pp. 385–396, 1983.

[5] K. van Kessel, R. Moss-Morris, E. Willoughby, T. Chalder, M. H. Johnson, and E. Robinson, "A randomized controlled trial of cognitive behavior therapy for multiple sclerosis fatigue," *Psychosomatic Medicine*, vol. 70, no. 2, pp. 205–213, 2008.

[6] D. A. Trojan, D. Arnold, J.-P. Collet et al., "Fatigue in multiple sclerosis: association with disease-related, behavioural and psychosocial factors," *Multiple Sclerosis*, vol. 13, no. 8, pp. 985–995, 2007.

[7] S. Cohen and G. Williamson, "Perceived stress in a probability sample of the United States," in *The Social Psychology of Health*, S. S. A. S. Oskamp, Ed., pp. 31–67, Sage, Newbury Park, Calif, USA, 1988.

[8] D. Y. P. Leung, T.-H. Lam, and S. S. C. Chan, "Three versions of perceived stress scale: validation in a sample of Chinese cardiac patients who smoke," *BMC Public Health*, vol. 10, article 513, 2010.

[9] E. Remor, "Psychometric properties of a European Spanish version of the Perceived Stress Scale (PSS)," *Spanish Journal of Psychology*, vol. 9, no. 1, pp. 86–93, 2006.

[10] E. Andreou, E. C. Alexopoulos, C. Lionis et al., "Perceived Stress Scale: reliability and validity study in Greece," *International Journal of Environmental Research and Public Health*, vol. 8, no. 8, pp. 3287–3298, 2011.

[11] R. Siqueira Reis, A. A. Ferreira Hino, and C. RomÉlio Rodriguez Añez, "Perceived stress scale: reliability and validity study in Brazil," *Journal of Health Psychology*, vol. 15, no. 1, pp. 107–114, 2010.

[12] D. M. Golden-Kreutz, M. W. Browne, G. M. Frierson, and B. L. Andersen, "Assessing stress in cancer patients: a second-order factor analysis model for the perceived stress scale," *Assessment*, vol. 11, no. 3, pp. 216–223, 2004.

[13] M. Ç. Örücü and A. Demir, "Psychometric evaluation of perceived stress scale for Turkish university students," *Stress and Health*, vol. 25, no. 1, pp. 103–109, 2009.

[14] K. J. Holzinger and F. Swineford, "The Bi-factor method," *Psychometrika*, vol. 2, no. 1, pp. 41–54, 1937.

[15] S. P. Reise, J. Morizot, and R. D. Hays, "The role of the bifactor model in resolving dimensionality issues in health outcomes measures," *Quality of Life Research*, vol. 16, no. 1, supplement, pp. 19–31, 2007.

[16] R. L. Spitzer, K. Kroenke, and J. B. W. Williams, "Validation and utility of a self-report version of PRIME-MD: the PHQ Primary Care Study," *Journal of the American Medical Association*, vol. 282, no. 18, pp. 1737–1744, 1999.

[17] K. Kroenke, R. L. Spitzer, and J. B. W. Williams, "The PHQ-9: validity of a brief depression severity measure," *Journal of General Internal Medicine*, vol. 16, no. 9, pp. 606–613, 2001.

[18] S. J. Ferrando, J. Samton, N. Mor et al., "Patient health questionnaire-9 to screen for depression in outpatients with multiple sclerosis," *International Journal of MS Care*, vol. 9, no. 3, pp. 99–103, 2007.

[19] J. Ware, M. Kosinski, J. E. Dewey, and B. Gandek, *How to Score and Interpret Measures: A Manual for Users of the SF-8 Health Survey*, QualyMetric, Boston, Mass, USA, 2001.

[20] C. B. Terwee, S. D. M. Bot, M. R. de Boer et al., "Quality criteria were proposed for measurement properties of health status questionnaires," *Journal of Clinical Epidemiology*, vol. 60, no. 1, pp. 34–42, 2007.

[21] B. S. Everitt, *The Cambridge Dictionary of Statistics*, Cambridge University Press, New York, NY, USA, 2nd edition, 2002.

[22] S. P. Reise and M. G. Haviland, "Item response theory and the measurement of clinical change," *Journal of Personality Assessment*, vol. 84, no. 3, pp. 228–238, 2005.

[23] S. K. Ostwald, M. P. Bernal, S. G. Cron, and K. M. Godwin, "Stress experienced by stroke survivors and spousal caregivers during the first year after discharge from inpatient rehabilitation," *Topics in Stroke Rehabilitation*, vol. 16, no. 2, pp. 93–104, 2009.

15

In Vivo Identification of Skeletal Muscle Dynamics with Nonlinear Kalman Filter: Comparison between EKF and SPKF

Mitsuhiro Hayashibe, David Guiraud, and Philippe Poignet

DEMAR Project, INRIA Sophia-Antipolis and LIRMM, CNRS, University of Montpellier, 34095 Montpellier, France

Correspondence should be addressed to Mitsuhiro Hayashibe; mitsuhiro.hayashibe@inria.fr

Academic Editors: A. Cappozzo and S. Park

Skeletal muscle system has nonlinear dynamics and subject-specific characteristics. Thus, it is essential to identify the unknown parameters from noisy biomedical signals to improve the modeling accuracy in neuroprosthetic control. The objective of this work is to develop an experimental identification method for subject-specific biomechanical parameters of a physiological muscle model which can be employed to predict the nonlinear force properties of stimulated muscle. Our previously proposed muscle model, which can describe multiscale physiological system based on the Hill and Huxley models, was used for the identification. The identification protocols were performed on two rabbit experiments, where the medial gastrocnemius was attached to a motorized lever system to record the force by the nerve stimulation. The muscle model was identified using nonlinear Kalman filters: sigma-point and extended Kalman filter. The identified model was evaluated by comparison with experimental measurements in the cross-validation manner. The feasibility could be demonstrated by comparison between the estimated parameter and the measured value. The estimates with SPKF showed 5.7% and 2.9% error in each experiment with 7 different initial conditions. It reveals that SPKF has great advantage especially for the identification of multiscale muscle model which accounts for the high nonlinearity and discontinuous states between muscle contraction and relaxation process.

1. Introduction

1.1. Muscle Modeling and FES. Functional electrical stimulation (FES) is an effective technique to evoke artificial contractions of paralyzed skeletal muscles. It has been employed as a general method in modern rehabilitation to partially restore motor function for patients with upper neural lesions [1, 2]. Recently, the rapid progress in microprocessor technology provided the means for computer-controlled FES systems [3–5]. A fundamental problem concerning FES is how to handle the high complexity and nonlinearity of the neuromusculoskeletal system [6, 7]. In addition, there is a large variety of patient situations depending on the type of neurological disorder. To improve the performance of motor neuroprosthetics beyond the current limited use of such system, subject-specific modeling is essential. The use of a mathematical model can improve the development of neuroprosthetics by optimizing their functionality for individual patients.

A mathematical model makes it possible to describe the relevant characteristics of the patient's skeletal muscle and to accurately predict the force as a function of the stimulation parameters. Indeed, synthesis of stimulation sequences or control strategies to achieve movement can be efficiently computed and optimized using numerical models [8]. Therefore, it can contribute to enhancing the design and function of controls applied to FES. Over the years, a great variety of muscle models have been proposed, differing in their intended application, mathematical complexity, level of structure considered, and fidelity to the biological facts. Some of them have attempted to exhibit the microscopic or macroscopic functional behavior, for instance Huxley [9] and Hill [10]. The distribution-moment model [11] constitutes a bridge between the microscopic and macroscopic levels. It is a model for sarcomeres or whole muscle which has been extracted via a formal mathematical approximation from Huxley crossbridge models. Models integrating geometry of the tendon and other macroscopic consideration can be found in [12]. A study by Bestel and Sorine [13], based on both microscopic Huxley and macroscopic Hill type model, proposed an explanation of how the beating of cardiac muscle is achieved through a chemical control input. It integrated the calcium dynamics in muscle cells that stimulate the contractile element of the model. Starting with this concept, we adapted it for striated muscle [14]. We proposed a musculotendinous model which considered the muscular masses and viscous frictions in muscle-tendon complex. This model is represented by differential equations where the outputs are the muscle's active stiffness and force. The model input represents the actual electrical signal as provided by the stimulator in FES.

1.2. In Vivo Identification for Subject-Specific Parameters. In actual FES system, the appropriate tuning is achieved empirically by intensively stimulating the patient's muscle for each task. If this adjustment could be calculated in the simulation, and if we could find the best signal pattern using virtual skeletal muscle, such method would be very helpful for movement synthesis for spinal cord injured (SCI) patients. However, in order to perform the simulation, an accurate skeletal muscle model is required to reproduce a well-predicted force for each muscle corresponding to the patient-specific characteristics.

For any biological systems, identification is a difficult problem due to the fact that (i) measurements must be as non-invasive, particularly on humans, (ii) some entities cannot be directly measured, (iii) an experimental setup and protocol have to be designed and certified, (iv) intersubject variations can be large, and (v) the large nonlinearity and complexity of the models cause some optimization algorithms to fail. Thus, few papers address biomechanical parameters identification in FES context, and they used macroscopic model for global force production [15]. Consequently, we described an approach for coupling the model with *in-vivo* measurements, that is, using a multiscale muscle model in an estimation procedure in order to perform the identification of the parameters, hence, giving access to physiologically meaningful parameters of the muscle. Preliminary result was reported in [16].

The skeletal muscle dynamics are in particular highly nonlinear, and we need to identify many unknown physiological parameters if a multiscale model is applied. The main objective of this paper is to develop an experimental computational method to identify unknown internal parameters from the limited information. For such identification of nonlinear system, extended Kalman filter (EKF) has often been used for skeletal muscle [17] and cardiac muscle identification [18]. It can work when the model is not complicated and not highly nonlinear. In this paper, a sigma-point Kalman filter (SPKF) was applied to the *in vivo* experimental data to identify internal states in the nonlinear dynamics of multiscale skeletal muscle model. SPKF has higher accuracy and consistency for nonlinear estimation than EKF theoretically. The feasibility of both identifications is verified by comparison. The computational performance is discussed.

The outline of the paper is as follows. The next section presents the formulation of the skeletal muscle model controlled by FES. The following section is devoted to the experimental identification of the model for isometric contraction, including the identification protocol. The experimental measurement was performed *in-vivo* on rabbits. Then, we present detailed results of the parameter estimation, the comparison with EKF, and cross-validation which illustrates the pertinence of the identification. Finally, we present some discussions, conclusions, and perspectives in the last sections.

2. Skeletal Muscle Model

Muscle modeling is complex, in particular when the model is based on biomechanics and physiological realities. Most of the muscle models have been based on phenomenological models derived from Hill's classic work [10] and well summarized by Zajac [12]. Hill macroscopic model is a standard muscle model for practical use. Recent work [19] performed the validation of Hill model during functionally relevant conditions. They concluded that model errors are large for different firing frequencies and largest at the low motor unit firing rates relevant to normal movement. They pointed out that the reason may come from the Hill model assumption to consider muscle activation, force-length, and force-velocity properties independently. It was suggested that more physiological coupling between activation and force-velocity properties can be demonstrated in microscopic crossbridge models incorporating a dependence between physiologically based activation and crossbridge attachment [19]. Thus, our approach is to provide a multiscale physiology-based model on the both micro- and macroscale fact to obtain meaningful internal parameters.

Our muscle model is composed of two elements of different nature: (i) an activation model which describes how an electrical stimulus generates an action potential (AP) and initiates the contraction and (ii) a mechanical model which describes the dynamics in force (Figure 1). For details of the muscle model, refer to the previously published article [14]. Here, a brief summary of the model and the information necessary for the identification are given.

2.1. Activation Model. The activation model describes the electrical activity of muscle which represents the excitation-contraction phenomena. In muscle physiology, it is known that two input elements dominate muscle contraction: fiber recruitment rates and temporal activation [20]. The recruitment rates determine the percentage of recruited motor units. In Hill model, it has only one input which corresponds to this recruitment rate. Hill model is mainly applied for voluntary contraction where temporal activation is not dominant. However, in FES, since all muscle fibers are synchronously activated, this temporal activation which occurs by every stimulation pulse, is important. The recruitment rates can be determined on the pulse width (PW) and pulse amplitude of signal I, generated by the stimulator [21]. The recruitment rate $\alpha(\mathrm{PW}, I)$ can be assumed to be a constant value when PW and I remain constant.

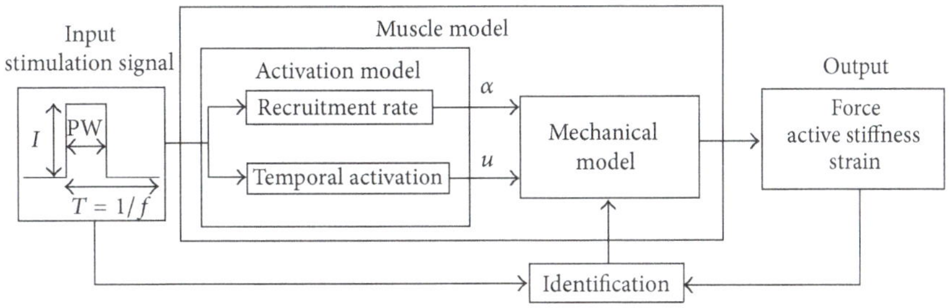

FIGURE 1: Outline of skeletal muscle model and its identification.

The temporal activation can be considered as the underlying physiological processes which describes the chemical input signal, u, that brings muscle cells into contraction as shown in Figure 2. Muscle contraction is initiated by an AP along the muscle fiber membrane, which goes deep into the cell through the T-tubules. It causes calcium releases that induce the contraction process when its concentration rises above a threshold and is sustained till the concentration drops back below this threshold once again. Hatze [22] gives an example of calcium dynamics (Ca^{2+}) modeling. Since we focus on the mechanical response in this paper, we choose a simple model that renders the main characteristics of the dynamics. The contraction-relaxation cycle is triggered by the (Ca^{2+}) associated with two phases: (i) contraction and, (ii) relaxation as in Figure 2. We use a delayed (τ) model to take into account the propagation time of the AP and an average time delay due to the calcium dynamics. The frequency of the chemical input, u, can be defined from the stimulation frequency. The time delay and the contraction time can be obtained from a twitch test by single stimulation pulse. A contraction takes place with a kinetics U_c then, if no other AP has been received in the mean time, an active relaxation follows indefinitely with a kinetics U_r. U_c is linked to the rate of actine-myosine cycle whereas U_r is related to the rate of crossbridge breakage. Finally, u can be written as follows, where $\Pi_c(t)$ is a trapezoidal switching function which connects relaxation and contraction state from 0 to 1:

$$u = \Pi_c(t) U_c + (1 - \Pi_c(t)) U_r. \quad (1)$$

2.2. Mechanical Model. The model is based on the macroscopic Hill-Maxwell type model and the microscopic description of Huxley [9]. For crossbridge modeling, Huxley [9] proposed an explanation of the crossbridge interaction in a sarcomere. A sarcomere model can be used to represent a whole muscle which is assumed to be a homogeneous assembly of identical sarcomeres. The distribution-moment model of Zahalak [11] is a model for sarcomeres or whole muscle which is extracted via a formal mathematical approximation from Huxley crossbridge models. This model constitutes a bridge between the microscopic and macroscopic levels. Based on Huxley and Hill-type models, Bestel and Sorine [13] proposed an explanation of how the beating of cardiac muscle may be performed, through a chemical control input, connected to the calcium dynamics in muscle cell, that stimulates the contractile element of the model.

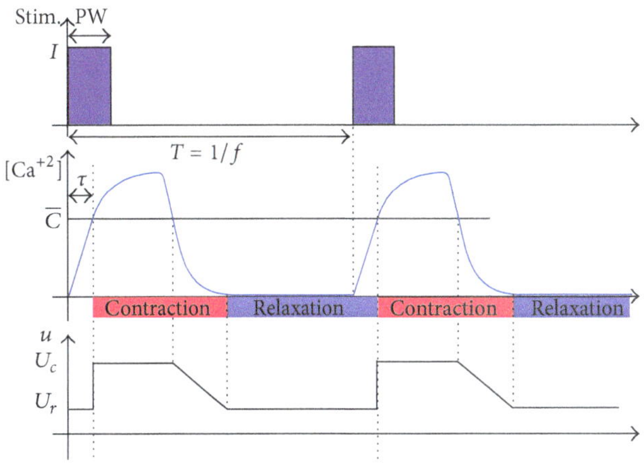

FIGURE 2: Chemical control input u for temporal activation.

The model is composed of macroscopic passive elements and a contractile element E_c controlled by input commands: the chemical input, u, as suggested by Bestel and Sorine [13] for the cardiac muscle on the sarcomere scale and the recruitment rate, α, on the fiber scale as shown in Figure 3. In order to express isometric contractions, whereas the skeleton is not actuated, our muscle model is introduced with masses m (kg) and linear viscous dampers λ_{s1}, λ_{s2} (Ns/m) to ensure energy dissipation. On both sides of E_c, there are elastic springs, k_{s1}, k_{s2} (N/m), and viscous dampers to express the viscoelasticity of the muscle-tendon complex. The parallel element, K_p, mainly represents surrounding tissues, but it can be omitted in isometric contraction mode. We assume the symmetric form with the two masses and passive elements identical. Here, $\varepsilon_s = \varepsilon_{s1} = \varepsilon_{s2}$, $k_s = k_{s1} = k_{s2}$, and $\lambda = \lambda_{s1} = \lambda_{s2}$. L_{c0} and L_{s0} (m) are the lengths of E_c and k_s in the rest state. Initially, we can define the relative length variation ε as positive when the length increases, as in (2). In particular, in the case of isometric contraction, the following relationship exists (3):

$$\varepsilon_s = \frac{L_s - L_{s0}}{L_{s0}} \qquad \varepsilon_c = \frac{L_c - L_{c0}}{L_{c0}}, \quad (2)$$

$$2L_{s0}\varepsilon_s + L_{c0}\varepsilon_c = 0. \quad (3)$$

The dynamical equation of one of the masses is given by (4). F_c and k_c express the force and the stiffness of E_c, respectively. The force F_e at the output of this muscle model is the sum

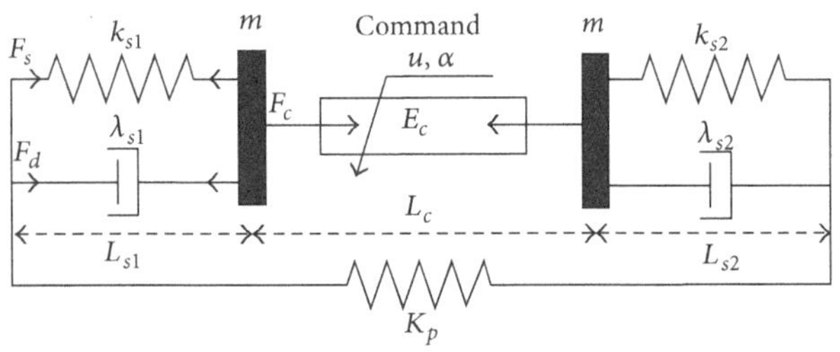

FIGURE 3: Macroscopic mechanical configuration of the muscle model.

of the spring force F_s and the damping force F_d. When we measure the tension of skeletal muscle under *in vivo* conditions, the experimentally measured force is equivalent to F_e. When we take the ratio of F_c and F_e, L_{s0} is offset and can be written as in (6). (7) is the relational equation in Laplace transform. From this relationship, the differential equation (8) can be obtained:

$$mL_{s0}\ddot{\varepsilon}_s = F_c - k_s L_{s0}\varepsilon_s - \lambda L_{s0}\dot{\varepsilon}_s, \tag{4}$$

$$F_e = F_s + F_d = k_s L_{s0}\varepsilon_s + \lambda L_{s0}\dot{\varepsilon}_s, \tag{5}$$

$$\frac{F_c}{F_e} = \frac{m\ddot{\varepsilon}_s + \lambda\dot{\varepsilon}_s + k_s\varepsilon_s}{\lambda\dot{\varepsilon}_s + k_s\varepsilon_s}, \tag{6}$$

$$\frac{\mathscr{L}[F_c]}{\mathscr{L}[F_e]} = \frac{ms^2 + \lambda s + k_s}{\lambda s + k_s}, \tag{7}$$

$$m\ddot{F}_e + \lambda\dot{F}_e + k_s F_e = \lambda\dot{F}_c + k_s F_c. \tag{8}$$

Finally, in isometric contraction, the differential equations of this model can be described as follows:

$$\dot{k}_c = -k_c u + \alpha k_m \Pi_c U_c - k_c |\dot{\varepsilon}_c| \tag{9}$$

$$\dot{F}_c = -F_c u + \alpha F_m \Pi_c U_c - F_c |\dot{\varepsilon}_c| + L_{c0} k_c \dot{\varepsilon}_c, \tag{10}$$

$$\ddot{F}_e = -\frac{\lambda}{m}\dot{F}_e - \frac{k_s}{m}F_e + \frac{\lambda}{m}\dot{F}_c + \frac{k_s}{m}F_c, \tag{11}$$

$$\ddot{\varepsilon}_c = -\frac{2F_c}{mL_{c0}} - \frac{k_s}{m}\varepsilon_c - \frac{\lambda}{m}\dot{\varepsilon}_c. \tag{12}$$

The dynamics of the contractile element correspond to (9) and (10). The terms k_m and F_m are the maximum values for k_c and F_c, respectively. From (3) and (4), the differential equation for ε_c is obtained as in (12). The internal state vector of this system should be set as $\mathbf{x} = [k_c \; F_c \; F_e \; \dot{F}_e \; \varepsilon_c \; \dot{\varepsilon}_c]$.

3. Experimental Identification

In this study, we have developed a method to identify the parameters in the mechanical part of a skeletal muscle model. The input controls of the model are set as the static recruitment rate α and the chemical control input u from the activation model. These two controls are computed from the FES input signal. Note that the identification was performed with constant FES parameters for pulse width and intensity of electrical stimulation so that the recruitment rate is constant. The amplitude and pulse width were selected to recruit 90% of the maximum muscular force; then α can be set as 0.9 for the fiber recruitment. In addition, the calcium dynamics in our model induce a time delay and an on/off control which represents contraction/relaxation so that correct data processing can avoid the detailed calcium dynamics. The trigger for signal u can be calculated from the timing of the electrical stimulation. U_c and U_r are set as 20 and 15, respectively, as in [23].

In isometric contraction, the differential equations of skeletal muscle dynamics are straightly given in (9)–(12). In this case, K_c, F_c, F_e, and ε_c are unknown time-varying values and m, λ_s, and L_{c0} are unknown static parameters to be estimated. For the identification of this model, it is a nonlinear state space model, and many state variables are not measurable. Moreover, *in-vivo* experimental data include some noise. Hence, we need an efficient recursive filter that estimates the state of a dynamic system from a series of noisy measurements.

3.1. Sigma-Point Kalman Filter. For this kind of nonlinear identification, extended Kalman filter (EKF) is the well-known standard method. In EKF, the nonlinear equation should be linearized to first order with partial derivatives (Jacobian matrix) around a mean of the state. The optimal Kalman filtering is then applied to the linearized system. When the model is highly nonlinear, EKF may give particularly poor performance and diverge easily. In skeletal muscle dynamics, its state-space is dramatically changed between the contraction and relaxation phases. At this time, partial derivatives would be incorrect due to the discontinuity. Therefore, we introduced the sigma-point Kalman filter (SPKF). The initial idea was proposed by Julier and Uhlmann [24] and has been well described by Merwe and Wan [25]. SPKF uses a deterministic sampling technique known as the unscented transform to pick a minimal set of sample points (called sigma points) around the mean. These sigma points are propagated through the true nonlinearity. This approach results in approximations that are accurate to at least second order in a Taylor series expansion. In contrast, EKF results in only first-order accuracy.

An outline of the SPKF algorithm is described. For details, the reader should refer to [25, 26]. The general Kalman framework involves estimation of the state of a discrete-time, nonlinear dynamic system,

$$\begin{aligned} \mathbf{x}_{k+1} &= \mathbf{f}(\mathbf{x}_k, \mathbf{v}_k), \\ \mathbf{y}_k &= \mathbf{h}(\mathbf{x}_k, \mathbf{n}_k), \end{aligned} \tag{13}$$

where $\mathbf{x}_k$ represents the internal state of the system to be estimated and $\mathbf{y}_k$ is the only observed signal. The process noise $\mathbf{v}_k$ drives the dynamic system, and the observation noise is given by $\mathbf{n}_k$. The filter starts by augmenting the state vector to L dimensions, where L is the sum of dimensions in the original state, model noise, and measurement noise. The corresponding covariance matrix is similarly augmented to an L by L matrix. In this form, the augmented state vector $\hat{\mathbf{x}}_k^a$ and covariance matrix $\mathbf{P}_k^a$ can be defined as

$$\hat{\mathbf{x}}_k^a = E[\mathbf{x}_k^a] = [\hat{\mathbf{x}}_k^T \ \bar{\mathbf{v}}_k^T \ \bar{\mathbf{n}}_k^T]^T, \quad \mathbf{P}_k^a = E[(\mathbf{x}_k^a - \hat{\mathbf{x}}_k^a)(\mathbf{x}_k^a - \hat{\mathbf{x}}_k^a)^T] = \begin{bmatrix} \mathbf{P}_{\mathbf{x}_k} & 0 & 0 \\ 0 & \mathbf{Q}_{\mathbf{v}_k} & 0 \\ 0 & 0 & \mathbf{R}_{\mathbf{n}_k} \end{bmatrix}, \tag{14}$$

where $\mathbf{P}_\mathbf{x}$ is the state covariance, $\mathbf{Q}_\mathbf{v}$ is the process noise covariance, and $\mathbf{R}_\mathbf{n}$ is the observation noise covariance.

In the process update, the $2L + 1$ sigma points are computed based on a square root decomposition of the prior covariance as in (15), where $\gamma = \sqrt{L+\lambda}$ and λ is found using $\lambda = \alpha^2(L+\kappa) - L$. α is chosen in $0 < \alpha < 1$ which determines the spread of the sigma points around the prior mean and κ is usually chosen equal to 0. The augmented sigma-point matrix is formed by the concatenation of the state sigma-point matrix, the process noise sigma-point matrix, and the measurement noise sigma-point matrix, such that $\mathcal{X}^a = [(\mathcal{X}^x)^T \ (\mathcal{X}^v)^T \ (\mathcal{X}^n)^T]^T$. The sigma-point weights to be used for mean and covariance estimates are defined as in (16). The optimal value of 2 is usually assigned to β:

$$\mathcal{X}_{k-1}^a = \left[\hat{\mathbf{x}}_{k-1}^a \ \ \hat{\mathbf{x}}_{k-1}^a + \gamma\sqrt{\mathbf{P}_{k-1}^a} \ \ \hat{\mathbf{x}}_{k-1}^a - \gamma\sqrt{\mathbf{P}_{k-1}^a}\right], \tag{15}$$

$$\omega_0^m = \frac{\lambda}{(L+\lambda)}, \quad \omega_0^c = \omega_0^m + (1 - \alpha^2 + \beta), \quad \omega_i^c = \omega_i^m = \frac{1}{(2(L+\lambda))} \quad (\text{for } i = 1,\ldots,2L). \tag{16}$$

And these sigma points are propagated through the nonlinear function. Predicted mean and covariance are computed as in (18) and (19) and predicted observation is calculated as follows:

$$\mathcal{X}_{k|k-1}^x = \mathbf{f}(\mathcal{X}_{k-1}^x, \mathcal{X}_{k-1}^v), \tag{17}$$

$$\hat{\mathbf{x}}_k^- = \sum_{i=0}^{2L} \omega_i^m \mathcal{X}_{i,k|k-1}^x, \tag{18}$$

$$\mathbf{P}_{\mathbf{x}_k}^- = \sum_{i=0}^{2L} \omega_i^c (\mathcal{X}_{i,k|k-1}^x - \hat{\mathbf{x}}_k^-)(\mathcal{X}_{i,k|k-1}^x - \hat{\mathbf{x}}_k^-)^T, \tag{19}$$

$$\mathcal{Y}_{k|k-1} = \mathbf{h}(\mathcal{X}_{k|k-1}^x, \mathcal{X}_{k-1}^n), \tag{20}$$

$$\hat{\mathbf{y}}_k^- = \sum_{i=0}^{2L} \omega_i^m \mathcal{Y}_{i,k|k-1}. \tag{21}$$

The predictions are then updated with new measurements by first calculating the measurement covariance and state-measurement cross-correlation matrices, which are then used to determine the Kalman gain. Finally, the updated estimate and covariance are determined from this Kalman gain as below:

$$\mathbf{P}_{\tilde{\mathbf{y}}_k} = \sum_{i=0}^{2L} \omega_i^c (\mathcal{Y}_{i,k|k-1} - \hat{\mathbf{y}}_k^-)(\mathcal{Y}_{i,k|k-1} - \hat{\mathbf{y}}_k^-)^T, \quad \mathbf{P}_{\mathbf{x}_k\mathbf{y}_k} = \sum_{i=0}^{2L} \omega_i^c (\mathcal{X}_{i,k|k-1}^x - \hat{\mathbf{x}}_k^-)(\mathcal{Y}_{i,k|k-1} - \hat{\mathbf{y}}_k^-)^T, \quad \mathbf{K}_k = \mathbf{P}_{\mathbf{x}_k\mathbf{y}_k}\mathbf{P}_{\tilde{\mathbf{y}}_k}^{-1}, \quad \hat{\mathbf{x}}_k = \hat{\mathbf{x}}_k^- + \mathbf{K}_k(\mathbf{y}_k - \hat{\mathbf{y}}_k^-), \quad \mathbf{P}_{\mathbf{x}_k} = \mathbf{P}_{\mathbf{x}_k}^- - \mathbf{K}_k\mathbf{P}_{\tilde{\mathbf{y}}_k}\mathbf{K}_k^T. \tag{22}$$

These process updates and measurement updates should be recursively calculated in $k = 1,\ldots,\infty$ until the end point of the measurement.

3.2. Experimental Measurement for Identification. Stimulation experiments were performed on two New Zealand white rabbits at Aarhus University Hospital in Aalborg, Denmark, as depicted in Figure 4. Anesthesia was induced and maintained with periodic intramuscular doses of a cocktail of 0.15 mg/kg Midazolam (DormicumR, Alpharma A/S), 0.03 mg/kg Fetanyl, and 1 mg/kg Fluranison (combined in HypnormR, Janssen Pharmaceutica) [14].

The left leg of the rabbit was anchored at the knee and ankle joints to a fixed mechanical frame using bone pins placed through the distal epiphyses of the femur and tibia. A tendon of the medial gastrocnemius (MG) muscle was attached to the arm of a motorized lever system (Dual mode system 310B Aurora Scientific Inc.). The position and force of the lever arm were recorded. An initial muscle-tendon length was established by flexing the ankle to 90°. A bipolar cuff electrode was implanted around the sciatic nerve, allowing the MG muscle to be stimulated. Data acquisition was performed at a 4.8 kHz sampling rate. The muscle force against the electrical stimulation was measured under isometric conditions.

4. Result of Identification

In order to facilitate the convergence of the identification, the estimation process has been split into two steps. In the first step, we only estimate geometrical parameter L_{c0}. In the second step, we estimate the dynamic parameters: m and λ. The biomechanical muscle model to be identified is presented as (9)–(12). We define the state vectors for geometric and dynamic estimations in SPKF as follows:

$$\mathbf{x_g} = [k_c \ F_c \ F_e \ \dot{F}_e \ \varepsilon_c \ \dot{\varepsilon}_c \ L_{c0}], \quad \mathbf{x_d} = [k_c \ F_c \ F_e \ \dot{F}_e \ \varepsilon_c \ \dot{\varepsilon}_c \ m \ \lambda]. \tag{23}$$

4.1. Parameter Estimation. Parameter estimation was performed using two rabbit experimental data. The stimulation signal input used for the estimation is composed of two

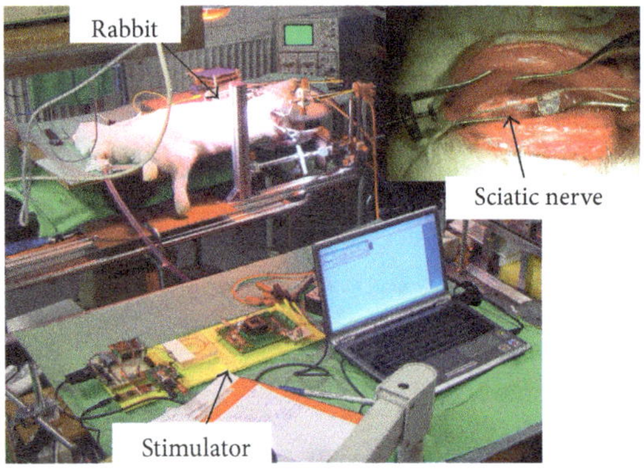

FIGURE 4: Overview of the rabbit experiment.

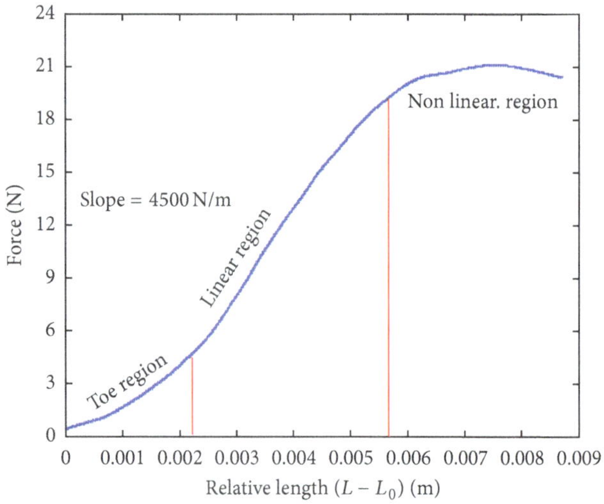

FIGURE 5: Force measurement for muscle passive stiffness.

successive pulses (doublet) at 16 Hz and 20 Hz with amplitude 105 μA and pulse width 300 μs. The stiffness k_s has been estimated separately, using the experiments performed on the isolated muscle. The isolated muscle was pulled with the motorized lever. The stiffness is taken as equal to the slope of the straight line of the passive length versus force relationship in the experimental measurement as shown in Figure 5. The k_s obtained was 4500 N/m. F_m and k_m can be obtained knowing the force response of muscle to a stimulation pattern with maximum signal parameter values (frequency, amplitude, pulse, and width). In this case, $k_m = 1000$ N/m and $F_m = 15$ N were obtained from the measurement.

The experimental muscle force against the doublet stimulation (20 Hz) was used for parameter estimation during measurement updates for F_e in SPKF. The covariance matrix has been initialized as in Table 1 for both geometric and dynamic parameter identifications. The evolutions of estimated internal states for k_c and ε_c are obtained as shown in Figure 6. From these behaviors, we can confirm that the contractile element of the model is successfully tracking the contraction represented by the dynamics of differential equations under the estimation process. Figure 7 shows the estimated parameter L_{c0} and the error covariance. The fact that the error covariace is being decreased during identification process shows stable convergence of the estimation. Even with the different initial values setting, parameter estimation results converged into a particular value in SPKF as shown in Figure 7(a). We tested the estimation from 7 different initial values with an interval of 5 mm from 55 mm to 85 mm. The color is changed from magenta to cyan in the plot.

As can be seen from the resultant computational behavior on the graphs, the internal state vectors of the muscle model converged well to stationary values even with different initial values. After the complete estimation process for geometric and dynamic parameters, the estimated values are summarized in Table 2. Normalized RMS errors between measured and estimated force were also computed for each case. Moreover, the estimated length of the contractile element with each stimulation showed values close to the actual measured lengths of the extracted muscle. The border between the contractile element and tendon is not so clear visually, but it was approximately 7 cm for both rabbit GM muscles.

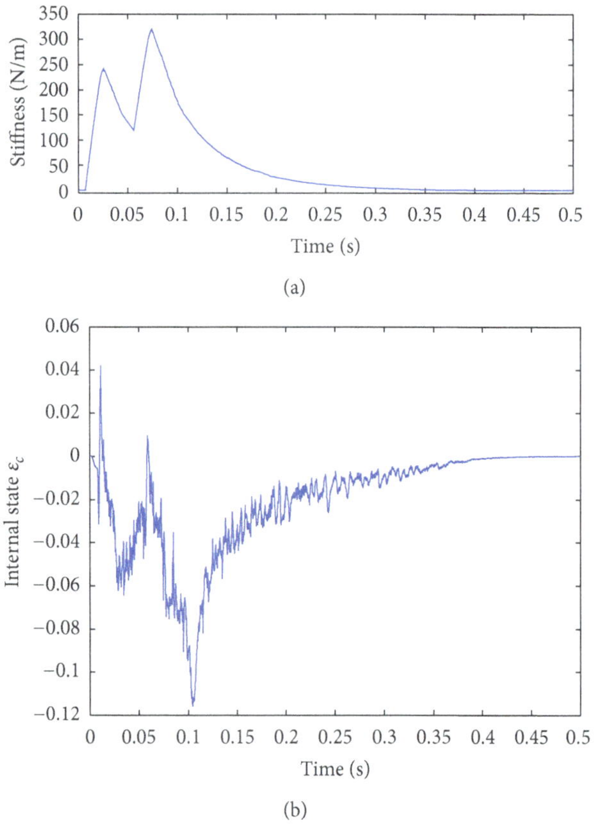

FIGURE 6: Estimated state of the stiffness K_c (a) and the strain ε_c (b) for the contractile element with SPKF.

The sizes of the two rabbits were similar; in particular, the estimated length of L_{c0} had good correspondence with the measured length for both rabbits and with different frequency stimulations. Physical parameters are impossible to make visual verification, but the estimated intrasubject property is maintained among the parameters obtained by different frequency stimulations from Table 2.

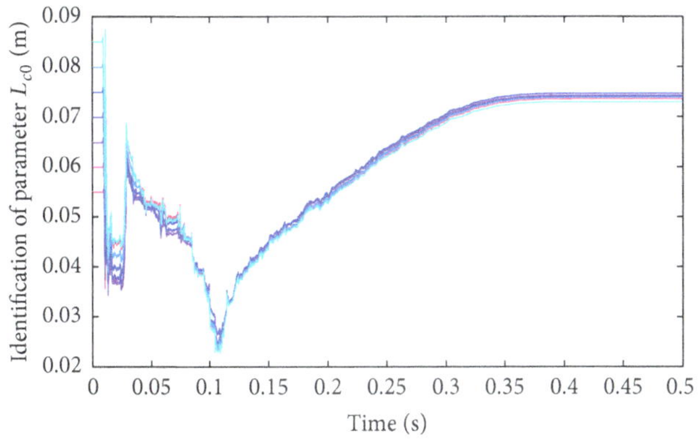

(a)

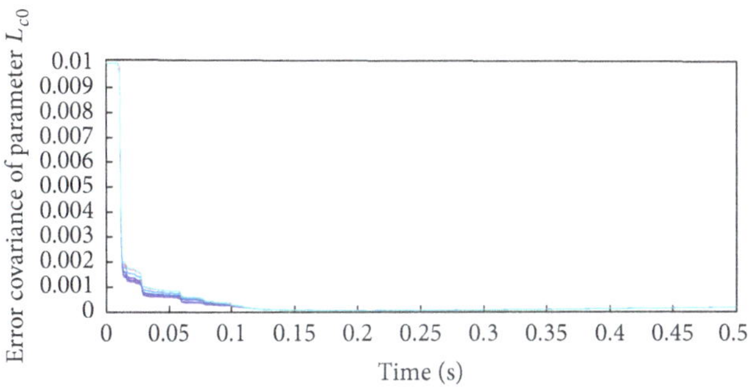

(b)

FIGURE 7: Estimated parameter for the original length of the contractile element L_{c0} (a) and its error covariance (b) with SPKF. The plot color is changed from magenta to cyan with 7 different initial values from 55 mm to 85 mm.

TABLE 1: The covariance matrix initialization.

Initial covariance matrix (geometric)
$\mathbf{P_x} = \text{diag}([1 \quad 0.1 \quad 0.1 \quad 1 \quad 1 \quad 10 \quad 10^{-2}])$
$\mathbf{Q_v} = \text{diag}([2.5 \quad 0.1 \quad 0.1 \quad 2.5 \quad 2.5 \quad 10 \quad 10^{-3}] \times 10^{-4})$
$\mathbf{R_n} = 2.5 \times 10^{-3}$
Initial covariance matrix for (dynamic)
$\mathbf{P_x} = \text{diag}([1 \quad 0.1 \quad 0.1 \quad 1 \quad 1 \quad 10 \quad 10^{-4} \quad 10])$
$\mathbf{Q_v} = \text{diag}([2.5 \quad 0.1 \quad 0.1 \quad 2.5 \quad 2.5 \quad 10 \quad 10^{-5} \quad 10^{-3}] \times 10^{-4})$
$\mathbf{R_n} = 2.5 \times 10^{-3}$

TABLE 2: Parameter estimation.

Parameters	Rabbit 1		Rabbit 2	
	16 Hz	20 Hz	16 Hz	20 Hz
L_{c0} (cm)	7.1	7.4	7.4	6.8
m (g)	16.5	19.8	36.5	39.8
λ (Ns/m)	19.7	19.4	19.7	19.2
NRMS (%)	0.60	0.46	1.02	0.82
Measured length of contractile element	7 cm		7 cm	
Body weight	4.5 kg		4.2 kg	

4.2. Comparison with the Extended Kalman Filter. The extended Kalman filter is generally chosen for nonlinear system identification. However, in EKF, first-order partial derivatives are used for the computation, which means that a matrix of partial derivatives (Jacobian) is computed around the estimate for each step. The detail of EKF is summarized in the appendix. When the process and measurement functions **f** and **h** are highly nonlinear, EKF can give particularly poor performance and diverge easily [25]. The estimate can have a bias due to the linear approximation especially for discontinuous systems.

Using the same computational conditions, such as initial values for states, parameters, and covariance matrices, parameter estimation was also performed with EKF to compare the estimation quality for this nonlinear system. The estimation results with EKF are shown in Figures 8 and 9. The numerical comparison for SPKF and EKF in 7 different initial conditions is summarized in Table 3 both for rabbit1 and rabbit2. With the observation noise covariance $R = 2.5 \times 10^{-3}$, the same as with SPKF, the result with EKF converged computationally as shown at the error covariance of EKF1 in the table. However, the matched result in force level does not mean directly that the estimated internal state and parameter are correct. The internal state ε_c in EKF estimation was not well estimated as the contracted strain variation. The difference can be observed by comparing the plots of Figures 9 and 6 for the EKF and SPKF estimates, respectively. In Figure 6, the estimated state of ε_c has two sharp peaks which correspond to the strain of the contractile element induced by muscle contraction by doublet stimulation. Thus, this internal state reflects the expected phenomenon in muscle dynamics. However, the estimated state in Figure 9 does not show sharp deformation induced by stimulation pulse.

The linear approximation in the EKF transformation matrix could be the cause of the lower quality of the state estimation. Finally, it resulted in a bias for parameter estimation. Thus, the converged value for L_{c0} under these conditions is not realistic. The EKF estimation was also performed with the observation noise covariance $R = 2.5 \times 10^{-2}$, giving more uncertainty to the measurement update. In this case, the estimated value became more realistic as the SPKF estimate did. However, the convergence became poor as in Figure 8(b) and it was highly dependent on the initial values as in Figure 8(a).

4.3. Model Cross-Validation. A cross-validation of the identified model was carried out to confirm the validity of this method. The resultant muscle force was calculated using the identified models with the control input generated by the stimulation frequency. Figure 10 shows the measured force response of the MG muscle of the rabbit and the simulated force with the identified model. The stimulation was three successive pulses in $I = 105\,\mu$A, PW $= 300\,\mu$s, and Freq $=$ 31.25 Hz. The red line indicates the measured muscle force, the blue and green dotted lines are the plots by the identified model with SPKF and EKF1, respectively. The model identified by SPKF could predict the nonlinear force properties of stimulated muscle quite well in this cross-validation. Figure 11

TABLE 3: Quantitative comparison on identification (SPKF versus EKF) in 7 different initial conditions.

Rabbit 1	SPKF	EKF1	EKF2
P for F_e	1.61×10^{-4}	1.61×10^{-4}	4.51×10^{-4}
P for L_{c0}	1.81×10^{-4}	2.47×10^{-4}	2.9×10^{-3}
Mean L_{c0} (cm)	7.4	4.7	7.5
Deviation L_{c0} (cm)	6.12×10^{-2}	7.67×10^{-3}	0.34
Average errors (%)	5.7	33.6	6.9
Rabbit 2	SPKF	EKF1	EKF2
P for F_e	1.72×10^{-4}	1.61×10^{-4}	4.53×10^{-4}
P for L_{c0}	8.97×10^{-4}	3.93×10^{-4}	2.5×10^{-3}
Mean L_{c0} (cm)	6.8	3.9	10.4
Deviation L_{c0} (cm)	8.92×10^{-2}	3.38×10^{-2}	6.49×10^{-2}
Average errors (%)	2.9	44.9	47.9

EKF1 and EKF2 represent EKF estimation with the observation noise covariance $R = 2.5 \times 10^{-3}$ and $R = 2.5 \times 10^{-2}$, respectively. P represents steady-state error covariance.

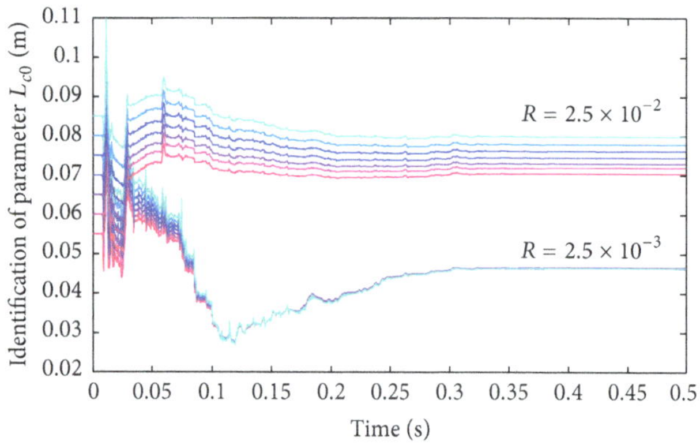

(a)

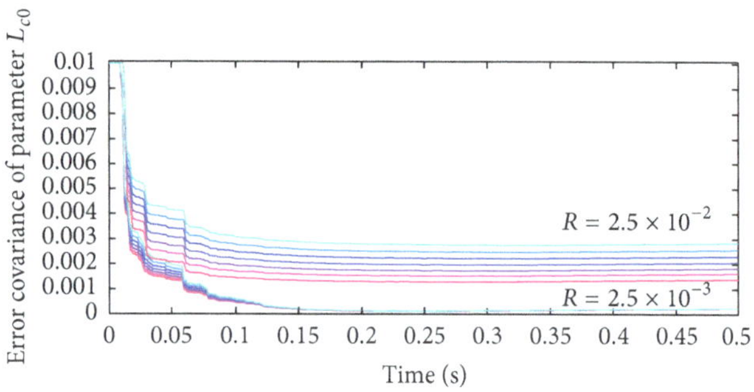

(b)

FIGURE 8: Estimated parameter for the original length of the contractile element L_{c0} (a) and its error covariance (b) with EKF. The plot color is changed from magenta to cyan with 7 different initial values from 55 mm to 85 mm. The results with two different settings for the observation noise covariance are shown.

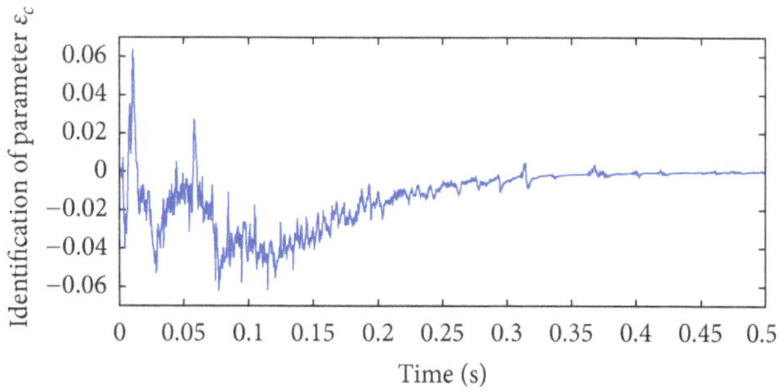

FIGURE 9: Estimated state of the strain of the contractile element ε_c with EKF.

is the result in the case of stimulation trains with six pulses in 20 Hz. There is a good agreement between the measured and the predicted force; however, when muscle fatigue appears, the experimental force is lower than that from the simulation. Particualrly, the difference between the measured and the estimated forces at the end can be considered as the error coming from modeling without considering muscle fatigue. Apart from the error coming from muscle fatigue, we could confirm the feasibility of the FES muscle modeling and the effectiveness of the identification. Normally, the muscle property varies greatly, being dependent on the type of muscle, and the force response is highly subject-specific. Therefore, the muscle force prediction by cross-validation is quite difficult even for the approximate prediction especially when force production is predicted for each stimulation pulse. The identification based on experimental response would contribute strongly to realistic force prediction in electrical stimulation and FES controller development. Further investigation is required for the expression of fatigue phenomena [27], for its reproducibility and identification.

5. Discussion

The skeletal muscle model used in this identification protocol is based on both macroscopic and microscopic physiology which is unlike the black-box or other approaches using simple Hill muscle model. The structured model requires more parameters in highly nonlinear dynamics, which have to be estimated by experiment. However, the great advantage of our model is the insight which it can give to a muscle's biomechanical and physiological connections, where the parameters have a physical significance such as length and mass. This paper describes an identification method which uses experimental response and a nonlinear, physiological muscle model to obtain subject-specific parameters. The advantage of animal experiment is to have direct access to extracted muscle for confirmation of the obtained parameter after the experiment.

This work was performed for application of FES stimulated muscles; however, since many living systems have nonlinear dynamics and subject specificity, this kind of identification approach itself could be applied to other organ models and clinical situations. In this work, both SPKF and EKF algorithms were applied for muscle dynamics identification. EKF showed a high dependency on initial settings of the computation and it was difficult to find the effective range of initial states and covariances. In SPKF, the obtained result was more consistent and robust with respect to various initial conditions. Moreover, for SPKF,

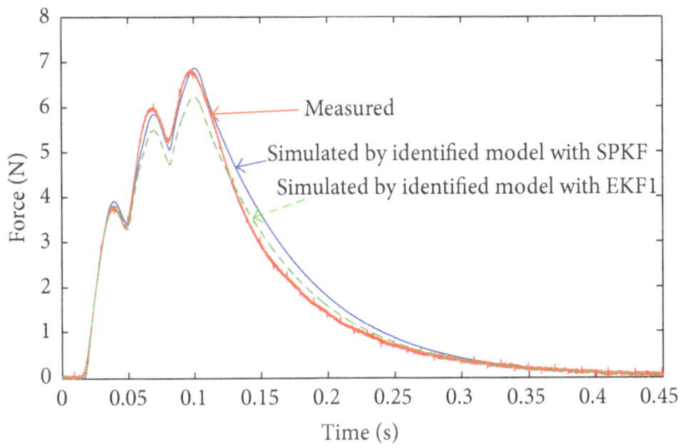

FIGURE 10: Measured and simulated isometric muscle force by the identified models with three successive stimulation pulses (in $I = 105\,\mu$A, PW = 300 μs, and Freq = 31.25 Hz).

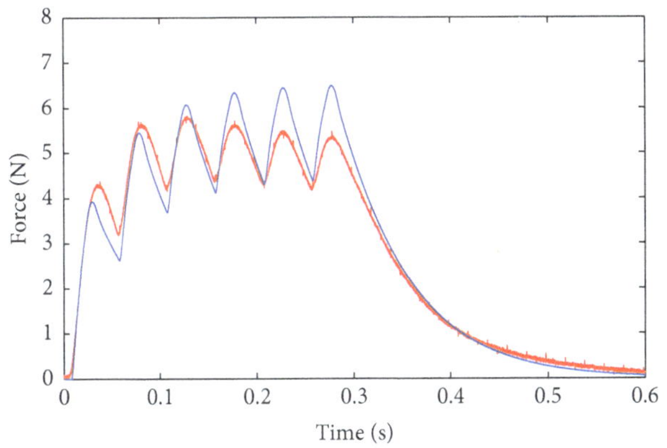

FIGURE 11: Measured (red) and simulated isometric muscle force by the identified model (blue) with six successive stimulation pulses (in $I = 105\,\mu$A, PW = 300 μs, and Freq = 20 Hz).

the computation of a Jacobian is not necessary, so it can easily be applied even to complex dynamics. SPKF results in approximations that are accurate to at least second order in Taylor series expansion. In contrast, EKF results in first-order accuracy. Further, the identification accuracy is clealy improved, especially for nonlinear systems, but the computation cost still remains the same as for EKF. Advanced and robust system identification, including designing experimental protocols, has a very important role to improve the control issues in neuroprosthetics. In addition, the main difficulty in understanding human systems is caused by their time-varying properties. The systems are not static and change over time. The function of a human being is not always the same; for example, muscle fatigue can easily change the expected force response. In order to deal with the time-varying characteristics of a human system, robust biosignal processing and model-based control which corresponded to nonlinearity and time variance would provide a breakthrough in the development of neuroprosthetics [28].

6. Conclusion

We have developed an experimental identification method for subject-specific biomechanical parameters of a skeletal muscle model which can be employed to predict the nonlinear force properties of stimulated muscle. The mathematical muscle model accounts for the multiscale major effects occurring during electrical stimulation. Thus, the identification method was required to deal with the high nonlinearity and discontinous states between muscle contraction and relaxation phase. The identified model was evaluated by comparison with experimental measurements in cross-validation. There was a good agreement between measured and simulated muscle force outputs. The result showed the performance which can contribute to the prediction of the nonlinear force of stimulated muscle under FES. The feasibility of the identification could be demonstrated by comparison between the estimated parameter and the measured value. In this study, the identification was performed by sigma-point Kalman filter and extended Kalman filter. The performance was compared and summarized under the same computational conditions. SPKF gives more stable performance than EKF. The internal state in EKF estimation was not well estimated as the contracted muscle strain. In SPKF estimation, keeping the realistic state transition and independence from initial conditions, it could realize converged solution for each identification trial.

SPKF is a Bayesian estimation algorithm which recursively updates the posterior density of the system state as new observations arrive online. This framework can allow us to calculate any optimal estimate of the state using newly arriving information. We believe that the proposed identification method has also the advantage for human muscle identification while it provides not only better accuracy in nonlinear dynamics but also adaptability to time-varying systems. The preliminary result is reported as in [29].

Appendix

Extended Kalman Filter

The extended Kalman filter [30] extends the scope of Kalman filter to nonlinear optimal filtering problems by forming a Gaussian approximation of the distribution of state $\mathbf{x}$ and measurements $\mathbf{y}$ using a Taylor series-based transformation. It is based on linear approximations to the transformation matrix. Assuming the same nonlinear system as in (13), EKF approximates a process with nonlinear difference and measurement relationships as follows:

$$\begin{gathered}\mathbf{x}_{k+1} \approx \mathbf{f}(\widehat{\mathbf{x}}_k, 0) + \mathbf{A}_k(\mathbf{x}_k - \widehat{\mathbf{x}}_k),\\ \mathbf{y}_k \approx \mathbf{h}(\widehat{\mathbf{x}}_k, 0) + \mathbf{C}_k(\mathbf{x}_k - \widehat{\mathbf{x}}_k),\\ \mathbf{A}_k = \left.\frac{\partial \mathbf{f}}{\partial \mathbf{x}}\right|_{\mathbf{x}=\widehat{\mathbf{x}}_k}, \qquad \mathbf{C}_k = \left.\frac{\partial \mathbf{h}}{\partial \mathbf{x}}\right|_{\mathbf{x}=\widehat{\mathbf{x}}_k}.\end{gathered} \tag{A.1}$$

Note that the difference between EKF and KF is that the matrices $\mathbf{A}_k$ and $\mathbf{C}_k$ in KF are replaced with Jacobian matrices which are partial derivatives around the estimate in EKF.

In order to avoid numerical problems, it is necessary to proceed the algorithm by using a square root factorization as a UD decomposition which ensures that the covariance matrix remains a positive definite matrix.

References

[1] A. Kralj and T. Bajd, *Functional Electrical Stimulation: Standing and Walking After Spinal Cord Injury*, CRC Press, Boca Raton, Fla, USA, 1989.

[2] R. Kobetic, R. J. Triolo, and E. B. Marsolais, "Muscle selection and walking performance of multichannel FES systems for ambulation in paraplegia," *IEEE Transactions on Rehabilitation Engineering*, vol. 5, no. 1, pp. 23–29, 1997.

[3] N. D. N. Donaldson, T. A. Perkins, and A. C. M. Worley, "Lumbar root stimulation for restoring leg function: stimulator and measurement of muscle actions," *Artificial Organs*, vol. 21, no. 3, pp. 247–249, 1997.

[4] R. Kobetic, R. J. Triolo, J. P. Uhlir et al., "Implanted functional electrical stimulation system for mobility in paraplegia: a follow-up case report," *IEEE Transactions on Rehabilitation Engineering*, vol. 7, no. 4, pp. 390–398, 1999.

[5] D. Guiraud, T. Stieglitz, K. P. Koch, J. Divoux, and P. Rabischong, "An implantable neuroprosthesis for standing and walking in paraplegia: 5-year patient follow-up," *Journal of Neural Engineering*, vol. 3, no. 4, pp. 268–275, 2006.

[6] W. K. Durfee, "Control of standing and gait using electrical stimulation: influence of muscle model complexity on control strategy," *Progress in Brain Research*, vol. 97, pp. 369–381, 1993.

[7] R. Riener, "Model-based development of neuroprostheses for paraplegic patients," *Philosophical Transactions of the Royal Society B*, vol. 354, no. 1385, pp. 877–894, 1999.

[8] D. Popovic and T. Sinkjaer, *Control of Movement for the Physically Disabled: Control for Rehabilitation Technology*, Spinger, London, UK, 2000.

[9] A. F. Huxley, "Muscle structure and theories of contraction," *Progress in Biophysics and Biophysical Chemistry*, vol. 7, pp. 255–318, 1957.

[10] A. V. Hill, "The heat of shortening and the dynamic constants in muscle," *Proceedings of the Royal Society of London B*, vol. 126, no. 843, pp. 136–195, 1938.

[11] G. I. Zahalak, "A distribution-moment approximation for kinetic theories of muscular contraction," *Mathematical Biosciences*, vol. 55, no. 1-2, pp. 89–114, 1981.

[12] F. E. Zajac, "Muscle and tendon: properties, models, scaling, and application to biomechanics and motor control," *Critical Reviews in Biomedical Engineering*, vol. 17, no. 4, pp. 359–411, 1989.

[13] J. Bestel and M. Sorine, "A differential model of muscle contraction and applications," in *Schloessmann Seminar on Mathematical Models in Biology, Chemistry and Physics*, Max Plank Society, Bad Lausick, Germany, 2000.

[14] H. El Makssoud, D. Guiraud, P. Poignet et al., "Multiscale modeling of skeletal muscle properties and experimental validations in isometric conditions," *Biological Cybernetics*, vol. 105, no. 2, pp. 121–138, 2011.

[15] R. Riener, M. Ferrarin, E. E. Pavan, and C. A. Frigo, "Patient-driven control of FES-supported standing up and sitting down: experimental results," *IEEE Transactions on Rehabilitation Engineering*, vol. 8, no. 4, pp. 523–529, 2000.

[16] M. Hayashibe, P. Poignet, D. Guiraud, and H. El Makssoud, "Nonlinear identification of skeletal muscle dynamics with sigma-point Kalman Filter for model-based FES," in *Proceedings of the IEEE International Conference on Robotics and Automation (ICRA '08)*, pp. 2049–2054, Pasadena, Calif, USA, May 2008.

[17] T. Schauer, N. Negård, F. Previdi et al., "Online identification and nonlinear control of the electrically stimulated quadriceps muscle," *Control Engineering Practice*, vol. 13, no. 9, pp. 1207–1219, 2005.

[18] O. Sayadi and M. B. Shamsollahi, "ECG denoising and compression using a modified extended Kalman filter structure," *IEEE Transactions on Biomedical Engineering*, vol. 55, no. 9, pp. 2240–2248, 2008.

[19] E. J. Perreault, C. J. Heckman, and T. G. Sandercock, "Hill muscle model errors during movement are greatest within the physiologically relevant range of motor unit firing rates," *Journal of Biomechanics*, vol. 36, no. 2, pp. 211–218, 2003.

[20] R. Riener and J. Quintern, "A physiologically based model of muscle activation verified by electrical stimulation," *Bioelectrochemistry and Bioenergetics*, vol. 43, no. 2, pp. 257–264, 1997.

[21] W. K. Durfee and K. E. MacLean, "Methods for estimating isometric recruitment curves of electrically stimulated muscle," *IEEE Transactions on Biomedical Engineering*, vol. 36, no. 7, pp. 654–667, 1989.

[22] H. Hatze, "A general mycocybernetic control model of skeletal muscle," *Biological Cybernetics*, vol. 28, no. 3, pp. 143–157, 1978.

[23] H. El Makssoud, *Modelisation et identification des muscles squelettiques sous stimulation electrique fonctionnelle [Ph.D. thesis]*, University of Montpellier II, 2005.

[24] S. J. Julier and J. K. Uhlmann, "A new extension of the Kalman filter to nonlinear systems," in *Proceedings of the 11th International Symposim on Aerospace, Defence Sensing, Simulation and Controls (AeroSence '97)*, 1997.

[25] R. Merwe and E. Wan, "Sigma-point Kalman filters for probabilistic inference in dynamic state-space models," in *Proceedings of the Workshop on Advances in Machine Learning*, Montreal, Canada, June 2003.

[26] S. J. Julier and J. K. Uhlmann, "Unscented filtering and nonlinear estimation," *Proceedings of the IEEE*, vol. 92, no. 3, pp. 401–422, 2004.

[27] E. Rabischong and D. Guiraud, "Determination of fatigue in the electrically stimulated quadriceps muscle and relative effect of ischaemia," *Journal of Biomedical Engineering*, vol. 15, no. 6, pp. 443–450, 1993.

[28] M. Hayashibe, Q. Zhang, D. Guiraud, and C. Fattal, "Evoked EMG-based torque prediction under muscle fatigue in implanted neural stimulation," *Journal of Neural Engineering*, vol. 8, no. 6, Article ID 064001, 2011.

[29] M. Hayashibe, M. Benoussaad, D. Guiraud, P. Poignet, and C. Fattal, "Nonlinear identification method corresponding to muscle property variation in FES—experiments in paraplegic patients," in *Proceedings of the 3rd IEEE RAS and EMBS International Conference on Biomedical Robotics and Biomechatronics (BioRob '10)*, pp. 401–406, Tokyo, Japan, September 2010.

[30] P. Maybeck, *Stochastic Models, Estimation and Control*, vol. 2, Academic Press, New York, NY, USA, 1982.

Can Written Disclosure Reduce Psychological Distress and Increase Objectively Measured Injury Mobility of Student-Athletes? A Randomized Controlled Trial

Elaine Duncan,[1] Yori Gidron,[2] and David Lavallee[3]

[1] *Department of Psychology and Allied Health Sciences, Glasgow Caledonian University, Glasgow G4 0BA, UK*
[2] *Faculty of Medicine & Pharmacy, Free University of Brussels (VUB), 1050 Brussels, Belgium*
[3] *School of Sport Stirling, University of Stirling, Stirling FK9 4LA, UK*

Correspondence should be addressed to David Lavallee; david.lavallee@stir.ac.uk

Academic Editors: K.-H. Lin, M. Schmitter-Edgecombe, and Y. Wu

Injured students-athletes took part in a randomized controlled trial to test whether written disclosure could reduce psychological distress and improve injury mobility. Writing took place alongside prescribed physical rehabilitation and consisted of three 20-minute writing sessions, once a week for three consecutive weeks. Participants in the experimental injury-writing group (n = 25) followed a structured form of written disclosure, called the guided disclosure protocol (GDP). They firstly, wrote about the onset of their injury in a chronological manner, secondly, they explicitly labelled their emotions and described the impact of the injury, finally they wrote about future coping and psychological growth. Controls (n = 21) wrote about nonemotional and noninjury related topics. In addition to self-report measures, a physiotherapist, blind to experimental condition, assessed mobility at the injury site. Although self-report indices remained unchanged, the GDP group evidenced a significant improvement in injury mobility compared to controls.

1. Introduction

Empirical work with athletes reveals that sports injury can cause considerable psychological distress [1–3] and that injured athletes have higher levels of emotional disturbance than noninjured controls [4]. The consequent withdrawal from training and competition can also be destabilizing [5]. Moreover, loss of athletic identity, withdrawal from the social climate of sport, and the possibility that an injury is career ending create an atmosphere of extreme anxiety and isolation which researchers and practitioners liken to a grief process [6–8]. There is also evidence that the emotional milieu of injury impacts upon an athletes' perceived and actual rehabilitation [9]. Moreover, models of injury coping and prevention suggest that poor psychological recovery may leave athletes more susceptible to reinjury [5, 10]. It is thus widely acknowledged that processing cognitive and emotional distress and helping athletes cope with sport-specific situational factors following injury are essential for adherence to treatment and eventual recovery [5, 11, 12].

Awareness of such factors has led to an increase in psychological interventions being implemented alongside standard physical rehabilitation protocols. Although, Reese and colleagues applauded such integrated practice they nevertheless queried the efficacy of psychological interventions in sports injury rehabilitation [13]. In a recent review they found that interventions consisting of guided imagery, relaxation, microcounselling skills, acceptance and commitment therapy, and written disclosure reduced various types of injury-related psychological distress. However, Reese and colleagues appealed for more systematic and better designed interventions on the grounds that study density was too low to make useful generalizations and that research was often atheoretical and/or lacked systematic use of randomized controlled trial methodology [13].

Of particular relevance to the present paper were the reviews' findings on written disclosure. For clarity, it is important to note that "written disclosure" may also be known as emotional expression and/or expressive writing. In this type of intervention participants are typically asked to write about emotionally upsetting and/or traumatic experiences for fixed time periods. Over 250 studies (including meta-analyses and systematic reviews) have shown that written disclosure interventions, and in particular those that provide guidance on what to write, reduce intrusive thoughts, improve overall mood, and boost immune functioning [14–16]. In addition, improved psychological and physical outcomes have also been found in such clinical populations as cancer patients [17], coronary patients [18], those undergoing a surgical procedure [19], chronic pelvic pain sufferers [20], and those with rheumatoid arthritis [21]. The mechanisms underpinning the effects of written disclosure are still a live debate but consensus that an interaction between biological, social, and psychological mechanisms is most likely [14, 15]. Given this robust evidence base, it is surprising that only three published studies have utilized written disclosure in a sports context, with only two of these directly related to sports injury rehabilitation. In a qualitative study, Hudson and Day [22] explored athletes' experiences of expressive writing about competitive sport stressors. The study outcomes suggested that expressive writing was a relatively cost efficient and approachable way of helping athletes reframe stressors and manage emotions. Directly related to sports injury rehabilitation are two studies conducted by Mankad and colleagues [23, 24]. In a single case study design written disclosure was used to facilitate coping with severe injury [23]. The participant, a male gridiron footballer, reported improved mood and self-esteem. Narrative analysis highlighted that his writing was suffused with emotion and cognitive understanding of his injury. In a repeated measures design, Mankad et al. [24] asked elite athletes to write about their negative thoughts and feelings surrounding their injury and rehabilitation experience for three consecutive days. Participants reported reduced levels of stress and mood disturbance and improved markers of immunity [24]. Linguistic word count analysis of the athletes' writings revealed fewer grief responses to injury across writing days. Mankad et al. [24] have argued that writing may act as the vehicle for the emotional and cognitive processing necessary for psychological adjustment to and recovery from injury [13, 25]. However, Mankad [26] recommended further experimental trials and in particular those that included objective measurement of injury status alongside assessment of psychological outcomes.

In sum, preliminary research suggests that written disclosure is associated with positive outcomes in a sports injury context and that the time is right for expansion of research in this area [22]. The present study hoped to add to research investigating the efficacy of psychological interventions in sports injury rehabilitation with particular focus on whether a guided instructions form of written disclosure could reduce psychological distress and improve objectively measured injury mobility. Evidence suggests that the potential benefits of written disclosure can be optimized when participants are offered guidance on what to write, [14, 27] so our participants adhered to a guided disclosure protocol (GDP) designed by Duncan and Gidron [28].

The GDP attempts to embody some of the positive findings from research on written disclosure. In particular that participants should receive specific instructions that encourage them to write an organized self-reflective narrative and that writing is best conducted under timed and controlled conditions. The design and rationale of the GDP is also rooted in the theoretical and empirical work on the dynamics of traumatic memory encoding. Specifically, the contention that shifting such memories from implicit and limbic to explicit and more cortical recall may be beneficial via cognitive processing of affective and somatic experiences [32, 33]. Finally, the GDP instructions incorporate the principles of reappraisal, benefit finding, and self-regulation. Specifically, adopting multiple perspectives of an event and reviewing its capacity to provide adaptive schemas and resources to deal with similar future events are useful [34–36].

The GDP has already been found to reduce clinic visits in frequent clinic attendees [37] and reduce psychological distress in parents of children with cancer [38]. We propose that the GDP offers a framework for the processing and alleviation of the emotional and cognitive consequences associated with injury in a sports context. Evidence, cited above, suggests that writing can also improve various physical parameters. Hence, the present study assessed mobility status of the presenting injuries. It was hypothesized that the GDP, injury-writing participants would report reduced levels of psychological distress and enhanced mobility in comparison to those writing about nonemotive and noninjury related topics.

To increase methodological rigour, the study was a randomized controlled trial. In addition to self-report indices of psychological distress, a physiotherapist, blind to experimental condition, objectively measured mobility at the injury site. Given the infancy of research on writing and sports injury, it was felt more appropriate to include a wide variety of injuries, as opposed to screening for one injury type only. The sample was injured student-athletes.

1.1. Participants and Recruitment. Participants were recruited from the student population attending a large university in the United Kingdom. Informed consent and local ethics committee procedures and practice were followed and established in full for all participants. Recruitment was achieved via the placement of leaflets within the university's rehabilitation facilities. These leaflets contained a brief outline of the study, the extent of participant commitment, and inclusion criteria. To be included participants had to be 18 years of age or over, to have been injured during competition and/or training, to have an injury that forced cessation of training and competition, and be attending physical rehabilitation. Participants were trusted to self-assess whether they fulfilled such inclusion criteria and to make contact with the researcher. One further inclusion criteria was that our participants should be those whose self-worth was highly invested in their sport. Previous research and theory suggest that athletes who define themselves primarily through their sport are likely to experience higher levels of distress than those whose perception of self-worth is not exclusively drawn from identification with the athletic role [39, 40]. Thus, only those with a strong and exclusive identification with the athlete role (i.e., by scoring above 30 on the athletic identity measurement scale; see description of scales below) were invited to continue into the writing intervention itself. Those not meeting this threshold continued with physical rehabilitation as normal but were excluded from the writing intervention. We made no attempt to select for particular sports.

2. Method

Forty-six participants were randomly assigned to the nonemotive, noninjury writing control group ($n = 21$) or the GDP, injury-writing group ($n = 25$). Participants completed preintervention (baseline) and postintervention outcome measures of psychological distress. The study physiotherapist, blind to experimental condition, measured mobility at five time points: prior to the writing (baseline), after each of the three writing sessions, (writing days, 1, 2, and 3) and after writing (postintervention). The study recruitment period spanned six months. The time lapse between injury onset, the start of physical rehabilitation and involvement in the writing intervention was two weeks.

2.1. Procedure. All consenting participants were invited to complete the athletic identity measurement scale (AIMS) [39]. Those scoring above 30 and giving consent to go forward into the intervention were randomly assigned to the GDP, injury-writing group or the nonemotive, noninjury writing control group. Those not reaching this threshold were debriefed, thanked for their time, and continued with their prescribed physical rehabilitation as normal.

In order to complete the various indices of emotional distress, writing participants met with a researcher on five separate occasions. These were timed to coincide with their scheduled physical treatment. On each occasion, participants were given oral and written instructions. These differed per group and for each of the three sessions (see intervention instructions below). For both groups, writing sessions took place once a week for three consecutive weeks on the day of and immediately prior to their prescribed physiotherapy treatment. Participants wrote at a desk in a private room adjacent to where physiotherapy took place. Each writing session lasted 20 minutes. All writing sessions were supervised and timed by a researcher and conducted on an individual, not group, basis. Fresh writing materials were provided at each writing session. Participants did not have access to their previous writings. The researcher collected the writings at the end of each session. Participants were assigned a unique participant number and advised to keep writing free of personal identifiers. Participants were reassured that the content of their stories would be kept confidential and viewed only by the research team should content analysis of actual writings be deemed appropriate at a later date.

All those taking part in the writing intervention itself completed a battery of self-report indices at preintervention (baseline), on each of the three writing days and at a postintervention stage. The time lapse between completion of outcome measures at baseline, the start and/or end of the intervention was no more than two weeks. At the postintervention stage, participants were also asked how valuable/meaningful the writing sessions were, how much they had talked to others about what they had written, and how much they had thought about what they had written. These were each rated on a 7-point Likert scale where, for example, 1 = very valuable/meaningful and where 7 = not at all valuable/meaningful. Experiential questions of this nature are a norm in written-disclosure studies, providing feedback on the experience of writing itself.

The self-report indices were the Reinjury Anxiety Inventory (RIAI) [41, 42]; 30-item mood questionnaires [43], and the centre for Epidemiological Studies on Depression Scale (CESD-10) [44]. In addition to pre and postintervention mood-sampling, participants completed the same mood questionnaire immediately following each of the three 20-minute writing sessions. This provided a measure of mood at five points: prior to the writing intervention, (baseline) immediately following each of the three writing sessions (writing days, 1, 2, and 3), and approximately two weeks after writing (postintervention).

Mobility at the injury site was measured at these same five time points. During the three-week writing phase, measurement was taken immediately after the timed writing sessions. When measuring mobility, the physiotherapist adhered to standard protocols, such as ensuring each participant had adequate time to warm up and cool down. No changes were made to the physiotherapists' prescribed treatment and/or their way of working with a client.

2.2. Intervention Instructions

2.2.1. Instructions to Participants in the GDP, Injury-Writing Group. As described in the procedure above, participants wrote on three separate occasions at weekly intervals. The sessions lasted 20 minutes. An outline of the instructions is provided, but for verbatim instructions please contact the first author. On the first day of writing (writing day 1) GDP participants wrote in a chronological and nonemotive manner about the occurrence of the injury. They were asked to provide an account of when the injury happened, the circumstances around its occurrence and to do so in a detached, objectively descriptive way. On writing day 2 (one week later), participants were asked to write about the emotions and feelings at the time of injury and its immediate impact on day-to-day life. Finally, in the third week of the intervention (writing day 3), participants were guided to write about their current perspective on the injury, possible psychological growth, and future coping.

2.2.2. Instructions to Participants in the Nonemotive, Noninjury Writing Group. Participants in the control group were also asked to engage in writing on three separate occasions spaced across a three-week period. Participants in this group were guided to write about nonemotive, noninjury related topics. Thus, on writing day 1, they were invited to write about what they had done since waking up that morning, on the second, to detail a recent social event, and on the third, their plans for the remainder of the day. On each occasion, it was stressed that they describe things exactly as they occurred or would occur, not to mention emotions, feelings, or opinions, but to be as objective as possible. Verbatim instructions for the control group are available by contacting the first author.

2.3. Description of Measures

2.3.1. Injury Mobility. We examined mobility across a range of injuries experienced by study participants. Mobility at the injury site was measured on five occasions with a Cybex 330 isokinetic exercise and monitoring machine. Isokinetic concentric peak torque measurements (in Newton-meters) were taken prior to the intervention, after each of the three writing sessions, and after the intervention.

2.3.2. Adherence to Rehabilitation. The physiotherapist also recorded the level of adherence to rehabilitation of each participant. This was simply recorded as the number of sessions actually attended, expressed as a percentage of total visits prescribed.

2.3.3. Psychological Measures

Athletic Identity Measurement Scale. This scale measures the strength and exclusivity of identification with the athletic role [39]. It is a 10-item scale with ratings on a 7-point Likert scale. The scale includes elements of athletic identity such as social (e.g., "Most of my friends are athletes"), cognitive (e.g., "I have many goals related to sport"), and affective (e.g., "I feel bad about myself when I do poorly in sport"). Final ratings were summed to provide an overall athletic identity score. The psychometric integrity of the AIMS has been provided through previous research [39]. This scale was used as part of the inclusion criteria as described above.

Reinjury Anxiety Inventory [41]. This scale probes the degree to which already injured athletes fear reinjury and has been shown to be a reliable and valid measure [42]. The inventory contains 28 items (on a 0–3 Likert scale, where 0 = not at all and 3 = very much so) and two subscales: reinjury anxiety in rehabilitation (RIA-R) and reinjury anxiety regarding reentry into competition (RIA-RE). The RIA-R has a range of 0–39, whereas the RIA-RE has a range of 0–45 with lower scores indicating less anxiety on both subscales.

Mood Questionnaire [43]. Positive and negative mood was measured at baseline and postintervention and following each writing session. This scale is a 30-item scale with equal numbers of positive and negative mood dimensions. Scoring is accomplished by summing points on a 5-point Likert scale for the 15 items pertaining to each mood dimension.

Centre of Epidemiological Studies Depression Scale [44]. This is designed to measure depressive symptomology in the general population. The original scale had 20 items, but the 10-item scale was chosen to lessen the burden on participants and because reliability statistics indicate that shorter versions of the scale do not sacrifice precision [45].

The decision to include indices of general mood, depressive symptomology, and fears around injury was not an arbitrary one, but informed by previous research into the experience and consequences of sports injury, cited above. For the purposes of this study these scales constituted our measure of psychological distress.

3. Results

3.1. Descriptive Statistics and Baseline Group Equality. Table 1(a) depicts the general categorical characteristics for the entire sample. Table 1(b) depicts the entire sample's data on continuous measures. The table lists the type of injuries presented in rehabilitation. Knee injury was the most common, followed by injuries sustained to the ankle area. Participants also presented with injuries to the shoulder, lower leg, and back.

Table 2 depicts the baseline and postintervention scores on the study outcomes, per group. At baseline, the GDP injury writing group's score on AIMS was significantly higher than that of controls ($t(44) = 2.48, P < .05$). Similarly, this group RAI-RE score was significantly higher than that of controls ($t(42) = 2.48, P < .05$). Thus, in the main outcome analyses, AIMS and RAI-RE were statistically controlled for. No other continuous background or outcome variable differed significantly between groups at baseline. Groups did not differ on gender or adherence to rehabilitation.

3.2. Main Outcome Analyses. Table 3 depicts the results of the mixed-design analyses of covariance (ANCOVA), controlling for baseline AIMS, and RAI-RE. A statistically significant time × group interaction was found for mobility, even when controlling for baseline mobility. Simple-effects analyses revealed that groups differed significantly on mobility at writing day 1 ($F(1, 32) = 10.8, P < .005$); at writing day 2 ($F(1, 31) = 17.6, P < .001$), at writing day 3 ($F(1, 33) = 22.2, P < .001$), and at the postintervention measurement ($F(1, 32) = 26.2, P < .001$). This interaction is depicted in Figure 1. In Figure 1, numbers 1, 2, 3, and 4 represent writing day 1 through to the postintervention measurement. Table 3 also depicts that time tended to interact with group in relation to depressive symptoms ($P = .06$) but this change was not statistically significant.

3.3. Post-Writing Evaluation. Participants in the GDP group reported significantly higher scores to the questions on how meaningful and how valuable the writing had been when compared to the controls. Though not statistically significant, GDP participants tended to think more about their writing than controls ($t(42) = 1.77, P < .10$) but did not differ on talking about the written content with others from controls ($t(42) = 1.04$).

4. Discussion

Evidence suggested that various forms of psychological interventions, including written disclosure could be useful adjuncts to standard physical rehabilitation in a sports context [13]. However, despite a strong evidence base only two

Table 1: Sample characteristics.

(a) Categorical data

Variable	%
Gender	
Men	58.7
Women	41.3
Locus of injury	
Knee	48.8
Ankle	30.2
Lower leg	11.6
Shoulder	7.0
Back	2.3
Adherence	
None	6.5
60%	6.5
80%	21.7
100%	65.2

(b) Continuous data (baseline)

Variable	Mean	SD
Age	21.5	2.9
AIMS	31.2	5.6
Mood—a	27.1	4.3
Mood—b	27.3	4.4
Depressive symptoms	20.8	3.7
RAI-R	15.5	8.1
RAI-RE	22.5	9.1
Mobility	30.1	14.1

Note. AIMS: athletic identity measurement scale; Mood—a: positive emotion; Mood—b: negative emotion; RAI-R: reinjury anxiety in rehabilitation; RAI-RE: reinjury anxiety reentry into competition.

Table 2: Baseline background information and pre- and postintervention results on outcomes per study group.

Variable	GDP		Control	
	Mean	SD	Mean	SD
Age	21.2	3.0	21.9	2.9
Adherence	87.2	22.3	85.7	30.4
AIMS	39.0	5.3	35.0	5.3*
Mood—a—baseline/preintervention	27.8	3.6	26.3	4.9
Mood—a—writing day 1	23.5	4.5	21.2	5.8
Mood—a—writing day 2	24.3	4.0	22.5	5.9
Mood—a—writing day 3	23.3	4.2	21.8	5.9
Mood—a—time 4/postintervention	26.8	5.0	28.4	6.1
Mood—b—baseline/preintervention	28.1	4.1	26.5	4.5
Mood—b—writing day 1	24.0	4.2	23.2	5.4
Mood—b—writing day 2	25.7	4.8	23.4	4.7
Mood—b—writing day 3	24.7	4.9	23.4	5.2
Mood—b—time 4/postintervention	26.0	5.9	25.9	5.4
Depression—baseline	9.2	4.5	8.8	4.7
Depression—post	9.3	5.8	7.7	3.7
RAI-R—baseline	16.8	7.5	13.7	8.7
RAI-R—post	16.9	7.6	13.2	9.8
RAI-RE—baseline	25.4	8.4	18.8	9.0*
RAI-RE—post	24.5	8.8	18.0	8.6
Mobility—baseline/preintervention	27.7	11.8	33.3	16.4
Mobility—writing day 1	3.8	2.5	1.8	1.4
Mobility—writing day 2	5.4	2.1	2.5	1.3
Mobility—writing day 3	8.4	3.3	3.2	1.5
Mobility—time 4/postintervention	9.7	4.4	3.6	1.5

Note: $^*P < .05$; $^{**}P < .01$.
GDP: Guided Disclosure Protocol. AIMS: athletic identity measurement scale; RAI-R: reinjury anxiety in rehabilitation; RAI-RE: reinjury anxiety reentry into competition; Mood—a: positive emotion; Mood—b: negative emotion.

Table 3: Results of analyses of covariance testing interaction effects of group (GDP, control) by time since writing on study outcomes, controlling for covariates.

Outcome	Effect	*F*	DF	Significance
Mobility	Time × Group	16.36	3,69	.000
Depression	Time × Group	3.73	1, 36	.06

studies to date had sought to use writing in a sports injury rehabilitation context [23, 24]. Aiming to extend research, the present study investigated whether a structured form of writing (GDP) could decrease psychological distress and increase injury mobility in student-athletes. Although, none of the self-report measures were differently affected by groups' mobility those in the GDP group improved almost three times compared to controls. These effects were independent of baseline AIMS, RAI-RE, and baseline mobility.

We believe that this is only the third study to have implemented written disclosure in a sports injury rehabilitation context. Although, the present study and those carried out by Mankad and colleagues found positive results major differences between the studies make direct comparison difficult. The sample in the present study was drawn from a population of student-athletes whereas those in Mankad's studies were described as elite level athletes. Although, each study contained measures of psychological and physical indices the types of instruments and procedures used varied as did the writing instructions. Unlike the others, the present study operationalized writing within randomized controlled trial methodology and included an objectively measured outcome. Despite such differences each study and the present provide evidence of gains from writing and how easy it is to implement such interventions.

Despite evidence that writing improves psychological outcomes in many diverse clinical and nonclinical samples, [14] our judgment of its ability to do so within a sports injury rehabilitation context would need to be a conservative one. More research is needed before declaring that written disclosure can be used alongside physical rehabilitation protocols to ameliorate psychological distress. Yet this study informed us that it possible to engage injured student athletes in the process of working through injury related emotions and cognitions via structured written disclosure.

It is also worth noting that evidence of positive change in physical but not psychological outcomes is not an unfamiliar

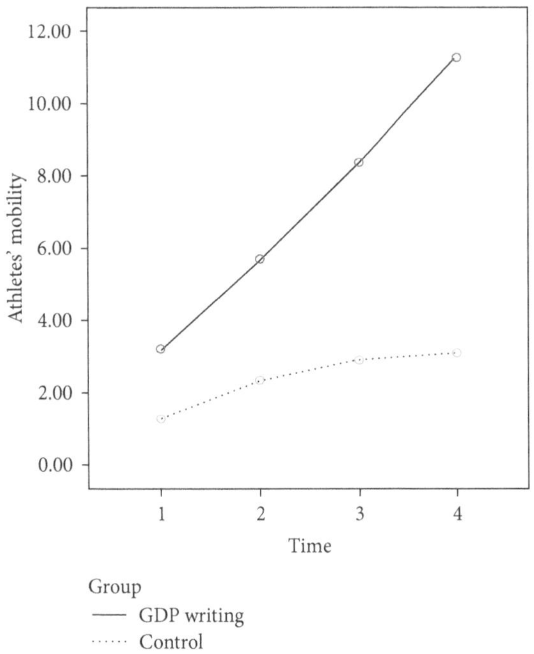

FIGURE 1: Effects of group and time on athletes' mobility.

pattern in writing studies [17, 21]. For example, Weinman and colleagues [46] investigated whether written disclosure could speed the progress of wound healing in healthy participants. All participants had agreed to have a 4 mm skin biopsy taken in the upper area of their nondominant arm. Participants in the emotional disclosure group evidenced significantly smaller wounds 14 and 21 days following the biopsy compared to participants who wrote about time management. Despite significant improvement in the main physical outcome, emotional disclosure had no effect on levels of the study's self-report outcomes, perceived stress, emotional distress, and health behaviours. Moreover, an authoritative review of 146 written disclosure studies noted that written disclosure does not always evidence changes in perceived stress or health behaviour even in the face of physical improvement [14]. Of course it is possible that the psychological inventories we used were not sensitive enough to capture any change in the psychological responses to injury in this particular sample. Yet our psychological measures were not atypical to those of previous sports injury studies where improved psychological outcomes have occurred [13]. It may also be the case that changes in such psychological indices would only be apparent in those who experienced much higher levels of injury-related distress than participants in our study.

It is the case that variation in such factors as dosage, the writing instructions, and the setting in which writing takes place moderate the outcomes of writing interventions [14]. It is therefore possible that our findings are an artefact of differences in the design and implementation of our intervention. For example, rather than three consecutive days of writing our participants adhered to a once a week for three weeks dosage. In addition our GDP instructions form part of a more structured form of disclosure than is typically seen in writing studies. In guiding our participants to write about day-to-day impact and possible psychological growth we encourage them to move beyond mere emotional catharsis and this may have implications for mood and other psychological processes. These factors may have contributed to the differential pattern of our outcomes but until we conduct a study with sufficient power and experimental conditions that address these factors we have no evidence that they moderated our main outcomes.

Nevertheless, the absence of effects on psychological outcomes makes accounting for the mechanisms underlying the improved mobility of our participants challenging. It is possible to speculate that mobility improvement was driven by upregulation of biological mediators. Indeed, one of the mechanisms by which expressive writing is said to work is that it lessens overall physiological stress, thereby promoting better physical functioning (15). We know that studies have shown that higher levels of psychological distress are related to slower wound healing [47]. This may occur due to the dysregulation of various derivatives of immunity such as insufficient interleukin-1 (IL-1) or matrix metalloproteinase [48], which are pivotal in wound healing [49]. Although psychological stress is related to inflammatory and molecular variables which influence healing [50], it is possible that the psychological tests used in the present study did not map onto such local molecular changes. However, the present study did not include measures of such biological mediators, consequently the proposal that writing aided immunity and inflammatory processes can be no more than speculation. In addition, we did not account for other factors that may impact on immunity and thereby tissue repair, such as health behaviours and sleep quality.

Although attendance at rehabilitation reached ceiling for both groups, it is possible that the GDP group adhered better to treatment protocols between sessions, but this was not assessed. Future studies may wish to track athletes adherence to treatment protocols between rehabilitation visits to test whether it may account for the changes in mobility observed in the present study. Nevertheless, our results add support to previous research on the positive association between rehabilitation adherence and rehabilitation outcome [51].

We took no account of preinjury psychological profile and previous history of injury and we do not know when, or if, these student-athletes returned to training and competition. Nevertheless, we observed significant improvements in mobility, using an independent rater, blind to group status, in a randomized controlled trial. In addition postintervention feedback informed us that writing about the thoughts and feelings surrounding injury was valuable and meaningful. The present study may have been enhanced by the inclusion of content analysis of the GDP participants' writing to check for linguistic markers of change in emotion and cognitions in relation to their injury.

5. Conclusion

Research into the benefits of written disclosure in a sports-injury context is in its infancy. The present study is the first to implement randomized controlled trial methodology in order to test the efficacy of written disclosure and the first to use objective measurement of mobility alongside writing. The findings of the present study, though positive with respect to mobility, did not provide direct evidence that the GDP alleviates self-reported psychological distress. Results showed significant change in injury status but the exact mechanisms of such changes are unclear. This study demonstrated that it is possible to engage injured athletes in a short-term, writing intervention in the early stages of prescribed physical rehabilitation. However, future writing studies that follow athletes to the end of rehabilitation and into the return to competition phase are needed. Including measures of immunity may provide more direct evidence of underlying mechanisms than are presently available. Finally, the GDP is not the only form of written disclosure thus future studies could compare its efficacy against other types of writing protocols within a sports injury and rehabilitation context.

References

[1] J. Tracey, "The emotional response to the injury and rehabilitation process," *Journal of Applied Sport Psychology*, vol. 15, no. 4, pp. 279–293, 2003.

[2] F. Carson and R. Polman, "Experiences of professional rugby union players returning to competition following anterior cruciate ligament reconstruction," *Physical Therapy in Sport*, vol. 13, no. 1, pp. 35–40, 2012.

[3] R. N. Appaneal, B. R. Levine, F. M. Perna, and J. L. Roh, "Measuring postinjury depression among male and female competitive athletes," *Journal of Sport and Exercise Psychology*, vol. 31, no. 1, pp. 60–76, 2009.

[4] B. W. Brewer, "Psychology of sport injury rehabilitation," in *Handbook of Sport Psychology*, R. N. Singer, H. A. Hausenblas, and C. M. Janelle, Eds., John Wiley & Sons, New York, NY, USA, 2001.

[5] M. Arvinen-Barrow and N. Walker, Eds., *The Psychology of Sport Injury and Rehabilitation*, Routledge, London, UK, 2012.

[6] L. Evans and L. Hardy, "Sport injury and grief responses: a review," *Journal of Sport and Exercise Psychology*, vol. 17, no. 3, pp. 227–245, 1995.

[7] P. Edouard, J. Pruvost, J. Edouard, and J. Morin, "Causes of dropouts in decathlon. A pilot study," *Physical Therapy in Sport*, vol. 11, no. 4, pp. 133–135, 2010.

[8] A. C. Cartoni, C. Minganti, and A. Zelli, "Gender, age and professional-level differences in the psychological correlates of fear of injury in Italian gymnasts," *Journal of Sport Behaviour*, vol. 28, no. 1, pp. 3–17, 2005.

[9] M. A. Morrey, M. J. Stuart, A. M. Smith, and D. M. Wiese-Bjornstal, "A longitudinal examination of athletes' emotional and cognitive responses to anterior cruciate ligament injury," *Clinical Journal of Sport Medicine*, vol. 9, no. 2, pp. 63–69, 1999.

[10] D. M. Wiese-Bjornstal, "Psychology and socioculture affect injury risk, response, and recovery in high-intensity athletes: a consensus statement," *Scandinavian Journal of Medicine and Science in Sports*, vol. 20, supplement 2, pp. 103–111, 2010.

[11] D. M. Wiese-Bjornstal, A. M. Smith, S. M. Shaffer, and M. A. Morrey, "An integrated model of response to sport injury: psychological and sociological dynamics," *Journal of Applied Scientific Medicine*, vol. 10, no. 1, pp. 46–69, 1998.

[12] M. S. Hagger, M. Griffin, N. L. D. Chatzisarantis, and J. Thatcher, "Injury representations, coping, emotions, and functional outcomes in athletes with sports-related injuries: a test of self-regulation theory," *Journal of Applied Social Psychology*, vol. 35, no. 11, pp. 2345–2374, 2005.

[13] L. M. S. Reese, R. Pittsinger, and J. Yang, "Effectiveness of psychological interventions following sport injury," *Journal of Sport and Health Science*, vol. 1, no. 2, pp. 71–70, 2012.

[14] J. Frattaroli, "Experimental disclosure and its moderators: a meta-analysis," *Psychological Bulletin*, vol. 132, no. 6, pp. 823–865, 2006.

[15] K. A. Baikie and K. Wilhelm, "Emotional and physical health benefits of expressive writing," *Advances in Psychiatric Treatment*, vol. 11, no. 5, pp. 338–346, 2005.

[16] J. E. Owen, E. R. Hanson, D. A. Preddy, and E. O. Bantum, "Linguistically-tailored video feedback increases total and positive emotional expression in a structured writing task," *Computers in Human Behavior*, vol. 27, no. 2, pp. 874–882, 2011.

[17] C. E. Mosher, K. N. DuHamel, J. Lam et al., "Randomised trial of expressive writing for distressed metastatic breast cancer patients," *Psychology and Health*, vol. 27, no. 1, pp. 88–100, 2012.

[18] G. M. Manzoni, G. Castelnuovo, and E. Molinari, "The WRITTEN-HEART study (expressive writing for heart healing): rationale and design of a randomized controlled clinical trial of expressive writing in coronary patients referred to residential cardiac rehabilitation," *Health and Quality of Life Outcomes*, vol. 9, article 51, 2011.

[19] L. Solano, V. Donati, F. Pecci, S. Persichetti, and A. Colaci, "Postoperative course after papilloma resection: effects of written disclosure of the experience in subjects with different alexithymia levels," *Psychosomatic Medicine*, vol. 65, no. 3, pp. 477–484, 2003.

[20] S. A. Norman, M. A. Lumley, J. A. Dooley, and M. P. Diamond, "For whom does it work? Moderators of the effects of written emotional disclosure in a randomized trial among women with chronic pelvic pain," *Psychosomatic Medicine*, vol. 66, no. 2, pp. 174–183, 2004.

[21] J. E. Kelley, M. A. Lumley, and J. C. C. Leisen, "Health effects of emotional disclosure in rheumatoid arthritis patients," *Health Psychology*, vol. 16, no. 4, pp. 331–340, 1997.

[22] J. Hudson and M. C. Day, "Athletes' experiences of expressive writing about sports stressors," *Psychology of Sport and Exercise*, vol. 13, no. 6, pp. 798–806, 2012.

[23] A. Mankad and S. Gordon, "Psycholinguistic changes in athletes' grief response to injury after written emotional disclosure," *Journal of Sport Rehabilitation*, vol. 19, no. 3, pp. 328–342, 2010.

[24] A. Mankad, S. Gordon, and K. E. Wallman, "Psycholinguistic analysis of emotional disclosure: a case study in sport injury," *Journal of Clinical Sports Psychology*, vol. 3, no. 2, pp. 182–196, 2009.

[25] D. Durso-Cupal, "Psychological interventions in sport injury prevention and rehabilitation," *Journal of Applied Sport Psychology*, vol. 10, no. 1, pp. 103–123, 1998.

[26] A. Mankad, *The role of inhibition and written disclosure in sport injury rehabilitation [Unpublished thesis]*, 2009.

[27] N. Vrielynck, P. Philippot, and B. Rimé, "Level of processing modulates benefits of writing about stressful events: comparing generic and specific recall," *Cognition and Emotion*, vol. 24, no. 7, pp. 1117–1132, 2010.

[28] E. Duncan and Y. Gidron, "Written emotional expression and health: evidence for a new guided-disclosure technique,"

Proceedings of the British Psychological Society, vol. 7, no. 1, p. 29, 1999.

[29] C. de Moor, J. Sterner, M. Hall et al., "A pilot study of the effects of expressive writing on psychological and behavioral adjustment in patients enrolled in a phase II trial of vaccine therapy for metastatic renal cell carcinoma," *Health Psychology*, vol. 21, no. 6, pp. 615–619, 2002.

[30] J. W. Pennebaker and J. R. Susman, "Disclosure of traumas and psychosomatic processes," *Social Science and Medicine*, vol. 26, no. 3, pp. 327–332, 1988.

[31] M. J. A. Schoutrop, A. Lange, G. Hanewald, U. Davidovich, and H. Salomon, "Structured writing and processing major stressful events: a controlled trial," *Psychotherapy and Psychosomatics*, vol. 71, no. 3, pp. 151–157, 2002.

[32] E. B. Foa, C. Molnar, and L. Cashman, "Change in rape narratives during exposure therapy for posttraumatic stress disorder," *Journal of Traumatic Stress*, vol. 8, no. 4, pp. 675–690, 1995.

[33] A. R. Moradi, M. R. Taghavi, H. T. N. Doost, W. Yule, and T. Dalgleish, "Performance of children and adolescents with PTSD on the Stroop colour-naming task," *Psychological Medicine*, vol. 29, no. 2, pp. 415–419, 1999.

[34] J. E. Bower, M. E. Kemeny, S. E. Taylor, and J. L. Fahey, "Finding positive meaning and its association with natural killer cell cytotoxicity among participants in a bereavement-related disclosure intervention," *Annals of Behavioral Medicine*, vol. 25, no. 2, pp. 146–155, 2003.

[35] M. A. Greenberg, C. B. Wortman, and A. A. Stone, "Emotional expression and physical health: revising traumatic memories or fostering self-regulation?" *Journal of Personality and Social Psychology*, vol. 71, no. 3, pp. 588–602, 1996.

[36] L. J. Warner, M. A. Lumley, R. J. Casey et al., "Health effects of written emotional disclosure in adolescents with asthma: a randomized, controlled trial," *Journal of Pediatric Psychology*, vol. 31, no. 6, pp. 557–568, 2006.

[37] Y. Gidron, E. Duncan, A. Lazar, A. Biderman, H. Tandeter, and P. Shvartzman, "Effects of guided written disclosure of stressful experiences on clinic visits and symptoms in frequent clinic attenders," *Family Practice*, vol. 19, no. 2, pp. 161–166, 2002.

[38] E. Duncan, Y. Gidron, E. Rabin, L. Gouchberg, A. M. Moser, and J. Kapelushnik, "The effects of guided written disclosure on psychological symptoms among parents of children with cancer," *Journal of Family Nursing*, vol. 13, no. 3, pp. 370–384, 2007.

[39] B. W. Brewer, J. L. van Raalte, and D. W. Linder, "Athletic identity: Hercules' muscles or Achilles' heel?" *International Journal of Sport Psychology*, vol. 24, pp. 237–254, 1993.

[40] P. D. Howe, *Sport, Professionalism and Pain: Ethnographies of Injury and Risk*, Routledge, London, UK, 2004.

[41] N. Walker, J. Thatcher, and D. Lavallee, "A preliminary development of the re-injury anxiety inventory (RIAI)," *Physical Therapy in Sport*, vol. 11, no. 1, pp. 23–29, 2010.

[42] N. Walker and J. Thatcher, "The emotional response to athletic injury: re-injury anxiety," in *Coping and Emotion in Sport*, J. Thatcher, D. Lavallee, and M. Jones, Eds., pp. 236–260, Routledge, Oxford, UK, 2012.

[43] M. A. Zevon and A. Tellegen, "The structure of mood change: an idiographic/nomothetic analysis," *Journal of Personality and Social Psychology*, vol. 43, no. 1, pp. 111–122, 1982.

[44] L. S. Radloff, "The CES-D scale: a self-report depression scale for research in the general population," *Applied Psychological Measurement*, vol. 1, pp. 385–401, 1977.

[45] E. M. Andresen, J. A. Malmgren, W. B. Carter, and D. L. Patrick, "Screening for depression in well older adults: evaluation of a short form of the CES-D," *The American Journal of Preventive Medicine*, vol. 10, no. 2, pp. 77–84, 1994.

[46] J. Weinman, M. Ebrecht, S. Scott, J. Walburn, and M. Dyson, "Enhanced wound healing after emotional disclosure intervention," *The British Journal of Health Psychology*, vol. 13, no. 1, pp. 95–102, 2008.

[47] L. V. Doering, D. K. Moser, W. Lemankiewicz, C. Luper, and S. Khan, "Depression, healing, and recovery from coronary artery bypass surgery," *The American Journal of Critical Care*, vol. 14, no. 4, pp. 316–324, 2005.

[48] Y. Y. Yang, H. F. Tsai, S. C. Lu, Y. F. Huang, and Y. C. Chang, "Regulation of tissue inhibitors of metalloproteinase-1 gene expression by cytokines in human gingival fibroblasts," *Journal of Endodontics*, vol. 28, no. 12, pp. 803–805, 2002.

[49] P. T. Marucha, J. K. Kiecolt-Glaser, and M. Favagehi, "Mucosal wound healing is impaired by examination stress," *Psychosomatic Medicine*, vol. 60, no. 3, pp. 362–365, 1998.

[50] M. Maes, C. Song, A. Lin et al., "The effects of psychological stress on humans: increased production of pro-inflammatory cytokines and a Th1-like response in stress-induced anxiety," *Cytokine*, vol. 10, no. 4, pp. 313–318, 1998.

[51] M. J. Satterfield, D. Dowden, and K. Yasumura, "Patient compliance for successful stress fracture rehabilitation," *Journal of Orthopaedic and Sports Physical Therapy*, vol. 11, no. 7, pp. 321–325, 1990.

17

Clinical Characteristics and Course of Patients Entering Cardiac Rehabilitation with Chronic Kidney Disease: Data from the Italian Survey on Cardiac Rehabilitation

Francesco Giallauria,[1] Francesco Fattirolli,[2] Roberto Tramarin,[3] Marco Ambrosetti,[4] Raffaele Griffo,[5] Carmine Riccio,[6] and Carlo Vigorito[1]

[1] *Department of Translational Medical Sciences, Cardiac Rehabilitation Unit, University of Naples "Federico II," Via S. Pansini 5, 80131 Naples, Italy*
[2] *Department of Critical Care Medicine and Surgery, Cardiac Rehabilitation Unit, University of Florence and Azienda Ospedaliero-Universitaria Careggi, Via delle Oblate 4, 50141 Florence, Italy*
[3] *Division of Cardiac Rehabilitation, Fondazione Europea di Ricerca Biomedica, Via Uboldo 56, 20063 Cernusco S/N, Italy*
[4] *Clinica "Le Terrazze," Via Foscolo 6/B, 21035 Cunardo, Italy*
[5] *Cardiac Rehabilitation Unit, Department of Cardiology, La Colletta Hospital, Via del Giappone, 16011 Arenzano, Italy*
[6] *Azienda Ospedaliera S. Anna e S. Sebastiano di Caserta, Via Gennaro Tescione 1, 81100 Caserta, Italy*

Correspondence should be addressed to Francesco Giallauria; giallauria@libero.it

Academic Editors: Y. Hu, Y. Laufer, and M. Probst

This survey shows the clinical risk profile, resource utilization, pharmacologic treatment, and course of cardiac rehabilitation (CR) programs in patients with chronic kidney disease (CKD). Data from 165 CR units in Italy were collected online from January 28 to February 10, 2008. The study cohort consisted of 2281 patients: 200 CKD patients and 2081 non-CKD patients. CKD patients were older and showed more comorbidity and complications during CR, a more complex clinical course and interventions with less functional evaluation, and a different pattern of drug therapy at hospital discharge. CKD patients had higher mortality during CR programs due to heart failure, respiratory insufficiency, and cognitive impairment. These findings suggest that patients with CKD should not be denied access to CR, provided careful attention to clinical status, possible complications, optimization of drug therapy, and close followup.

1. Introduction

Chronic kidney disease (CKD) is a major public health problem, strongly associated with a high cardiovascular mortality [1]. The high prevalence of established traditional risk factors for atherosclerosis such as diabetes, hypertension, and older age and nontraditional risk factors such as high level of homocysteine, lipoprotein (a), fibrinogen, and C-reactive protein in patients with CKD contributes to an accelerated rate of coronary heart disease (CHD) [2].

The American Heart Association scientific statement on kidney disease and cardiovascular disease has recommended that patients with CKD be placed in the highest-risk group for prevention, detection, and treatment of CHD risk factors [3]. CKD is prevalent in patients with CHD and is associated with a poor prognosis [4].

Exercise training alone or as core component of cardiac rehabilitation (CR) programs has several beneficial effects reducing long-term morbidity and mortality [5], preventing cardiac remodelling [6, 7], and improving cardiovascular functional capacity, cardiac symptoms, and quality of life [8]. The improvement of endothelial function [9], the anti-inflammatory properties [10], the improvement of neurohormonal and autonomic balance [11–14], and the reduction of oxidative stress [15] might be some of the putative mechanisms by which exercise training exerts its beneficial effects.

TABLE 1: Demographics characteristics of the study population (n, %).

	CKD (n = 200)	Non-CKD (n = 2081)	P value
Age (years) (mean ± SD)	73.6 ± 9.9	66.3 ± 11.7	<0.0001
Gender (male)	141 (70.5)	1536 (73.8)	0.31
Cardiovascular risk factors[1]			
0–2 (low)	57 (28.5)	854 (41.0)	0.0003
3–5 (medium)	113 (56.5)	1046 (50.3)	
>5 (high)	30 (15.0)	181 (8.7)	

[1]Smoking, family history of early coronary heart disease, high blood pressure, hypercholesterolemia, body mass index >27, diabetes, sedentary lifestyle, and early menopause.

Of note, some of the 1 beneficial effects of exercise-based CR observed in the general population of CHD patients have also been reported in CKD patients [16, 17]. To our knowledge, there are no data that specifically describe in large population of patients the prevalence of CKD in patients with CHD undergoing CR programs, their clinical characteristics, and course during the CR program.

The present survey aimed at providing an insight in the clinical characteristics and course of a CKD population in the real world of CR in Italy.

2. Methods

2.1. Study Design. The multicenter, prospective observational study design of the ISYDE-2008 has been described in detail elsewhere [18, 19]. In summary, the primary purpose of this study was to take a snapshot on current organization, settings, and provision of CR in Italy and to describe the patient population referred to CR, giving a comprehensive and detailed description of clinical characteristics, risk profile, diagnostic procedures, exercise and educational program, discharge modalities, treatment at discharge, and follow-up schedules. The enrolment period lasted from January 28 to February 10 2008. Data were collected on a web-based case report form, which reported data on clinical characteristics, diagnostic procedures, exercise and educational programs, treatment, and follow-up plans of all the consecutive patients discharged from CR programs in the 2-week study period. The present study focused on CKD patients. As suggested by the National Kidney Foundation Kidney Disease Outcome Quality Initiative, CKD was prospectively defined and considered present if the estimated glomerular filtration rate (eGFR) was <60 mL/min/1.73 m^2 for 3 months at study entry [20]. The eGFR was calculated using the abbreviated Modification of Diet in Renal Disease Study Equation [21]: eGFR (mL/min/1.73 m^2 of body surface area) = 186 × (serum creatinine in mg/dL) − 1.154 × (age in years) − 0.203 × 0.742 in female subjects. As a part of geriatric multidimensional evaluation, performed in about one-fourth of our population, cognitive function was evaluated by MMSE [22], and cognitive impairment was assigned when corrected MMSE value was <21.

2.2. Participating Centers. The survey was designed to be carried out in all Italian residential and outpatient CR centers. Centers were invited to participate in the survey on a purely voluntary basis by the executive board of the study and by the regional GICR-IACPR coordinator, who was responsible for interfacing with the investigators in each of the participating centers and overlooked the implementation of the survey protocol. Data collected in the study refer to 165 CR units (87% of all invited facilities). These CR units, representative of national CR organization, were subdivided in 103 (62.4%) residential units, 18 (10.9%) facilities with day-hospital care, and 33 (20%) facilities with outpatient CR (information not available in 11 CR units (6.7%)). The complete list of ISYDE-2008 investigators and participating centers with names of the directors or contact physicians is reported in the Acknowledgments.

2.3. Role of the Funding Source. No funding sources had any role in the study design, conduct, data collection, analysis, data interpretation, or writing of this paper. The GICR-IACPR coordinated the study, managed the data, and undertook all analyses. All members of the scientific board and writing committees had full access to the database and assumed final responsibility for the results submitted for publication.

2.4. Statistical Analysis. The main analysis was performed subdividing the study cohort into two groups, according to the diagnosis of CKD. Data are expressed as means ± standard deviation (SD) or proportions. Comparisons between groups were performed by unpaired t-test, χ^2 or Fisher exact test as required. Correlations between variables were assessed with Pearson's correlation coefficient. Predictors of death were evaluated with multivariate logistic regression analysis. All analyses were performed using SAS (version 9.1, Cary, NC) with significance set at $P < 0.05$.

3. Results

Table 1 summarizes the demographic characteristics of the study population. The study cohort consisted of 2281 patients (66.9±11.8 yrs): 200 (71.3±12.2 yrs, 66% male) CKD patients and 2081 (66.3±11.6 yrs, 74% male) non-CKD patients. CKD patients showed a significantly higher cardiovascular risk factors score (including smoking, history, hypertension, dyslipidemia, obesity, diabetes, sedentary lifestyle, and early menopause) compared to the non-CKD cohort (P = 0.0003).

Table 2: Previous interventions and comorbidities (n, %).

	CKD (n = 200)	Non-CKD (n = 2081)	P value
Previous myocardial infarction	77 (38.5)	426 (20.5)	<0.0001
Previous percutaneous transluminal coronary angioplasty	37 (18.5)	188 (9.0)	<0.0001
Previous cardiac surgery	33 (16.5)	217 (10.4)	0.008
Heart failure	69 (24.2)	131 (6.6)	<0.0001
Carotid arteries atherosclerosis[1]	20 (10.0)	140 (6.7)	0.08
Peripheral artery disease[2]	25 (12.5)	126 (6.0)	0.0005
Chronic obstructive pulmonary disease	52 (26.0)	246 (11.8)	<0.0001
Respiratory insufficiency	19 (9.5)	93 (4.5)	0.002
Hepatic disease	11 (5.5)	52 (2.5)	0.01
Stroke	12 (6.0)	71 (3.4)	0.06
Cognitive impairment	21 (10.5)	43 (2.1)	<0.0001
Diabetes	97 (48.5)	378 (18.2)	<0.0001
Orthopedic/joints/immune-related disease	29 (14.5)	178 (8.5)	0.005

[1]Stenosis >70% or previous revascularization; [2]Fontaine stage >1 or previous revascularization.

Table 3: Complications during cardiac rehabilitation programs (n, %).

	CKD (n = 200)	Non-CKD (n = 2081)	P value
Atrial fibrillation	49 (24.5)	403 (19.4)	0.08
Severe ventricular arrhythmias[1]	11 (5.5)	79 (3.8)	0.23
Permanent pacemaker implantation	13 (6.5)	57 (2.7)	0.003
Acute myocardial infarction	4 (2.0)	31 (1.5)	0.57
Cerebrovascular events[2]	5 (2.5)	36 (1.7)	0.43
Cognitive impairment*	7 (2.5)	31 (1.5)	0.03
Anemia[3]	38 (19.0)	275 (13.2)	0.02
Worsening of CKD or new onset of renal failure[4]	63 (31.5)	56 (2.7)	<0.0001
Hepatic insufficiency	4 (2.0)	14 (0.7)	0.04
Sternal revision	7 (3.5)	27 (1.3)	0.01
Massive pleural effusion needing thoracenthesis	6 (3.0)	51 (2.5)	0.63
Inotropic support/mechanical assistance	24 (12.0)	88 (4.2)	<0.0001
Respiratory assistance[5]	17 (8.5)	78 (3.7)	0.0001
Systemic infections	16 (8.0)	62 (3.0)	0.0002
Death	4 (2)	11 (0.5)	0.02

[1]>30 sec or symptomatic ventricular tachycardia; [2]stroke, transient ischemic attack; [3]Hb ≤10 g/dL or ≥3 g/dL reduction with respect to the preindex event value; [4]creatinine increase ≥1 mg/dL; [5]including oxygen therapy, mechanical ventilation, continuous positive airway pressure (cPAP), bilevel positive airway pressure (biPAP) >96 h. *Worsening of cognitive impairment or new onset of cognitive impairment.

Compared to non-CKD, CKD patients showed a greater frequency of previous interventions and comorbidities such as myocardial infarction, percutaneous coronary intervention (PCI), cardiac surgery, heart failure, diabetes, peripheral artery disease (PAD), chronic obstructive pulmonary disease (COPD), cognitive impairment, and orthopedic/immunological diseases (Table 2).

During CR programs, CKD patients underwent more permanent pacemaker implantation or developed more complications such as anemia, systemic infections, and worsening of CKD and required more frequently inotropic support or respiratory assistance compared to non-CKD patients (Table 3).

Differences between CKD and non-CKD patients were also detected in diagnostic or therapeutic procedures during CR (Table 4). Compared to non-CKD, CKD patients less likely underwent diagnostic procedures such as exercise stress testing on admission or at discharge, whereas no significant differences were found among groups in six-minute walking test (6MWT) on admission or at discharge and cardiopulmonary exercise stress tests at discharge (Table 4). As many as 77 CKD patients (38%) received no physical performance test (nor 6MWT, exercise stress testing, or cardiopulmonary exercise testing); this proportion was significantly greater than that in non-CKD patients (20%, $P < 0.0001$). Compared to non-CKD not performing any physical performance testing, CKD patients not performing any physical performance testing showed a higher percentage of comorbidities such as myocardial infarction (36% versus 16%, $P < 0.0001$), percutaneous coronary intervention (PCI) (16% versus 5%,

Table 4: Diagnostic and therapeutic procedures during cardiac rehabilitation programs (n, %).

	CKD (n = 200)	Non-CKD (n = 2081)	P value
6-minute walking test on admission	79 (39.5)	904 (43.4)	0.28
6-minute walking test at discharge	83 (41.5)	864 (41.5)	0.99
Exercise stress testing on admission	9 (4.5)	437 (21.0)	<0.0001
Exercise stress testing at discharge	27 (13.5)	678 (32.6)	<0.0001
Cardiopulmonary exercise stress testing on admission	4 (2.0)	118 (5.7)	0.02
Cardiopulmonary exercise stress testing at discharge	16 (8.0)	141 (6.8)	0.51
Holter electrocardiogram	88 (44.0)	832 (40.0)	0.27
Venous infusions	68 (23.9)	171 (8.6)	<0.0001
Thoracentesis	6 (3.0)	26 (1.2)	0.04
Blood transfusions	9 (4.5)	13 (0.6)	<0.0001
Geriatric multidimensional evaluation	58 (29.0)	396 (19.0)	0.0007
Computed tomography	16 (8.0)	73 (3.5)	0.002
Ultrasounds	44 (22.0)	330 (15.6)	0.02
Individual exercise sessions	92 (46.0)	495 (23.8)	<0.0001

Table 5: Drug therapy at hospital discharge after cardiac rehabilitation programs.

	CKD (n = 200)	Non-CKD (n = 2081)	P value
Inhibitors of angiotensin-converting enzyme	86 (43.0)	1171 (56.3)	0.0003
Angiotensin II receptor blockers	46 (23.0)	341 (16.4)	0.02
Beta-blockers	133 (66.5)	1433 (68.9)	0.49
Nitrates	68 (34.0)	372 (17.9)	<0.0001
Diuretics	156 (78.0)	1012 (48.6)	<0.0001
Statins	119 (59.5)	1391 (66.8)	0.03
Omega-3 fatty acids	26 (13.0)	352 (16.9)	0.15
Oral anticoagulant therapy	72 (36.0)	532 (25.6)	0.001
Aspirin	100 (50.0)	1408 (67.7)	<0.0001
Digitalis	23 (11.5)	101 (4.8)	<0.0001
Amiodarone	25 (12.5)	107 (5.1)	<0.0001
Calcium channel blockers	51 (25.5)	385 (18.5)	0.01
Antidepressant	21 (10.5)	120 (5.8)	0.008

$P = 0.0008$), carotid arteries atherosclerosis (13% versus 6%, $P = 0.02$), peripheral artery disease (PAD) (14% versus 6%, $P = 0.006$), heart failure (32% versus 12%, $P < 0.0001$), chronic obstructive pulmonary disease (COPD) (31% versus 13%, $P < 0.0001$), diabetes (54% versus 16%, $P < 0.0001$), hepatic disease (6% versus 2%, $P = 0.02$), cognitive impairment (16% versus 5%, $P = 0.0005$), and orthopedic disease (26% versus 14%, $P = 0.007$) and a higher percentage of complications during the CR program such as anemia (21% versus 9%, $P = 0.003$), worsening of CKD (30% versus 3%, $P < 0.0001$), need of inotropic support (5% versus 1%, $P = 0.007$) or respiratory assistance (8% versus 3%, $P = 0.02$), infections (12% versus 4%, $P = 0.007$), and blood transfusions (8% versus 2%, $P = 0.005$), respectively.

Echocardiography showed a lower percentage of CKD patients with preserved left ventricular ejection fraction (LVEF > 50%) compared to non-CKD patients (37% versus 61%, $P < 0.0001$, resp.) and a higher percentage of moderate (LVEF = 30–49%, 37% versus 26%, $P < 0.0001$, resp.) and severe (LVEF < 30%, 17% versus 5%, $P < 0.0001$, resp.) compromise of LVEF compared to the non-CKD cohort.

Patients with CKD also underwent more frequent geriatric multidimensional evaluation, and CT or ultrasound diagnosis, venous infusion, blood transfusion, or thoracentesis. They also performed preferentially more individually tailored rather than group exercise training session.

At discharge, compared to non-CKD, CKD patients were less frequently prescribed angiotensin-converting enzyme inhibitors, statins, and aspirin. Conversely, CKD patients were more frequently prescribed angiotensin II receptor blockers, nitrates, diuretics, oral anticoagulant therapy, digitalis, amiodarone, insulin, oral hypoglycemic drugs, and calcium channel blockers (Table 5). No significant differences were observed in beta-blockers or omega-3 fatty acids discharge prescription among the 2 groups (Table 5).

CKD patients were less likely discharged home (88% versus 91%, $P = 0.05$) and more likely transferred to intensive care units (8% versus 4%, $P = 0.005$). CKD patients had higher death rate during CR programs (2.0% versus 0.5%, $P = 0.02$). After adjusting for age, ejection fraction, comorbidities (acute myocardial infarction, percutaneous coronary intervention, cardiac surgery, carotid artery critical lesions, peripheral artery disease, respiratory insufficiency, heart failure, diabetes, stroke, and cognitive impairment), and complications during CR program (atrial fibrillation and severe ventricular arrhythmias), multivariate logistic analysis showed that heart failure (OR 1.6, 95% CI, 1.1 to 2.4, $P = 0.04$), respiratory insufficiency (OR 2.4, 95% CI, 1.4 to 4.0, $P = 0.0007$), and cognitive impairment (OR 4.5, 95% CI, 2.5 to 8.1, $P < 0.0001$) were significant predictors of death in CKD patients.

4. Discussion

To the best of our knowledge, the present study is the first to explore the characteristics of the "real world" CKD patients admitted to CR programs in Italy. The principal findings of this study were the higher burden of cardiovascular risk factors and comorbidities associated with a worse clinical course during CR in patients with CKD compared to patients without CKD.

This survey revealed that only about 9% of patients admitted to CR had diagnosed CKD, a number significantly lower than that reported in a cohort of patients with post-myocardial infarction followed at the Mayo Clinic (29.6%), among patients enrolled in the Valiant Trial (33.6%), among a national cohort of elderly patients with myocardial infarction (37%), and in a other cohorts of patients referred for CR (25.6%) [4, 23–25]. The lower percentage of CKD patients found in our study, compared to previous reports in CR environment [25], may reflect indication bias, with a the tendency of deny referral to CR programs of patients with CKD in Italy. In addition, in agreement with previously reported studies, our patients with CKD had a greater burden of comorbidities and cardiovascular risk factors than their non-CKD counterparts.

This survey showed the higher prevalence of CKD patients participating to CR programs with previous PCI or coronary artery bypass graft (CABG). Patients with CKD undergoing myocardial revascularization have worse survival than other CAD patients [26, 27]. Several studies have reported that PCI in patients with CKD may be associated with poor long-term results [28, 29]. In a large retrospective analysis of patients undergoing elective PCI with balloon angioplasty or/and bare-metal stent implantation, CKD was found to have a negative prognostic impact, similar to that of diabetes, on cardiovascular morbidity and mortality [30]. Recently, Ashrith et al. [31] showed that in patients with CKD and multivessel CAD, CABG led to better survival than PCI with drug-eluting stents, but CABG patients had a greater short-term risk of requiring permanent hemodialysis. In our study, despite the worsening of CKD observed in many patients, no patient required hemodialysis. This might be a consequence of a selection bias, since our observational study likely represents a selected population of patients with CKD after an acute cardiac event, where the worst patients requiring hemodialysis immediately after coronary revascularization were not addressed to CR. Future prospective studies are needed in order to evaluate the effect of CR in CKD patients undergoing PCI or CABG in terms of post-procedure hemodialysis dependence and mortality.

Compared to non-CKD patients, we found a roughly doubled prevalence of symptomatic PAD in CKD patients enrolled to CR programs (12.5% versus 6%, $P = 0.0005$). Selvin and Erlinger [32] reported that low kidney function (OR 2.00, 95% CI 1.08 to 3.70) was positively associated with prevalent PAD. In patients with CAD, the prevalence of previously unrecognized PAD is 15% [33]. In this survey, 7% of CKD patients had coexisting diabetes and PAD, thus representing a very high-risk patient population referred to CR programs.

This survey also highlighted the higher prevalence of diabetes in CKD patients participating to CR programs compared to the non-CKD cohort (48% versus 18%, $P < 0.0001$, resp.). This high prevalence of diabetes in our CKD patients is not surprising, since diabetes is one of the major risk factor for CKD and for CHD [34].

Despite the fact that geriatric multidimensional evaluation was performed in less than one-third of the patients, the present survey showed that cognitive impairment prevalence (10 versus 2%) and worsening of cognitive impairment during CR (2.5 versus 1.5%) were significantly higher in CKD patients compared to the non-CKD cohort. In fact, CKD is known to independently affect cognitive status: recent studies have shown impaired kidney function to be associated with greater prevalence of cognitive impairment [35], a more-rapid rate of cognitive decline [36], and incident cognitive impairment [37, 38].

A previous study showed that in patients with mild cognitive impairment of heterogeneous etiology including vascular, metabolic, or endocrine factors, CKD was an independent risk factor for cognitive impairment [39], and it showed that CKD in older adults with mild cognitive impairment was a potentially modifiable risk factor.

An additional cause of mental deterioration in our CKD patients was the frequent association with CHF. In our survey, 24.2% of CKD patients had CHF. It is well recognized that CHF is an independent factor affecting cognitive impairment [40], and cognitive dysfunction and heart failure are common conditions in the elderly [41]. Mild cognitive impairment, a subtle but measurable deficit usually involving the memory domain, is the most commonly reported dysfunction in elderly patients with heart failure, being detectable in more than half of the patients [40]. Potential underlying mechanisms for cognitive dysfunction in heart failure may involve low cardiac output status with consequent cerebral hypoperfusion as well as increased risk of cerebrovascular ischemic events [40]. Therefore, these findings suggest that an initial evaluation of cognitive performance should be implemented in CKD patients, especially in older patients and those with CHF.

The present survey showed higher prevalence of anemia in CKD patients compared to the non-CKD cohort (19% versus 13%, $P = 0.02$). It is well known that anemia is a very common feature of CKD patients [42], and it is not surprising that in patients with CKD undergoing CABG surgery or other invasive procedures anemia may be even more frequent. Reduced hemoglobin levels and CKD are common and interrelated factors in CHF [43, 44].

Chronic kidney disease can contribute to the development and exacerbation of heart failure and progressive heart failure contributes to renal hypoperfusion and activation of inflammatory factors, which can lead to the development or worsening of kidney dysfunction. These findings suggest that in CKD patients during CR hemoglobin level should be closely monitored and raised to acceptable levels, especially in older and CHF patients [43]. It is also recommended that in CHF patients with CKD the hemoglobin values should not be raised beyond 12 mg/dL, in order to avoid risk of thrombosis [45].

The present survey also highlighted that larger proportion of CKD patients did not perform any type of physical performance test compared to the non-CKD cohort. This might have prognostic relevance, since the lack of referral to exercise stress testing is by itself a negative prognostic indicator [46].

The present survey revealed also interesting differences relatively to drugs use. The rather low discharge indication to statin in the total populations is a consequence of the difficulties of adopting in the real clinical world the recommendations of international guidelines regarding secondary prevention [47] or of the presence of many patients after noncoronary surgery not requiring statins (59.5% (CKD) versus 66.8% (non-CKD patients), $P = 0.03$). Moreover, CKD patients showed a higher use of diuretics that might have precipitated in some patient in the worsening of CKD [48].

Finally, complications (particularly arrhythmias, pump failure requiring inotropic support, respiratory insufficiency, worsening of CKF, or infections) and mortality during CR were higher in CKD patients compared to the non-CKD cohort, reflecting the higher clinical risk profile of these patients after an acute cardiac event. In patients with CHD or CHF, CKD has been identified as an important predictor of adverse outcome and increased morbidity [4, 23, 24]. Anavekar et al. [4] reported a 10% increase in the hazard of death and nonfatal cardiovascular outcomes after myocardial infarction for every 10-unit decrease in GFR below 81 mL/min per 1.73 m^2. Wright et al. [23] reported a 3-fold increase in in-hospital mortality after myocardial infarction in individuals with mild renal failure (GFR = 51–75 mL/min per 1.73 m^2), a 7-fold increase among those with moderate renal failure (GFR = 35–50 mL/min per 1.73 m^2), and a >10-fold increase among patients with severe renal failure. Bruch et al. [49] reported a 3-fold increase of cardiac events in CHF patients with CKD; and outcome was significantly worse in CKD patients than in patients without CKD (event-free survival rate 51% versus 87% in those without CKD, $P = 0.001$). Therefore, more attention to the clinical stabilization of these patients is required during CR.

Our study has several limitations. The observational nature of the study cannot rule out that the more severely compromised patients with CKD were not addressed to CR and, therefore, those described in our study may represent a selected relatively healthy minority. The number of patients with CKD reported in the present survey is very small (about 9% of the overall population). This makes the study underpowered for a deepened interpretation. This probably depends on the very small time of the enrolment period (only two weeks). The combination of data from CR centers offering very different cardiac rehabilitation regimens (e.g., residential versus outpatients) is another confounder. The observational nature of the study cannot rule out that the more severely compromised patients with CKD were not addressed to CR and, therefore, those described in our study may represent a selected more relatively healthy minority. Moreover, according to recent evidence [50–52], the present survey did not collect data regarding modality of exercise training regimen (interval versus continuous) or the dose of exercise (in terms of volume and intensity) that can greatly affect the functional and clinical parameters (together with outcome) of CKD patients. Another major limitation of the present study was the lack of reporting some important functional and clinical parameters of possible interest; this was due to the short-term survey type of study, which collected the essential data in order to characterize the demographic and clinical course of the patients. Despite these limitations, the survey successfully highlighted crucial differences in the clinical characteristics, risk profile, management, and short term outcome in CKD patient population entering CR programs in Italy, compared to non-CKD patients.

In conclusion, this survey shows in a large population the clinical risk profile, resource utilization, pharmacologic treatment, and course of CR programs in CKD patients, compared to non CKD patients. In the future, prospective studies are needed in order to identify the best strategies for expanding referral to CR in more compromise patients, fostering the application of tailored functional evaluation, optimization of pharmacological and nonpharmacological treatment, and adherence to secondary prevention guidelines, with the aim of reducing in-hospital complications and improving functional recovery, long-term mortality, morbidity, and quality of life in CKD patients. Therefore, patients with CKD should not be denied access to CR, provided careful attention to clinical status, possible complications, optimization of drug therapy, and close followup.

Acknowledgments

On behalf of the ISYDE-2008 Investigators of the Italian Association for Cardiovascular Prevention and Rehabilitation (GICR-IACPR). *ISYDE-2008 Study Investigators. Scientific Board.* R. Tramarin (Cernusco S/N-MI), R. Griffo (Arenzano, GE), C. Riccio (Caserta), R. Carlon (Cittadella, PD), A. Castello (Palermo), M. Ferratini (Milano), C. Schweiger (Milano), C. Chieffo (Napoli), C. Vigorito (Napoli). *Writing Committee.* R. Tramarin (Cernusco S/N-MI), C. Vigorito (Napoli); M. Ambrosetti (Cunardo, VA), S. De Feo (Peschiera del Garda, VR), R. Griffo (Arenzano, GE), M. Piepoli (Piacenza), C. Riccio (Caserta). *Executive Committe.* M. Ambrosetti (Cunardo, VA), S. De Feo (Peschiera del Garda, VR), T. Diaco (Rivolta d'Adda, CR). Delegati Regionali del

Gruppo Italiano di Cardiologia Riabilitativa e Preventiva: Abruzzo: C. Ciglia (Chieti), Basilicata: A. Lapolla (Policoro, MT), Calabria: F. Pietropaolo (Soriano Calabro, VV), Campania: G. Furgi (Telese Terme, BN), Friuli Venezia Giulia: G. Martin (Sacile, PN), Emilia Romagna: P. Semprini (Rimini), Lazio: A. Avallone (Roma), Liguria: D. Bertoli (Sarzana, SP), Lombardia: T. Diaco (Rivolta d'Adda, CR), Marche: R. Belardinelli (Ancona), Piemonte: F. Soffiantino (Lanzo Torinese, TO), Puglia: D. Scrutinio (Cassano Murge, BA), Sardegna: P. Maxia (Cagliari), Sicilia: R. Coco (Catania), Toscana: C. Giustarini (Volterra, PI), Umbria: P. Anniboletti (Perugia), Veneto: G. Favretto (Motta di Livenza, TV). *Technical Support.* P. Vaghi (Saronno), P. Calisi (Arenzano, GE), C. Chiavetta (Genova), Aristea S.p.A. (Genova), Segno & Forma S.p.A. (Milano). *ISYDE-2008 Investigators (Italian Regions in Italic). Abruzzo:* Leonello Guarracini, Presidio Ospsaledaliero Tagliacozzo, Tagliacozzo; Carlo Ciglia, Casa di Cura Villa Pini D'Abruzzo, Chieti; Giorgio, Marcellini, Presidio Ospedaliero S. Omero, S. Omero. *Calabria:* M. Iannopollo, Presidio Ospedaliero Siderno, USL 9 Locri (RC), Siderno; Gennarino Borrello, Azienda Ospedaliera Mater Domini, Catanzaro; Milena Matta, Presidio Ospedaliero di Cetraro, Cetraro; N. Peccerillo, Ospedale di Mormanno, ASL 2 Castrovillari, Mormanno; Franco Boncompagni, Ospedale dell'Annunziata, Cosenza; Achille Amici, Casa di Cura "San Francesco", Mendicino (CS), Mendicino; Francesco Pietropaolo, Presidio Ospedaliero, Soriano Calabro; Emidio Feraco, IRCCS INRCA, Cosenza; G. Pulitano, Presidio Ospedaliero Policlinico Madonna della Consolazione, Reggio Calabria; Ermete Tripodi, ASP 5 Regione Calabria, Scilla. *Campania:* Giuseppe Furgi, IRCCS Fondazione Salvatore Maugeri, Telese Terme; Carmelo Chieffo, Casa di Cura Clinical Center, Napoli; Soccorso Capomolla, Presidio Ospedaliero Polispecialistico Don Gnocchi Onlus, Sant'Angelo dei Lombardi; Paolo Golino, Azienda Ospedaliera di Caserta, Dipartimento di Cardiologia, Caserta; Gennaro Parrilli, Campolongo Hospital S.p.A. Casa di Cura, Eboli; Antonio Di Patria, Casa di Cura Villa delle Magnolie, Castel Morrone; Claudio Di Gioia, Casa di Cura Privata Villa Margherita, Istituto S. Giuseppe Moscati, Benevento; Domenico Micieli, Azienda Ospedaliera V. Monaldi, Napoli; Carlo Vigorito, Azienda Universitaria Policlinico, Università di Napoli Federico II, Napoli; Silvio Perrotta, ASL Napoli 1, Napoli; Alessandro Rubino, Azienda S. G. Moscati, Avellino; Vincenzo Aulitto, Centro Serapide S.p.A., Pozzuoli; Gerardo Riccio, Ospedale di Nocera, Nocera Inferiore. *Emilia Romagna:* Luciano Codec, Azienda Universitaria Ospedale S. Anna, Ferrara; Paolo Coruzzi, Fondazione Don Carlo Gnocchi, Onlus, Parma; Enrico Violi, Azienda Ospedaliera di Reggio Emilia, Castelnovo Monti; Massimo Nardini, Ospedale Regina Margherita, Castelfranco Emilia; Stefano Urbinati, Azienda USL di Bologna, Bologna; Sylvia Dcruz, Casa di Cura Privata ad Indirizzo Riabilitativo San Giacomo srl, Ponte dell'Olio; Pierluigi Semprini, Ospedale Infermi Rimini, Rimini; Massimo Piepoli, Azienda Unità Sanitaria Locale di Piacenza, Piacenza; Alessandro Fucili, Ospedale Sant'Anna, Ferrara; Massimo Cerulli, Ospedale Privato Accreditato Villa Pineta, Gaiato di Pavullo N/F; Bini Roberto, Azienda USL Cesena, Cesenatico; Guido Balestra, Villa Maria Cecilia Hospital, Cotignola. *Friuli Venezia Giulia:* Dulio Tuniz, IMFR Udine, ASS N. 4, Udine; Giovanni Martin, Azienda Ospedaliera Santa Maria degli Angeli Pordenone, Sacile; Pierpaolo Gori, Casa di Cura Pineta del Carso, Aurisina; Roberto Marini, ASS N. 2 Isontina, Gorizia; Tullio Morgera, Ospedale San Polo, Monfalcone. *Lazio:* Franco Di Mario, Istituto Clinico Riabilitativo Villa delle Querce, Nemi; Maurizio Volterrani, IRCCS San Raffaele Pisana, Roma; Alfonso Galati, Presidio Ospedaliero Santo Spirito, Presidio Villa Betania, ASL Roma E, Roma; Alessandro Salustri, Policlinico Luigi Di Liegro, Roma; Anna Patrizia Jesi, Presidio Ospedaliero Salus Infirmorum, Roma; Augusto Lacch, Azienda Ospedaliera San Camillo, Forlanini, Roma; Francesco Loperfido, Complesso Integrato Columbus. Università Cattolica del Sacro Cuore, Roma. *Liguria:* Luca Corsiglia, Istituto Cardiovascolare Camogli, Ruta di Camogli; Raffaele Griffo, ASL 3 Genovese, Arenzano; Paolo Pantaleo, Struttura Ospedaliera Privata Accreditata Villa Azzurra, Rapallo; Guido Gigli, Regione Liguria ASL 4, Centro Regionale di Riabilitazione Cardiologica, Sestri Levante; Daniele Bertoli, ASL 5 Spezzino, Sarzana. *Lombardia:* Diego Marchesi, Clinica Domus Salutis Ancelle della Carità, Brescia; Oreste Febo, IRCCS Fondazione Salvatore Maugeri, Montescano; Franco Cobelli, IRCCS Fondazione Salvatore Maugeri Pavia, Pavia; Claudio Malinverni, Azienda Ospedaliera "Bolognini", Seriate; Maurizio Ferratini, Fondazione Don Gnocchi Onlus, Milano; Norman Jones, Ospedale Trabattoni Ronzoni, Seregno; Claudio Anzà, Multimedica Holding, Presidio Ospedaliero di Castellanza, Castellanza; R. Frizzelli, Azienda Ospedaliera C. Poma di Mantova, Bozzolo; Paolo Gei, Spedali Civili di Brescia, Gardone Riviera; Flavio Acquistapace, Policlinico di Monza, Monza; Roberto Pedretti, IRCCS Fondazione Salvatore Maugeri, Tradate; Roberto Tramarin, Fondazione Europea di Ricerca Biomedica, Onlus, Cernusco S/N, Milano; Stefano Carugo, Centro di Cardiologia Riabilitativa, Pio Albergo Trivulzio, Milano; Gabriella Malfatto, Istituto Auxologico Italiano IRCCS, Milano; Tommaso Diaco, Azienda Ospedale Maggiore di Crema, Rivolta D'Adda; Marco Ambrosetti, Clinica Le Terrazze, Cunardo; Carlo, Meloni, Ospedale San Raffaele IRCCS U.O. Riabilitazione Cardiaca, Milano; Amerigo Giordano, IRCCS Fondazione Salvatore Maugeri, Lumezzane; Alberto Schizzarotto, Azienda Ospedaliera S. Antonio Abate di Gallarate, Somma Lombardo; Renzo Zanettini, Azienda Ospedaliera Istituti Clinici di Perfezionamento, Milano; Roberto Bosco, Ospedale Romano di Lombardia, Romano di Lombardia; Giuseppe Occhi, Azienda Ospedaliera della Valtellina e Valchiavenna, Sondalo; Stefano Aglieri, Istituto Clinico Humanitas, Rozzano; Giuseppe Caprioli, Humanitas, Cliniche Gavazzeni S.p.A., Bergamo; Nicola Cuocina, Azienda Ospedaliera Ospedali Riuniti di Bergamo, Bergamo; Luciano Lazzaroni, Aurelio Lorenzi, Centro di Cardiologia Riabilitativa di Cesano Boscone, Casa di Cura Ambrosiana, Cesano Boscone; Cinzia Savonelli, Cof Lanzo Hospital S.p.A. Clinica Ortopedica e Fisiatrica., Lanzo D'Intelvi; Marco Veniani, Azienda G. Salvini Garbagnate Milanese, Rho; Giovanni Corda, Azienda Ospedaliera ed Universitaria: Ospedale di Circolo ed Università dell'Insubria, Varese, Cuasso al Monte; Claudia Meinecke, Azienda Istituti Ospitalieri di Cremona, Cremona; Giuseppe Castiglioni, ASL Prov. Milano, Presidio

Ospedaliero Cassano D'Adda, Cassano D'Adda; Ravizza Pierfranco, Azienda Ospedaliera Ospedale di Lecco, Merate; Paolo Giani, Fondazione Europea di Ricerca Biomedica Onlus, Trescore Balneario; Fabio Robustelli della Cuna-Ospedale di Morbegno, ASL Provincia di Sondrio, Morbegno; Giuseppe Gullace, Azienda Provinciale Ospedale di Lecco, Lecco; Federico Passoni, Azienda Ospedaliera di Legnano, Cuggiono; Maria Vittoria Barelli, Centro Fisioterapico Riabilitativo Club Francesco Conti, Milano; Italo Richichi, Ospedale San Matteo U.O. di Riabilitazione, Belgioioso; Angelo Rossi, Casa di Cura Villa Esperia, Salice Terme; Alessandro Politi, Ospedale Generale di Zona, Gravedona. *Marche:* Romualdo Belardinelli, Azienda Ospedaliero, Universitaria Umberto I, Ancona; Casa di Cura Villa Serena, Jesi; Mauro Persico, ASUR Marche Zona Territoriale 12, San Benedetto del Tronto, Area Vasta N. 5, San Benedetto del Tronto. *Piemonte e Valle d'Aosta:* Pantaleo Giannuzzi, IRCCS Fondazione Salvatore Maugeri, Clinica del Lavoro e della Riabilitazione, Veruno; Gianmauro Mazzucco, Casa di Cura Villa Serena, Centro Medico di Riabilitazione Cardiologica e Pneumologica, Piossasco; Enzo Bosimini, Casa di Cura Major, Sede Distaccata IRCCS Fondazione Maugeri Veruno, Torino; Giuseppe Riva, Casa di Cura Riabilitativa Stella del Mattino, Boves; Francesco Soffiantino, Presidio Ospedaliero di Lanzo, Lanzo Torinese; Nicola Massobrio, Ospedale Evangelico Valdese di Torino, Torino; Luca Gondoni, Unità Operativa ad indirizzo Cardiologico, IRCCS Istituto Auxologico Italiano, Piancavallo di Oggebbio; Franco Aina, Azienda Ospedaliero-Universitaria Ospedale Maggiore della Carità di Novara, Novara; Biagio Ingignoli, Ospedale Ss Trinità, Fossano; Maria Vincenza Cal, Ospedale di Acqui Terme, Acqui Terme; Aillon Costante, Azienda USL Valle D'Aosta, Ospedale Regionale "Umberto Parini", Aosta. *Puglie:* Domenico Scrutinio, IRCCS Fondazione Salvatore Maugeri, Cassano Murge; Massimo Villella, IRCCS Casa Sollievo della Sofferenza, San Giovanni Rotondo; Concetta La Rosa, Casa di Cura Villa Verde snc, Taranto. *Sardegna:* Luigi Sannia, ASL Sassari, Sassari. *Sicilia:* Paolo Barbanto, Presidio Ospedaliero M. Ascoli, S. Tommaselli, Azienda Ospedaliera, Catania; Antonio Castello, Ospedale Buccheri La Ferla Fatebenefratelli, Palermo; Rosario Coco, Azienda Ospedaliera Cannizzaro, Dipartimento Cardiovascolare, Catania; Renato Rametta, Azienda Ospedaliera "San Giovanni di Dio", Agrigento; Daniele Albanese, Unità di Valutazione Funzionale e Riabilitazione del Cardiopatico, Ospedale Civico A.R.N.A.S., Palermo; Antonio Circo, Casa di Cura Carmide Villa l'Ulivo, Catania; Rosaria Raciti, Centro Cuore Morgagni, Pedara; Luigi Scarnato, Casa di Cura Regina Pacis, San Cataldo; Flavia Dispensa, Fondazione Istituto San Raffaele Giglio, Cefalù; Leondardo La Spina, Centro Ionico di Cardiologia, Riposto; Alfio Stuto, Star For Life c/o Poliambulatorio di Cardiologia Dr. Armaro Biagio s.a.s., Siracusa; Calogero Vasco, Azienda Ospedaliera Umberto I, Enna; Salvatore Gibiino, Diagnostica Cardiovascolare del Dr. S. Gibiino & C. snc., Catania; Michele Gabriele, Ospedale di Mazara Del Vallo, Mazara Del Vallo; Claudio Dispensieri, Azienda Ospedaliera Piemonte, Messina; Vittorio Carini, Casa di Cura Riabilitativa "Villa Sofia", Acireale. *Toscana:* Michele Provvidenza, ASL 12 Versilia, Presidio Ospedaliero di Viareggio, Lido di Camaiore; Alessandro Scalzini, ASL 6 Livorno, Presidio Ospedaliero di Cecina, Cecina; Carlo Giustarini, Auxilium Vitae Volterra S.p.A., Volterra; Claudio Macchi, Fondazione Don Gnocchi Onlus, IRCCS, Impruneta; Francesco Fattirolli, Azienda Ospedaliero Universitaria Careggi, Firenze; Mauro Vannucci, IFCA Villa Ulivella e Glicini, Firenze; Luciana Iacopetti, ASL 3 Pistoia, Presidio Ospedaliero Pescia, Pescia; Mario Cordoni, ASL 6 Livorno, Presidio Ospedaliero di Piombino, Piombino. *Trentino e Alto Adige:* Ferrario Gabriele, Casa di Cura Eremo, Arco; Renato Santoni, Ospedale Classificato San Pancrazio, Arco; Walter Pitscheider, Centro di Riabilitazione del Cardiopatico, Salus Center, Bolzano; Roberto Bettini, Ospedale di Trento, Mezzolombardo; Daniela Girardini, S. Maria del Carmine, Rovereto, Centro di Riabilitazione Cardiologica Ospedale di Ala, Ala. *Umbria:* Sara Mandorla, ASL 1, Gualdo Tadino, Gualdo Tadino; Fabrizio Anniboletti, ASL 2 Servizio di Cardiologia Ex Ospedale Grocco Perugia, Perugia; Federico Patriarchi, UO Cardiologia Ospedale di Foligno, Nocera Umbra. *Veneto:* Giuseppe Favretto, Ospedale Riabilitativo di Alta Specializzazione S.p.A., Motta di Livenza; Pier Luigi Baroni, Casa di Cura Villa Garda, Garda; Fede Bordin, ASL N. 4, Presidio Ospedaliero di Thiene, Thiene; Pietro Biondi, ULSS 8, Montebelluna; Fabio Bellotto, Istituto Riabilitativo, Cortina D'Ampezzo; Albino Zanocco, Azienda Ospedaliera, Mirano; Andrea Ponchia, ULSS 16, Padova; Enzo Mantovani, Azienda ULSS 15, Camposampiero; Ennio Li Greci, Ospedale Don L. Chiarenzi, AALSS 21 Legnago (Verona), Zevio; Roberto Carlon, Azienda ALSS 15 Presidio Ospedaliero di Cittadella, Cittadella; Leopoldo Celegon, UO di Cardiologia, Riabilitazione Cardiologica, Castelfranco Veneto; Stefano Baracchi, Ospedale al Mare Lido di Venezia, Lido di Venezia; Grazia Pizzolato, AUSSL N. 10, San Donà di Piave; Lorenzo Peroni, Policlinico San Marco, Mestre; Enzo Apolloni, Ospedale di Asiago, Asiago; Gianmarco Mosele, Casa di Cura Privata Villa Margherita S.r.l., Arcugnano; Mario Guarnerio, Ospedale di Feltre, Feltre; Loris Roncon, Ospedale di Rovigo, Rovigo.

References

[1] A. J. Collins, R. N. Foley, B. M. Chavers et al., "Excerpts from the US renal data system 2009 annual data report," *The American Journal of Kidney Diseases*, vol. 55, no. 1, supplement 1, pp. A6–A7, 2010.

[2] P. Muntner, L. L. Hamm, J. W. Kusek, J. Chen, P. K. Whelton, and J. He, "The prevalence of nontraditional risk factors for coronary heart disease in patients with chronic kidney disease," *Annals of Internal Medicine*, vol. 140, no. 1, pp. 9–17, 2004.

[3] M. J. Sarnak, A. S. Levey, A. C. Schoolwerth et al., "Kidney disease as a risk factor for development of cardiovascular disease: a statement from the American heart association councils on kidney in cardiovascular disease, high blood pressure research, clinical cardiology, and epidemiology and prevention," *Circulation*, vol. 108, no. 17, pp. 2154–2169, 2003.

[4] N. S. Anavekar, J. J. V. McMurray, E. J. Velazquez et al., "Relation between renal dysfunction and cardiovascular outcomes after myocardial infarction," *The New England Journal of Medicine*, vol. 351, no. 13, pp. 1285–1295, 2004.

[5] R. S. Taylor, A. Brown, S. Ebrahim et al., "Exercise-based rehabilitation for patients with coronary heart disease: systematic

review and meta-analysis of randomized controlled trials," *The American Journal of Medicine*, vol. 116, no. 10, pp. 682–692, 2004.

[6] F. Giallauria, P. Cirillo, R. Lucci et al., "Left ventricular remodelling in patients with moderate systolic dysfunction after myocardial infarction: favourable effects of exercise training and predictive role of N-terminal pro-brain natriuretic peptide," *European Journal of Cardiovascular Prevention and Rehabilitation*, vol. 15, no. 1, pp. 113–118, 2008.

[7] F. Giallauria, G. Galizia, R. Lucci et al., "Favourable effects of exercise-based cardiac rehabilitation after acute myocardial infarction on left atrial remodeling," *International Journal of Cardiology*, vol. 136, no. 3, pp. 300–306, 2009.

[8] F. Giallauria, R. Lucci, M. D'Agostino et al., "Two-year multicomprehensive secondary prevention program: favorable effects on cardiovascular functional capacity and coronary risk profile after acute myocardial infarction," *Journal of Cardiovascular Medicine*, vol. 10, no. 10, pp. 772–780, 2009.

[9] F. Tarro Genta, E. Eleuteri, P. L. Temporelli et al., "Flow-mediated dilation normalization predicts outcome in chronic heart failure patients," *Journal of Cardiac Failure*, vol. 19, no. 4, pp. 260–267, 2013.

[10] F. Giallauria, P. Cirillo, M. D'Agostino et al., "Effects of exercise training on high-mobility group box-1 levels after acute myocardial infarction," *Journal of Cardiac Failure*, vol. 17, no. 2, pp. 108–114, 2011.

[11] F. Giallauria, A. de Lorenzo, F. Pilerci et al., "Long-term effects of cardiac rehabilitation on end-exercise heart rate recovery after myocardial infarction," *European Journal of Cardiovascular Prevention and Rehabilitation*, vol. 13, no. 4, pp. 544–550, 2006.

[12] F. Giallauria, A. de Lorenzo, F. Pilerci et al., "Reduction of N terminal-pro-brain (B-type) natriuretic peptide levels with exercise-based cardiac rehabilitation in patients with left ventricular dysfunction after myocardial infarction," *European Journal of Cardiovascular Prevention and Rehabilitation*, vol. 13, no. 4, pp. 625–632, 2006.

[13] F. Giallauria, R. Lucci, A. de Lorenzo, M. D'Agostino, D. Del Forno, and C. Vigorito, "Favourable effects of exercise training on N-terminal pro-brain natriuretic peptide plasma levels in elderly patients after acute myocardial infarction," *Age and Ageing*, vol. 35, no. 6, pp. 601–607, 2006.

[14] N. A. Smart, T. Meyer, J. A. Butterfield et al., "Individual patient meta-analysis of exercise training effects on systemic brain natriuretic peptide expression in heart failure," *European Journal of Preventive Cardiology*, vol. 19, no. 3, pp. 428–435, 2012.

[15] B. Rinaldi, G. Corbi, S. Boccuti et al., "Exercise training affects age-induced changes in SOD and heat shock protein expression in rat heart," *Experimental Gerontology*, vol. 41, no. 8, pp. 764–770, 2006.

[16] G. Byrne and F. Murphy, "Cardiac rehabilitation for patients with chronic kidney disease," *Journal of Renal Care*, vol. 36, supplement 1, pp. 154–162, 2010.

[17] S. Heiwe and S. H. Jacobson, "Exercise training for adults with chronic kidney disease," *Cochrane Database of Systematic Reviews*, no. 10, Article ID CD003236, 2011.

[18] F. Giallauria, C. Vigorito, R. Tramarin et al., "Cardiac rehabilitation in very old patients: data from the Italian survey on cardiac rehabilitation-2008 (ISYDE-2008)—official report of the Italian association for cardiovascular prevention, rehabilitation, and epidemiology," *Journals of Gerontology A*, vol. 65, no. 12, pp. 1353–1361, 2010.

[19] F. Giallauria, F. Fattirolli, R. Tramarin et al., "Cardiac rehabilitation in chronic heart failure: data from the Italian SurveY on carDiac rEhabilitation (ISYDE-2008)," *Journal of Cardiovascular Medicine*, 2013.

[20] "National kidney foundation: clinical practice guidelines for chronic kidney disease: evaluation, classification, and stratification," *The American Journal of Kidney Diseases*, vol. 2, supplement1, pp. S46–S47, 2002.

[21] A. S. Levey, J. P. Bosch, J. B. Lewis, T. Greene, N. Rogers, and D. Roth, "A more accurate method to estimate glomerular filtration rate from serum creatinine: a new prediction equation," *Annals of Internal Medicine*, vol. 130, no. 6, pp. 461–470, 1999.

[22] M. F. Folstein, S. E. Folstein, and P. R. McHugh, "'Mini-mental state': a practical method for grading the cognitive state of patients for the clinician," *Journal of Psychiatric Research*, vol. 12, no. 3, pp. 189–198, 1975.

[23] R. S. Wright, G. S. Reeder, C. A. Herzog et al., "Acute myocardial infarction and renal dysfunction: a high-risk combination," *Annals of Internal Medicine*, vol. 137, no. 7, pp. 563–570, 2002.

[24] M. G. Shlipak, P. A. Heidenreich, H. Noguchi, G. M. Chertow, W. S. Browner, and M. B. McClellan, "Association of renal insufficiency with treatment and outcomes after myocardial infarction in elderly patients," *Annals of Internal Medicine*, vol. 137, no. 7, pp. 555–562, 2002.

[25] R. Venkataraman, B. Sanderson, and V. Bittner, "Outcomes in patients with chronic kidney disease undergoing cardiac rehabilitation," *The American Heart Journal*, vol. 150, no. 6, pp. 1140–1146, 2005.

[26] W. A. Cooper, S. M. O'Brien, V. H. Thourani et al., "Impact of renal dysfunction on outcomes of coronary artery bypass surgery: results from the society of thoracic surgeons national adult cardiac database," *Circulation*, vol. 113, no. 8, pp. 1063–1070, 2006.

[27] P. J. M. Best, R. Lennon, H. H. Ting et al., "The impact of renal insufficiency on clinical outcomes in patients undergoing percutaneous coronary interventions," *Journal of the American College of Cardiology*, vol. 39, no. 7, pp. 1113–1119, 2002.

[28] G. Y. H. Lip, V. S. Rathore, R. Katira, S. P. Singh, and R. D. S. Watson, "Changes in renal function with percutaneous transluminal coronary angioplasty," *International Journal of Cardiology*, vol. 70, no. 2, pp. 127–131, 1999.

[29] R. Y. Zhang, Z. B. Zhu, Q. Zhang et al., "Impact of moderate or severe renal insufficiency on long-term outcomes in patients undergoing drug-eluting stent based coronary intervention," *International Journal of Cardiology*, vol. 136, no. 1, pp. 72–79, 2009.

[30] P. J. M. Best, P. B. Berger, B. R. Davis et al., "Impact of mild or moderate chronic kidney disease on the frequency of restenosis: results from the PRESTO trial," *Journal of the American College of Cardiology*, vol. 44, no. 9, pp. 1786–1791, 2004.

[31] G. Ashrith, V. Lee, M. A. Elayda, R. M. Reul, and J. M. Wilson, "Short- and long-term outcomes of coronary artery bypass grafting or drug-eluting stent implantation for multivessel coronary artery disease in patients with chronic kidney disease," *The American Journal of Cardiology*, vol. 106, no. 3, pp. 348–353, 2010.

[32] E. Selvin and T. P. Erlinger, "Prevalence of and risk factors for peripheral arterial disease in the United States: results from the national health and nutrition examination Survey, 1999-2000," *Circulation*, vol. 110, no. 6, pp. 738–743, 2004.

[33] I. D. Moussa, M. R. Jaff, R. Mehran et al., "Prevalence and prediction of previously unrecognized peripheral arterial disease in patients with coronary artery disease: the peripheral arterial

disease in interventional patients study," *Catheterization and Cardiovascular Interventions*, vol. 73, no. 6, pp. 719–724, 2009.

[34] P. Fioretto, M. L. Caramori, and M. Mauer, "The kidney in diabetes: dynamic pathways of injury and repair. The Camillo Golgi lecture 2007," *Diabetologia*, vol. 51, no. 8, pp. 1347–1355, 2008.

[35] K. Yaffe, L. Ackerson, M. K. Tamura et al., "Chronic kidney disease and cognitive function in older adults: findings from the chronic renal insufficiency cohort cognitive study," *Journal of the American Geriatrics Society*, vol. 58, no. 2, pp. 338–345, 2010.

[36] A. S. Buchman, D. Tanne, P. A. Boyle, R. C. Shah, S. E. Leurgans, and D. A. Bennett, "Kidney function is associated with the rate of cognitive decline in the elderly," *Neurology*, vol. 73, no. 12, pp. 920–927, 2009.

[37] S. L. Seliger, D. S. Siscovick, C. O. Stehman-Breen et al., "Moderate renal impairment and risk of dementia among older adults: the cardiovascular health cognition study," *Journal of the American Society of Nephrology*, vol. 15, no. 7, pp. 1904–1911, 2004.

[38] T. Etgen, D. Sander, M. Chonchol et al., "Chronic kidney disease is associated with incident cognitive impairment in the elderly: the INVADE study," *Nephrology Dialysis Transplantation*, vol. 24, no. 10, pp. 3144–3150, 2009.

[39] T. L. Nickolas, M. Khatri, B. Boden-Albala et al., "The association between kidney disease and cardiovascular risk in a multiethnic cohort: findings from the Northern manhattan study (NOMAS)," *Stroke*, vol. 39, no. 10, pp. 2876–2879, 2008.

[40] R. L. C. Vogels, P. Scheltens, J. M. Schroeder-Tanka, and H. C. Weinstein, "Cognitive impairment in heart failure: a systematic review of the literature," *European Journal of Heart Failure*, vol. 9, no. 5, pp. 440–449, 2007.

[41] L. Trojano, R. A. Incalzi, D. Acanfora, C. Picone, P. Mecocci, and F. Rengo, "Cognitive impairment: a key feature of congestive heart failure in the elderly," *Journal of Neurology*, vol. 250, no. 12, pp. 1456–1463, 2003.

[42] B. C. Astor, P. Muntner, A. Levin, J. A. Eustace, and J. Coresh, "Association of kidney function with anemia: the third national health and nutrition examination survey (1988–1994)," *Archives of Internal Medicine*, vol. 162, no. 12, pp. 1401–1408, 2002.

[43] A. S. Go, J. Yang, L. M. Ackerson et al., "Hemoglobin level, chronic kidney disease, and the risks of death and hospitalization in adults with chronic heart failure—the anemia in chronic heart failure: outcomes and resource utilization (ANCHOR) study," *Circulation*, vol. 113, no. 23, pp. 2713–2723, 2006.

[44] P. R. Kalra, A. P. Bolger, D. P. Francis et al., "Effect of anemia on exercise tolerance in chronic heart failure in men," *The American Journal of Cardiology*, vol. 91, no. 7, pp. 888–891, 2003.

[45] F. Locatelli, P. Aljama, B. Canaud et al., "Target haemoglobin to aim for with erythropoiesis-stimulating agents: a position statement by ERBP following publication of the trial to reduce cardiovascular events with aranesp therapy (TREAT) study," *Nephrology Dialysis Transplantation*, vol. 25, no. 9, pp. 2846–2850, 2010.

[46] P. H. Stone, Z. G. Turi, J. E. Muller et al., "Prognostic significance of the treadmill exercise test performance 6 months after myocardial infarction," *Journal of the American College of Cardiology*, vol. 8, no. 5, pp. 1007–1017, 1986.

[47] M. F. Piepoli, U. Corrà, W. Benzer et al., "Secondary prevention through cardiac rehabilitation: from knowledge to implementation. A position paper from the cardiac rehabilitation section of the european association of cardiovascular prevention and rehabilitation," *European Journal of Cardiovascular Prevention and Rehabilitation*, vol. 17, no. 1, pp. 1–17, 2010.

[48] R. G. Hawkins and M. C. Houston, "Is population-wide diuretic use directly associated with the incidence of end-stage renal disease in the United States? A hypothesis," *The American Journal of Hypertension*, vol. 18, no. 6, pp. 744–749, 2005.

[49] C. Bruch, M. Rothenburger, M. Gotzmann et al., "Chronic kidney disease in patients with chronic heart failure—impact on intracardiac conduction, diastolic function and prognosis," *International Journal of Cardiology*, vol. 118, no. 3, pp. 375–380, 2007.

[50] N. A. Smart, G. Dieberg, and F. Giallauria, "Intermittent versus continuous exercise training in chronic heart failure: a meta-analysis," *International Journal of Cardiology*, vol. 166, no. 2, pp. 352–358, 2013.

[51] N. A. Smart, G. Dieberg, and F. Giallauria, "Functional electrical stimulation for chronic heart failure: a meta-analysis," *International Journal of Cardiology*, vol. 167, no. 1, pp. 80–85, 2013.

[52] N. A. Smart, F. Giallauria, and G. Dieberg, "Efficacy of inspiratory muscle training in chronic heart failure patients: a systematic review and meta-analysis," *International Journal of Cardiology*, 2012.

18

Quality of Life in Mothers of Children with Cerebral Palsy

Halim Yilmaz, Gulten Erkin, and Alparslan Ali İZKİ

The Department of Physical Medicine and Rehabilitation, Konya Education and Research Hospital, 42090 Konya, Turkey

Correspondence should be addressed to Halim Yilmaz; drhalimyilmaz@hotmail.com

Academic Editors: W. Liu, K. Nakazawa, and Y. Wu

Objective. To investigate health-related quality of life (HRQoL) in mothers of children with cerebral palsy (CP) and to determine factors into HRQoL. *Materials and Method*. Participants comprised 137 mothers of children with spastic-type CP, and controls comprised 140 mothers with healthy children. Functional levels of children with CP were evaluated using Gross Motor Function Classification System (GMCFS). HRQoL of mothers with CP children and control groups was assessed with 36-Item Short-Form Health Survey (SF-36) and depression levels with Beck Depression Inventory (BDI). *Results*. Social function, mental health, role limitation emotional, and vitality as subscale of mental component of SF-36 were found to be lower in CP children's mothers than controls. BDI scores were higher in CP children's mothers than controls. Among mothers with CP children, a negative correlation was detected between BDI scores and all subscale scores of SF-36 and age rate of mothers and physical function, bodily pain, and physical component scale scores, among subscales of SF-36. *Conclusion*. Our study indicates that HRQoL is impaired in CP children's mothers, and depression is a significant symptom affecting HRQoL of mothers with CP children. Therefore, to increase HRQoL, mothers of children with CP should be motivated to join social activities related to their interests, and mothers with depressive symptoms should be psychologically supported.

1. Introduction

Quality of life (QoL) has been described as an individual's perception of own his/her status in life as to cultural features and value system. Health-related quality of life (HRQoL), however, is a subcomponent of QoL including physical, social, and emotional status of wellbeing. HRQoL is the happiness and satisfaction of individuals in different parts of life influencing or influenced by individuals' health [1–3]. QoL is one of the signs of health. Similar to traditional mortality and morbidity rates, QoL is also among considerable factors essential to be taken into account while individuals' health status is determined [4]. Seen in brains of those from fetal to early childhood periods with symptoms such as ataxia, spasticity, walking with one foot or leg dragging or on toes, crouched or scissored gait, and muscle tone, cerebral palsy (CP) is a neurologic nonprogressive disorder permanently affecting body movement and muscle coordination and leading to limitations in activities [5]. Functional deficits developing due to physical, cognitive, emotional, and social disorders prevent children with CP from performing their roles in society [6, 7]. Families of children with CP fail to be into the children and themselves because of children's continuous requirements for special care, frequent medical checkups, and continuous physiotherapy treatment modalities and to take over their roles in society. Therefore, HRQoL of family members undertaking medical care of children with CP is influenced negatively [4, 8, 9]. In our study, it was aimed to determine HRQoL of mothers of children with CP and to investigate factors affecting HRQoL.

2. Material and Method

The study was performed in the Physical Medicine and Rehabilitation Department of Konya Training and Research Hospital in Konya, Turkey, between September 2011 and January 2013, and 137 mothers with CP children and 140 with healthy children were included into the study. An approval was obtained from the local ethical board of Meram Medical School of Selcuk University. Those accepting to participate were informed, and written consents were obtained. Demographic, medical, and developmental histories of children with CP were taken from families, and age, gender, clinical type, and body involvement of children were defined. Subjects were categorized under Swedish classification. Mothers with CP children are put into classifications as spastic (diplegic, quadriplegic, and hemiparetic), ataxic, dyskinetic (including athetosis and dystonia), and mixed type according to this classification [10]. Only spastic-type children were enrolled into our study. Functional level of children with CP was assessed using Gross Motor Function Classification System (GMFCS). Sociodemographic data of mothers in both groups were determined. HRQoL of mothers was assessed with 36-Item Short-Form Health Survey (SF-36) and depression level with Beck Depression Inventory (BDI).

Inclusion criteria of mothers were composed of having a child with CP, living with the child, not having chronic disorder, not having a rheumatologic, orthopedic, and neurologic problem that will markedly affect HRQoL, not being pregnant, having no history of psychological disorders, not using antidepressant and anxiolytic drugs, and not have another patient or disabled individual along with the CP child. On the other hand, inclusion criteria of controls consisted of having a healthy child and living together, not living with another patient or disabled individual, lacking a history of psychological disorders, not using of antidepressant and anxiolytic drugs, without chronic disorders, not using assisted device, not having pregnanct and not having a rheumatologic, orthopedic and neurologic problem that will markedly affect HRQoL.

Assessing the last 4-week period, SF-36 is a valid and frequently used scale to evaluate HRQoL, specific for no groups of age, disorder, and treatment, includes general health concepts, and composed of 36 questions with 8 subscales as physical function, role limitation physical, role limitation emotional, bodily pain, social function, mental health, vitality, and general health. Scores of items are encoded for each subscale and formed as a scale ranging from 0 (poorest health status) to 100 (best health status). SF-36 has two summary measures as physical component scale (PCS) and mental component scale (MCS). PCS is comprised of subscales of physical function, role physical, bodily pain, and general health, and MCS is comprised of subscales of vitality, social function, role emotional, and mental health [11, 12]. BDI consists of 21 self-evaluating items, scored between 0–3 and including depressive symptoms. A BDI score of 17 and over is evaluated in favour of depression [13]. Likewise, the score of 17 and over was assessed in favour of depression in our study. As the total score increases, depression becomes severe [13]. GMFCS used to define functional levels in individuals with CP is a classification system scored between level 1 and 5. While performing comfortably indoor and outdoor activities with no requirements for assisted devices in level 1, a patient is completely dependent as to mobility in level 5. Differentiation between levels is determined according to the functional restrictions and use of assisted devices [14, 15].

3. Statistical Analyses

For statistical analyses, SPSS 20 package software was used. Descriptive statistical findings were given as mean ± SD. In comparison of parameters, Student's t- and chi-square tests were used. Educational status, level of income, and type of family were assessed using crosstabs. Whether a difference was present between groups as to such frequencies was detected via chi-square or Fisher's exact tests. Analyses were performed with Spearman's rho correlation test. Statistically significance rate and confidence interval were accepted as $P < 0.05$ and 95%, respectively. As correlation coefficients, the correlations between 0 and 0,25 were assessed as "none", between 0,25 and 0,50 as "weak-moderate," between 0,50 and 0,75 as "severe," and between 0,75 and 1,00 as "much severe."

4. Results

Mean age rate of children with CP was 9.27 ± 5.34, and 54.8% ($n = 74$) were girls and 46.0% ($n = 63$) were boys. Of CP children, 40.2% ($n = 55$) were determined to be dyplegic, 39.4% ($n = 54$) to be quadriplegic, and 20.4% ($n = 28$) to be hemiplegic. GMFCS levels were as follows: 16.1% ($n = 22$), level 1; 17.5% ($n = 24$), level 2; 17.5% ($n = 24$), level 3; 19.0% ($n = 26$), level 4; and 29.9% ($n = 41$), level 5. All mothers in both groups were housewives, and sociodemographic and clinical features of all mothers were presented in Table 1. No statistically significant difference was found between participants in the two groups as to educational level, type of family, number of living children, and level of income ($P > 0.05$) (Table 1). On the evaluation of those with BDI ≥17 in favour of depression, the rates of depression were determined as 48.9% in mothers with CP children and 13.6% in controls ($P < 0.001$). In mothers with CP children, scores of social function, mental health, role limitation emotional, vitality, and mental component among subscales of SF-36 were statistically and significantly lower, compared to controls (Table 2). BDI scores, however, were statistically and significantly higher in mothers with CP children than controls ($P < 0.001$). When those with BDI ≥17 were evaluated in favour of depression in mothers with CP children, all subscale scores of SF-36, mental component scale, and physical component scale scores were found to be lower in depressive mothers with CP children than those without (Table 3). In mothers with CP children, a negative correlation was detected between BDI scores and SF-36 subscales such as physical function ($r = -0.464$), bodily pain ($r = -0.307$), role limitation physical ($r = -0.441$), health perception ($r = -0.295$), social function ($r = -0.433$), mental health ($r = -0.489$), role limitation emotional ($r = -0.525$), vitality ($r = -0.393$), mental component scale ($r = -0.538$), and physical component scale scores ($r = -0.501$). Additionally, no correlation was found between all subscales of SF-36, mental and physical component scale scores, GMCFS, and body involvement of CP in mothers with CP children ($P > 0.05$). A negative correlation was observed between the age level of mothers with CP children, and SF-36 subscales like physical function ($r = -0.255$), bodily pain ($r = -0.233$), and physical component scale scores ($r = -0.228$). No correlation was present between all subscale scores of SF-36 and GMCFS, body involvement of CP, educational status, level of income, and number of living children ($P > 0.05$).

TABLE 1: Sociodemographic data of CP children's mothers and controls.

	CP children's mothers (n = 137)	Controls (n = 140)	χ^2	P
Age (year)	35.96 ± 9.02	37.22 ± 8.91		0.254
BMI (kg/m^2)	27.35 ± 5.22	28.27 ± 5.01		0.135
Level of income (dollar/month)	612.97 ± 394.19	715.72 ± 771.99		0.165
Number of living children	2.75 ± 1.20	2.56 ± 1.27		0.229
BDI scores	18.29 ± 12.79	9.85 ± 7.34		<0.001
Type of family				
Core family n (%)	105 (76.6%)	99 (70.7%)	1.254	0.263
Combined family n (%)	32 (23.4%)	41 (29.3%)		
Educational status				
Illiterate	34 (24.8%)	35 (25%)		
Primary (8 years)	79 (57.7%)	73 (52.1%)	1.946	0.584
High school (11 years)	11 (8%)	18 (12.9%)		
College (12 years and over)	13 (9.5%)	14 (10%)		

BMI: body mass index. BDI: Beck Depression Inventory.
SF-36: 36-Item Short-Form Health Survey.

TABLE 2: SF-36 subscale scores in CP children's mothers and controls.

	CP children's mothers (n = 137)	Controls (n = 140)	P
SF-36-physical component	51.83 ± 23.10	56.52 ± 21.55	0.101
Physical function	59.10 ± 29.14	63.04 ± 25.16	0.169
Bodily pain	54.07 ± 33.32	56.85 ± 27.03	0.445
Role limitation physical	50.11 ± 39.24	53.53 ± 38.16	0.462
Health perception	44.08 ± 19.45	52.64 ± 21.92	0.001
SF-36-mental component scale	51.20 ± 24.49	65.63 ± 17.87	<0.001
Social function	52.33 ± 26.36	65.06 ± 20.30	<0.001
Mental health	53.62 ± 22.50	67.49 ± 19.90	<0.001
Role limitation emotional	45.44 ± 40.41	61.93 ± 37.36	<0.001
Vitality	53.39 ± 26.07	68.06 ± 19.96	<0.001

SF-36: 36-Item Short-Form Health Survey.

5. Discussion

In the literature, studies investigating HRQoL and related factors in mothers of children with CP report different findings. Some studies report that HRQoL of mothers with CP children is affected negatively [4, 9, 16–19]. While HRQoL of mothers is reported to be associated with depression [4, 16, 18, 19], anxiety [19], educational status [9, 19, 20], and functional levels [9], others assert that no correlation is present between HRQoL of mothers and functional levels of CP children [4]. In a study performed by Diwan et al. [16], 70% of mothers with CP children were reported to have mild-to-moderate depression, and the depression was reported to have a negative effect on HRQoL of mothers. Erdoganoglu and Gunel [9] reported that, HRQoL of mothers with CP children is affected at a higher rate, compared to fathers, and HRQoL is influenced due to motor and functional levels of CP children. In a similar study, Oneş et al. suggested that, HRQoL of mothers with CP children is affected negatively; HRQoL is negatively correlated with levels of depression and education in mothers, and no correlation is present between HRQoL and functional levels [4]. In their study, Bumin et al. [19] emphasized that HRQoL of disabled children is associated with depression and anxiety levels, and a negative association is also present between HRQoL and mothers' educational status. Kaya et al. [17] reported that the deterioration of mental health in mothers with CP children gives rise to experiencing further low back pain by mothers, leading to more deterioration in HRQoL. In a study by Keller et al. [21], disability in children was reported to decrease social activities of mothers and to have an influence on routine deterioration.

Disability in a child, the basic component of a family, and accompanying challenges affect profoundly other members of the family and may be an intensive source of anxiety. In members of family having to take care of the disabled child all day and for ages, physical and psychosocial health is influenced in a negative way [9, 22]. As a result of cultural impacts in Turkey, mothers mostly take over the responsibility for disabled children and have to be interested in the challenges stemming from the disability alone for a long time. Therefore, we consider that physical and emotional health status of mothers is poorly affected. Present studies indicate that HRQoL of mothers of CP children is affected negatively, but the factors concerning HRQoL and related

TABLE 3: SF-36 subscale scores in those with depression (BDI ≥ 17) and without depression (BDI < 17) in CP children's mothers.

	BDI score < 17	BDI score ≥ 17	*P*
SF-36-physical component scale	63.01 ± 20.68	40.15 ± 19.53	<0.001
Physical function	72.85 ± 24.85	44.66 ± 26.31	<0.001
Bodily pain	64.29 ± 31.50	43.40 ± 32.0	<0.001
Role limitation physical	64.93 ± 36.94	34.63 ± 35.64	<0.001
Health perception	50.00 ± 18.11	35.13 ± 15.53	<0.001
SF-36-mental component scale	63.04 ± 21.78	37.91 ± 20.00	<0.001
Social function	62.97 ± 23.02	41.22 ± 25.14	<0.001
Mental health	62.62 ± 20.41	44.20 ± 20.78	<0.001
Role limitation emotional	64.36 ± 37.26	25.67 ± 33.74	<0.001
Vitality	62.21 ± 24.81	44.18 ± 24.26	<0.001

SF-36: 36-Item Short-Form Health Survey.
BDI: Beck Depression Inventory.

factors are controversial. In our study, it was determined that, as consistent with the literature, HRQoL especially mental components of mothers with CP children is definitely deteriorated, and high levels of depression affect negatively HRQoL of mothers. However, we could detect no association between HRQoL of mothers and functional level of CP children, body involvement of CP, educational status of mothers, level of income, and number of children.

We consider that comprehensive studies including numerous participants are needed to determine HRQoL of mothers with CP children and related factors. Our study includes several limitations. Firstly, our study involves no findings generalized to whole society in that it was a single-centered study. Another limitation is that only spastic-type cerebral palsied children were included into the study. In order to obtain more comprehensive results, mothers of children with ataxic, dyskinetic, and mixed involvements, as well as those with spastic-type, should also be included into studies.

In light of the literature and our findings, HRQoL of mothers with CP children is considered to be affected negatively. Therefore, in planning a rehabilitation program for CP children, HRQoL of mothers should also be evaluated in detail, as well as that of CP children, and as to problems defined, solutions should be produced. Additionally, mothers should be encouraged to take part in social activities related to their interests, and those with depressive symptoms should be supported psychologically. Therefore, it is considered that mothers, undertaking the most significant role in the rehabilitation and caring for the child, should be interested in CP children in a better way.

References

[1] The WHOQOL Group, "The development of the World Health Organisation quality of life assessment instrument (the WHO-QOL)," in *Quality of Life Assessment: International Perspectives*, J. Orley and W. Kuyken, Eds., pp. 41–57, Springer, Heidelberg, Germany, 1994.

[2] Quality Of Life Instruments Database, January 2013, http://www.qolid.org/.

[3] N. Dayapoglu and M. Tan, "Quality of life in stroke patients," *Neurology India*, vol. 58, no. 5, pp. 697–701, 2010.

[4] K. Oneş, E. Yilmaz, B. Cetinkaya, and N. Caglar, "Assessment of the quality of life of mothers of children with cerebral palsy (primary caregivers)," *Neurorehabilitation and Neural Repair*, vol. 19, no. 3, pp. 232–237, 2005.

[5] M. C. Bax, "Terminology and classification of cerebral palsy," *Developmental Medicine and Child Neurology*, vol. 6, pp. 295–297, 1964.

[6] C. Morris, J. J. Kurinczuk, and R. Fitzpatrick, "Child or family assessed measures of activity performance and participation for children with cerebral palsy: a structured review," *Child: Care, Health and Development*, vol. 31, no. 4, pp. 397–407, 2005.

[7] G. Erkin, C. Aybay, M. Kurt, I. Keles, A. Cakci, and S. Ozel, "The assessment of functional status in Turkish children with cerebral palsy (a preliminary study)," *Child: Care, Health and Development*, vol. 31, no. 6, pp. 719–725, 2005.

[8] G. S. Liptak and P. J. Accardo, "Health and social outcomes of children with cerebral palsy," *Journal of Pediatrics*, vol. 145, no. 2, pp. S36–S41, 2004.

[9] Y. Erdoganoglu and M. K. Gunel, "Serebral paralizili çocukların ailelerinin sağlıkla ilgili yaşam kalitelerinin araştırılması," *Toplum Hekimliği Bülteni*, vol. 2, no. 6, pp. 35–39, 2007.

[10] L. Mutch, E. Alberman, B. Hagberg, K. Kodama, and M. V. Perat, "Cerebral palsy epidemiology: where are we now and where are we going?" *Developmental Medicine and Child Neurology*, vol. 34, no. 6, pp. 547–551, 1992.

[11] J. E. Ware, "SF-36 health survey update," *Spine*, vol. 25, no. 24, pp. 3130–3139, 2000.

[12] J. E. Ware Jr., M. Kosinski, M. S. Bayliss, C. A. McHorney, W. H. Rogers, and A. Raczek, "Comparison of methods for the scoring and statistical analysis of SF-36 health profile and summary measures: summary of results from the Medical Outcomes Study," *Medical Care*, vol. 33, no. 4, pp. AS264–279, 1995.

[13] N. Hisli, "Beck depresyon envanterinin geçerliliği üzerine bir çalışma," *Psikoloji Dergisi*, vol. 22, pp. 118–126, 1988.

[14] R. Jahnsen, G. Aamodt, and P. Rosenbaum, "Gross Motor Function Classification System used in adults with cerebral palsy: agreement of self-reported versus professional rating," *Developmental Medicine and Child Neurology*, vol. 48, no. 9, pp. 734–738, 2006.

[15] A. McCormick, M. Brien, J. Plourde, E. Wood, P. Rosenbaum, and J. McLean, "Stability of the Gross Motor Function Classification System in adults with cerebral palsy," *Developmental Medicine and Child Neurology*, vol. 49, no. 4, pp. 265–269, 2007.

[16] S. Diwan, H. Chovatiya, and J. Diwan, "Depression and quality of life in mothers of children with cerebral palsy," *National Journal of Integrated Research in Medicine*, vol. 2, no. 4, pp. 11–13, 2011.

[17] K. Kaya, S. Unsal-Delialioglu, N. K. Ordu-Gokkaya et al., "Musculo-skeletal pain, quality of life and depression in mothers of children with cerebral palsy," *Disability and Rehabilitation*, vol. 32, no. 20, pp. 1666–1672, 2010.

[18] L. Eker and E. H. Tüzün, "An evaluation of quality of life of mothers of children with cerebral palsy," *Disability and Rehabilitation*, vol. 26, no. 23, pp. 1354–1359, 2004.

[19] G. Bumin, A. Günal, and Ş. Tükel, "Anxiety, depression and quality of life in mothers of disabled children," *SDÜ Tıp Fakültesi Dergisi*, vol. 15, no. 1, pp. 6–11, 2008.

[20] G. H. S. Singer, L. K. Irvin, and N. Hawkins, "Stress management training for parents of children with severe handicaps," *Mental Retardation*, vol. 26, no. 5, pp. 269–277, 1988.

[21] D. Keller and A. S. Honig, "Maternal and paternal stress in families with school-aged children with disabilities," *American Journal of Orthopsychiatry*, vol. 74, no. 3, pp. 337–348, 2004.

[22] V. McManus, S. I. Michelsen, K. Parkinson et al., "Discussion groups with parents of children with cerebral palsy in Europe designed to assist development of a relevant measure of environment," *Child: Care, Health and Development*, vol. 32, no. 2, pp. 185–192, 2006.

19

Rehabilitation of Back Extensor Muscles' Inhibition in Patients with Long-Term Mechanical Low-Back Pain

Chidozie Emmanuel Mbada,[1] Olusola Ayanniyi,[2] Samuel Olusegun Ogunlade,[3] Elkanah Ayodele Orimolade,[4] Ajibola Babatunde Oladiran,[4] and Abiola Oladele Ogundele[5]

[1] *Department of Medical Rehabilitation, College of Health Sciences, Obafemi Awolowo University, Ile-Ife, Nigeria*
[2] *Department of Physiotherapy, College of Medicine, University of Ibadan, Ibadan, Nigeria*
[3] *Department of Orthopaedic and Trauma, College of Medicine, University of Ibadan, Ibadan, Nigeria*
[4] *Department of Orthopaedic Surgery and Traumatology, Obafemi Awolowo University Teaching Hospitals Complex, Ile-Ife, Nigeria*
[5] *Department of Physiotherapy, Obafemi Awolowo University Teaching Hospitals Complex, Ile-Ife, Nigeria*

Correspondence should be addressed to Chidozie Emmanuel Mbada; doziembada@yahoo.com

Academic Editors: K. Hashimoto, J. D. Kingsley, J. J. Sosnoff, M. Syczewska, and M. Yu

This study investigated the effect of static or dynamic back extensors endurance exercise in combination with McKenzie Protocol (MP) in patients with Long-term Mechanical Low-Back Pain (LMLBP). This randomized controlled trial involved 84 patients, who were assigned into MP Group (MPG), MP plus Static Back Extensors Endurance (SBEE) Exercise Group (MPSBEEG), or MP plus Dynamic Back Extensors' Endurance (DBEE) Exercise Group (MPDBEEG). Twenty-five, 22, and 20 participants in MPG, MPSBEEG, and MPDBEEG, respectively, completed the thrice weekly eight-week study (drop-out rate = 20.2%) and outcomes were measured in terms of SBEE, DBEE, and Back Muscles Fatigue (BMF) at the 4th and 8th week, respectively. There were significant differences in groups mean change scores on SBEE (14.6 ± 8.44, 45.7 ± 17.0 and 17.1 ± 10.2 sec), DBEE (2.88 ± 1.88, 12.9 ± 11.1, and 10.7 ± 6.51 rep), and BMF (12.6 ± 2.16, 10.1 ± 2.08, and 10.8 ± 2.19) at week 4, and SBEE (29.6 ± 8.44, 60.7 ± 17.1, and 32.1 ± 10.2 sec), DBEE (8.36 ± 2.22, 18.1 ± 10.1, and 16.6 ± 6.24 reps), BMF (3.88 ± 1.67, 5.41 ± 2.32, and 4.35 ± 1.63) at week 8, respectively ($P < 0.05$). It was concluded that MP alone, or in combination with SBEE or DBEE, exercise was effective in the rehabilitation of back extensors' endurance and fatigability in patients with LMLBP. However, the addition of SBEE to MP led to significantly higher positive effects.

1. Introduction

Long-term mechanical low-back pain (LBP) results in inhibition and atrophy of the deep segmental muscles such as multifidus and overactivity of the longer superficial muscles of the trunk with resultant decreased dynamic activity and increased fatiguibility [1–4]. Long-term mechanical LBP is more difficult to treat [5–7] and treatment outcomes give variable results [8–10] and it consequently results in both physical and psychological deconditionings that trap the patient in a vicious circle characterized with decreased physical performance, exacerbated nociceptive sensations, depression, impaired social functioning, and work disability [11].

One of the more commonly used physical therapy approaches in the management of long-term mechanical LBP with documented effectiveness is the McKenzie Protocol (MP) [12–15]; However, there seems to be inconclusive evidence whether the MP addresses the accompanying back muscles inhibition in patients with long-term mechanical LBP. Some studies considered the McKenzie's extension exercises as passive and presumably opined that it may not counter the back muscles' inhibition and atrophy resulting from long-term LBP [16–18], however, a study by Fiebert and Keller [19] among apparently healthy individuals demonstrated that the McKenzie's extension exercises were not truly passive for lumbar back extensor muscles.

On the other hand, back endurance exercise is believed to enhance muscle reactivation and reconditioning [20–23]. There is emerging evidence to suggest that endurance training of the low-back extensors in patients with LBP can be effective in reducing pain, disability, and work loss, and improving fatigue threshold and physical performance [24–27]. Pain-related muscular inhibition of the back muscles characteristically leads to loss of muscle motor units, muscle atrophy, iatrogenic muscular inhibition, and decreased strength and endurance [20–22, 28, 29]. Unfortunately, assessment and training of endurance of the back extensor muscles compared with muscular strength have been reported to be less frequently carried out [30], though, endurance capabilities of these muscles may be as important or even more important than strength in the treatment and prevention of LBP [31]. Furthermore, there seems to be a dearth of studies involving dynamic endurance exercise of the back extensor muscles compared with a chronicle of studies that have investigated the effect of static muscular endurance exercise training in patients with acute [24], subacute [27], and long-term LBP [32], respectively. Meanwhile, dynamic endurance may be needed more than static endurance as most of the daily tasks involve dynamic movement [33, 34]. Therefore, the objective of this study was to investigate the effect of static or dynamic back extensors endurance exercise in combination with McKenzie Protocol on static and dynamic back extensor muscles' endurance and fatigability in patients with long-term mechanical LBP.

2. Materials and Methods

A single-blind randomized controlled trial involving 84 patients with LMLBP was conducted. Long-term LBP was defined as a history of LBP of not less than 3 months. Mechanical LBP refers to back pain of musculoskeletal origin that results from inflammation caused by irritation or trauma to the disk, the facet joints sufficient enough to stress, deform, or damage the ligaments, or the muscles of the back [35, 36] in which symptoms vary with physical activity [37]. The participants were patients attending the physiotherapy department, Obafemi Awolowo University (OAU) Teaching Hospitals Complex and the OAU Health Centre, Ile-Ife, Nigeria, respectively. Eligibility to participate in the study was carried out with the McKenzie Institute's Lumbar Spine Assessment Format (MILSAF). The MILSAF was used to recruit a homogenous sample of participants who demonstrated directional preference (DP) for extension.

Exclusion criteria for this study were as follows:

(1) red flags indicative of serious spinal pathology with signs and symptoms of nerve root compromise (with at least two of these signs: dermatomal sensory loss, myotomal muscle weakness, and reduced lower limb reflexes),

(2) any obvious spinal deformity or neurological disease,

(3) a reported history of cardiovascular diseases contraindicated to exercise; or individuals who were with elevated blood pressure (>140/90 mmHg),

(4) pregnancy or previous spinal surgery,

(5) previous experience of McKenzie method,

(6) directional preference for flexion, lateral or no directional preference based on the McKenzie assessment.

Permuted block randomization was used to assign participants to one of three treatment groups. Viz- the McKenzie Protocol Group (MPG) (n = 29), MP plus Static Back Endurance Exercise Group (MPSBEEG) (n = 27), and MP plus Dynamic Back Endurance Exercise Group (MPDBEEG) (n = 28). Sixty seven (32 males (47.8%) and 35 females (52.2%)) participants completed the 8-week study. Twenty five participants completed the study in MPG, 22 in MPSBEEG, and 20 in MPDBEEG. A total drop-out rate of 20.2% was observed in the study. Each group received treatment thrice weekly for eight weeks and outcomes were assessed at the end of 4th and 8th weeks of study. Ethics and Research Committee of the Obafemi Awolowo University Teaching Hospitals Complex (Reg no.: ERC/2010/01/02) and the joint University of Ibadan/University College Hospital Institutional Review Committee (Ref no.: UI/UC/10/0194), respectively, gave approval for the study.

2.1. Instruments. A height meter (Seca 240—made in UK) calibrated from 0 to 200 cm was used to measure the height of each participant to the nearest 0.1 cm. A weighing scale (Hana weighing Scale—made in China) calibrated from 0 to 120 kg was used to measure the body weight of participants in kilograms to the nearest 1.0 kg. A metronome (Wittner Metronome system Maelzel, Made in Germany) was used to set the tempo for dynamic back endurance muscles endurance. A Quartz stop watch (Quartz USA) was used to determine the endurance time or the isometric holding time in seconds (i.e., from the onset of the BSME to volitional fatigue). A plinth that could be inclined at angles 30°, 45°, and 60° was used for the purpose of conducting the BSME and RAUT and the McKenzie Protocol, static and dynamic back endurance exercise, respectively. Two nonelastic straps were used to ensure stability during the BSME and RAUT tests, respectively. A towel was positioned beneath the ankle straps to reduce the strain on the distal aspect of the tendo calcaneus (Achilles tendon) and thereby ensure comfort of the participants during the tests. The Borg scale of perceived exertion [38] was used to assess level of fatigue to both BSME and RAUT, respectively. The scale was translated into the Yoruba language. The translation was done at the Department of Linguistics and African Languages of Obafemi Awolowo University, Ile Ife. Pearson product moment correlation coefficient (r) of 0.84 was obtained for the criterion validity of the back translation of the Yoruba version.

2.2. Physical Performance Test. Physical performance assessment for both static and dynamic back extensors endurance was conducted prior the commencement of treatment intervention and at the 4th and 8th weeks of treatment, respectively. Physical performance tests used in this study included the modified Biering-Sørensen test of Static Muscular Endurance (BSME) and Repetitive Arch-Up Test (RAUT) for dynamic endurance, respectively. Prior to the endurance tests, the participants were instructed in detail on the study procedures. The test was preceded by a low-intensity warm-up phase of five minutes that comprised stretches and strolling at a self-determined pace around the research venue.

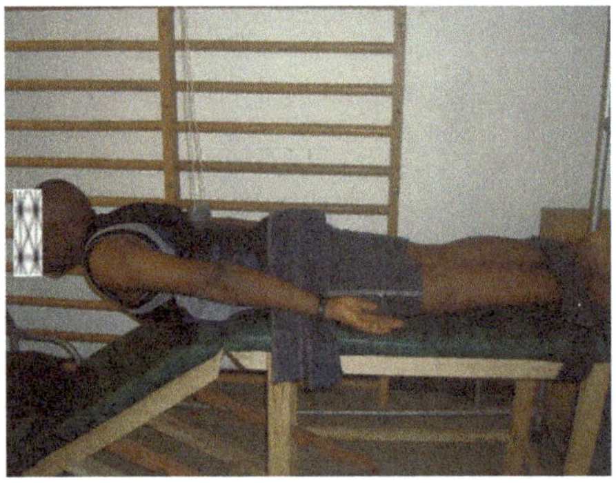

Figure 1: The modified Biering-Sorensen test of static muscular endurance position.

The modified BSME and RAUT were performed in random order among the participants with a 15-minute interval provided between both tests. The tests ended with a cool-down phase, comprising the same low-intensity stretches and strolling around the research venue for about five minutes.

2.2.1. Assessment of Static Back Extensors' Endurance. The BSME was used to assess the static back endurance. During the test the participant laid on the plinth in the prone position with the upper edge of the iliac crests aligned with the edge of the plinth with their hands held by their sides. The lower body was fixed to the plinth by two nonelastic straps located around the pelvis and ankles. Horizontality in the test position was ensured by asking the participant to maintain contact between his/her back and a hanging weighted ball. Once a loss of contact for more than 10 seconds was noticed, the participant was encouraged once to immediately maintain contact again. Once the participant could not immediately correct or hold the position or claimed to be fatigued the test was terminated [20, 39] (Figure 1).

2.2.2. Assessment of Dynamic Back Extensors' Endurance. Repetitive Arch-Up Test (RAUT) was used to assess the static back endurance. During the test, the participant lay in a prone position on the plinth with the arms positioned along the sides. The iliac crest was positioned at the edge of the plinth. The lower body was fixed to the plinth by two non-elastic straps located around the pelvis and ankles. With the arms held along the sides touching the body, the subject was asked to flex the upper trunk downward to 45° as indicated by a board. The participant then raised the upper trunk upwards to the horizontal position followed by returning back downward to 45 degrees to complete a cycle. The repetition rate was one repetition per two to three seconds. The movement was repeated as many times as possible at a constant pace synchronous to a metronome count. Once the movement becomes jerky or nonsynchronous, or did not reach the horizontal level, the subject was encouraged once to immediately correct the motion again. The test was terminated once the participant could not go on with the tempo of the motion or reported fatigue or exhaustion [39] (Figures 2 and 3).

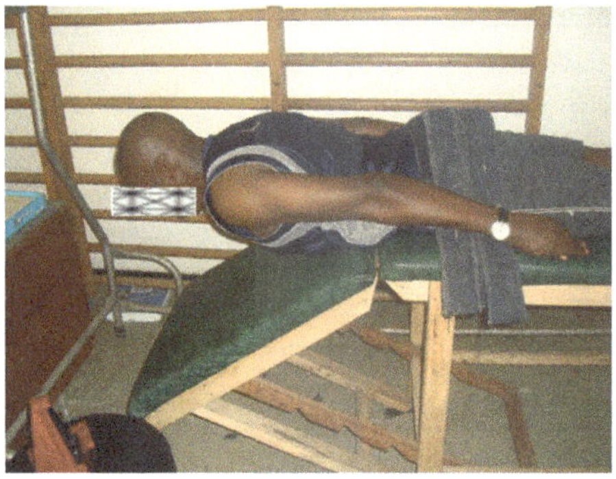

Figure 2: Horizontal phase of the Repetitive Arch-Up Test.

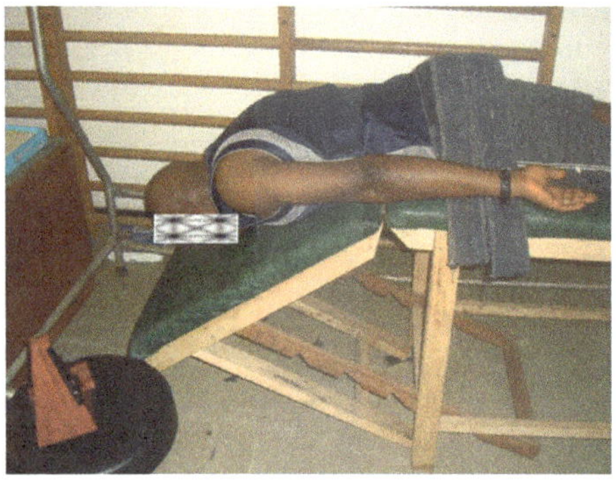

Figure 3: Downward phase of the Repetitive Arch-Up Test.

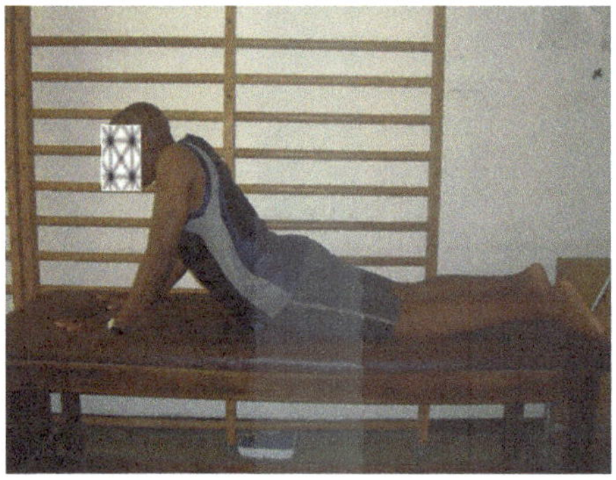

Figure 4: McKenzie's extension exercise posture in lying.

2.3. Treatment. The participants were instructed in details on the procedures of study at inclusion. Treatment for the different groups was in three phases comprising warmup, main exercise, and cooldown, respectively. The warm-up phase involved a low-intensity activities comprising stretches and strolling at self-determined pace around the research venue for aduration of five minutes. Treatment also ended with a cool-down phase comprising of the same low-intensity exercise as the warm-up for about five minutes.

The McKenzie Protocol (MP) involved a course of specific lumbosacral repeated movements in extension that cause the symptoms to centralize, decrease, or abolish. The determination of the direction preference for extension was followed by the main MP activities including "Extension lying prone," "Extension In Prone" and "Extension in standing" (Figures 4 and 5). The MP also included a set of back care education

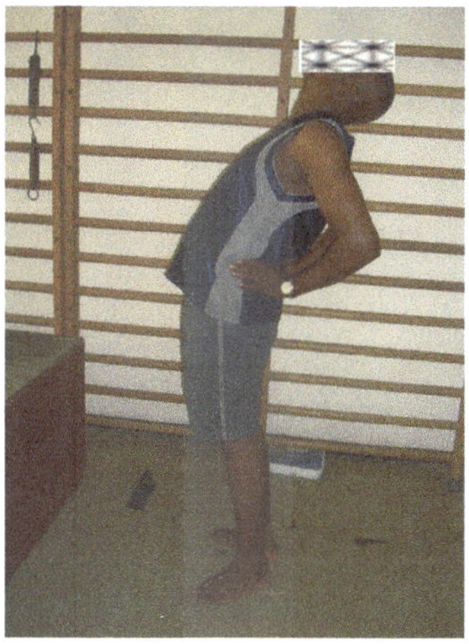

FIGURE 5: McKenzie's extension exercise posture in standing.

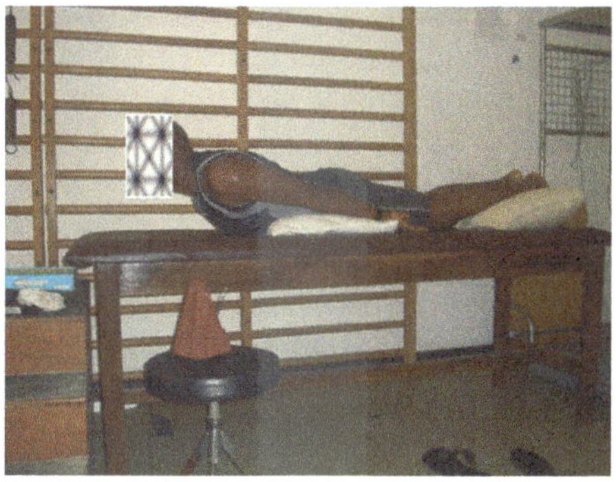

FIGURE 6: Exercise position 1: prone position with arms by the sides of the body, and head and trunk lifted off the plinth from neutral to extension for static and Dynamic Back Extensors' Endurance exercise.

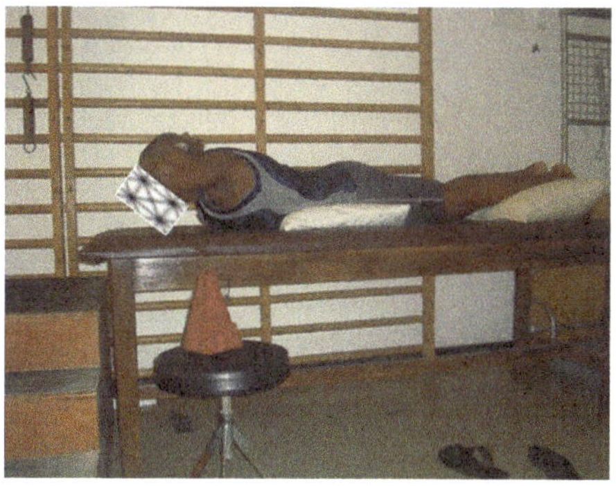

FIGURE 7: Exercise position 2: prone position with hands interlocked at occiput so shoulders are abducted to 90° and elbows flexed, and head and trunk lifted off the plinth from neutral to extension for static and dynamic back extensors endurance exercise.

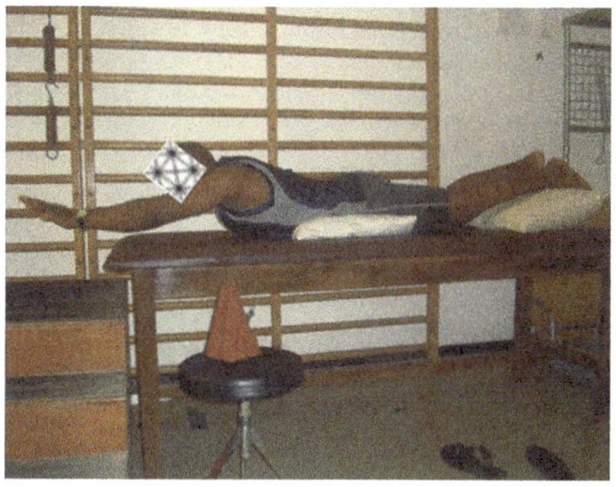

FIGURE 8: Exercise position 3: prone position with both arms elevated forwards, and head and trunk lifted off the plinth from neutral to extension for static and dynamic back extensors endurance exercise.

instructions which comprised a 9-item instructional guide on standing, sitting, lifting, and other activities of daily living for home exercise for all the participants.

2.3.1. Static Back Extensors Endurance Exercise. In addition to completing the MP (i.e., back extension exercises plus the back care education), static back extensors endurance exercise included five different exercises of increasing level of difficulty where the positions of the upper and lower limbs were altered. The participants began the exercise training programme with the first exercise position but progressed to the next exercises at their own pace when they could hold a given position for 10 seconds. On reaching the fifth progression, they continued with the fifth progression until the end of the exercise programme.

2.3.2. Dynamic Back Extensors Endurance Exercise. In addition to completing the MP, dynamic back extensors endurance exercise included five different exercises. The dynamic back endurance exercise was an exact replica of the static back extensors endurance exercise protocol in terms of exercise positions, progressions, and duration. However, instead of static posturing of the trunk in the prone lying position and holding the positions of the upper and lower limbs suspended in the air during all the five exercise progressions for the 10 seconds, the participant was asked to move the trunk and the suspended limbs 10 times (Figures 6, 7, 8, 9, and 10).

The details of the treatment procedure for MPG, MPSBEEG, and MPDBEEG have been published elsewhere by the authors [40].

2.4. Data Analysis. Data were analyzed using descriptive and inferential statistics of one-way analysis of variance (ANOVA) and multiple comparisons post hoc tests at $P = 0.05$. The data analyses were carried out using SPSS 13.0 version software (SPSS Inc., Chicago, IL, USA).

3. Results

The mean age, height, weight, BMI, and pain intensity of all the participants were 51.8 ± 7.35 years, 1.66 ± 0.04 m, 76.2 ± 11.2 kg, $27.2 \pm 4.43\,\text{kg/m}^2$, and 6.55 ± 1.75, respectively. Across group comparison of participants' baseline anthropometric and clinical parameters is presented in Table 1. The result indicates that the participants' baseline measures across the MPG, MPSBEEG, and MPDBEEG were comparable ($P > 0.05$). Repeated measures ANOVA and post hoc multiple

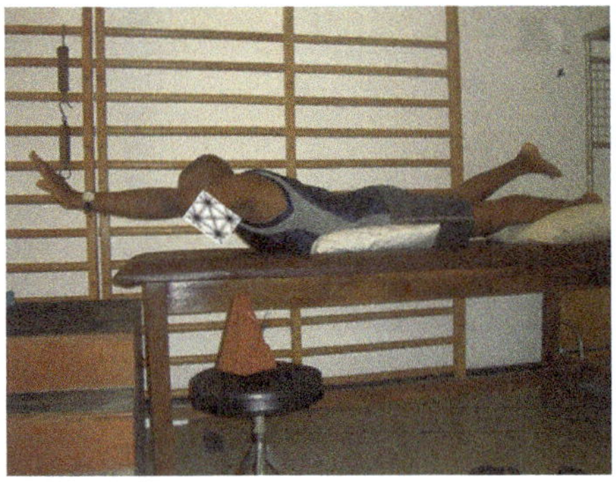

Figure 9: Exercise position 4: prone position and head, trunk and contralateral arm and leg lifted off the plinth from neutral to extension for static and dynamic back extensors endurance exercise.

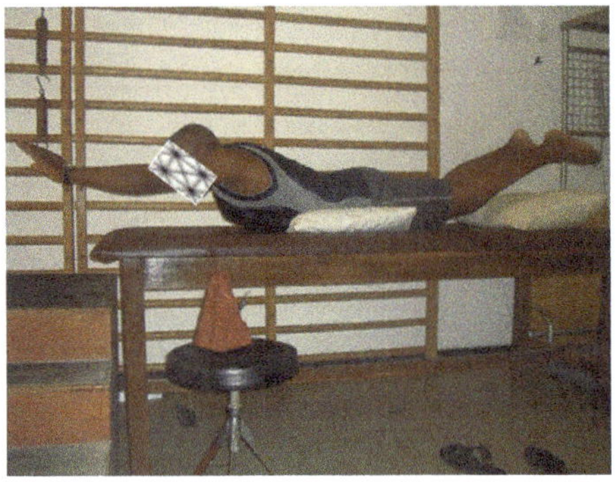

Figure 10: Exercise position 5: prone position with both arms elevated forwards and both legs (with knees extended) lifted off the plinth from neutral to extension for static and dynamic back extensors endurance exercise.

comparisons of the participants' clinical variables across the 3 time points of the study are presented in Table 2.

Results among the different groups showed that there were significant differences ($P < 0.05$) in the participants' outcome parameters across the 3 timepoints of the study.

One-way ANOVA and least Significant difference post hoc multiple comparison of the participants' treatment outcomes (mean change) at weeks four and eight of the study are presented in Table 3. From the result, there were significant differences in groups' mean change scores on static endurance (14.6 ± 8.44, 45.7 ± 17.0, and 17.1 ± 10.2 sec), dynamic endurance (2.88 ± 1.88, 12.9 ± 11.1, and 10.7 ± 6.51 rep), and muscle fatigue (12.6 ± 2.16, 10.1 ± 2.08, and 10.8 ± 2.19) at week 4, and static endurance (29.6 ± 8.44, 60.7 ± 17.1, and 32.1 ± 10.2 sec), dynamic endurance (8.36 ± 2.22, 18.1 ± 10.1, and 16.6 ± 6.24 resp.), muscle fatigue (3.88 ± 1.67, 5.41 ± 2.32, and 4.35 ± 1.63) at week 8, respectively. Least significant difference (LSD) post hoc analysis was used to elucidate where the differences within between groups lie.

4. Discussion

This study investigated the effect of static or dynamic back extensors endurance exercise in combination with McKenzie Protocol on back extensor muscles' endurance and fatiguability in patients with long-term mechanical LBP. From the result of this study, no significant difference in physical characteristics and baseline outcome parameters of the participants in the different treatment groups was observed. Baseline characteristics are believed to be predictors of response to treatment in clinical trials for LBP [41–43]. Comparability in baseline measure in clinical trials is reported to reduce the chances of cofounders other than the intervention in predicting outcomes. In this study, the groups were comparable in their general characteristics and baseline clinical parameters. Therefore, it is implied that the results obtained at different point in the course of the study could have been large due to the effects of the various treatment regimens.

Within-group comparison across the 3 timepoints (weeks 0–4, 4–8, and 0–8) of the study revealed that the MP had significant effects on muscle fatigue and static and dynamic endurance, respectively. Studies on the effect of the MP on muscle fatigability and endurance (static or dynamic) seem to be not available in the literature. However, this present study found that patients that were treated with the MP only had significant reduction in back muscles' fatigability level and increased static and dynamic back extensor muscles' endurance, respectively. It is opined that the effect of MP on muscle fatigue and endurance might be due to the relationship between pain and each of muscle fatigue and endurance. MP has been reported from previous studies to significantly ameliorate pain in patients with long-term LBP [12, 14, 44, 45]. It is believed that chronic pain and fatigue often occur together in majority of individuals with musculoskeletal pain and that muscle pain and fatigue are not independent conditions and may share a common pathway that is disrupted in chronic muscle pain conditions [46]. Similarly, pain in itself has been reported to precipitate decreased muscle endurance resulting from increased muscle metabolite from prolonged muscle tension and spasm [47], muscle deconditioning [48] and inhibition of the paraspinal muscles [48]. It is adduced that the MP may not have a direct effect on muscle fatigue and endurance but a consequence of its effect on pain. However, this speculation is open to empirical investigation.

Within-group comparison across the 3 timepoints (weeks 0–4, 4–8, and 0–8) of the study revealed that the MP plus Static Back Endurance Exercise (MPSBEE) had significant effects on muscle fatigue and static and dynamic endurance, respectively. There seems to be a scarcity of similar studies to which the result obtained in this study can be compared directly. However, there are other reports that indicate that endurance training of the low-back extensors can be effective to elevate fatigue threshold and improve performance, thus reduce disability [24, 25, 27, 49], and decrease work loss [26, 50, 51]. Furthermore, endurance training is believed to cause mechanical loading of the muscles [52] which in turn leads to tissue adaptation [53].

The orientation and posture for the static back extensor endurance exercise in this study were extension in sagittal plane while in prone lying. It is believed that an increase in sagittal curvature and change in spinal shape may alter physiologic loading through the spine as a consequence of

TABLE 1: Comparison of participants' baseline anthropometric and clinical parameters.

Variable	MPG (n = 25) $\bar{x} \pm$ SD	MPSBEEG (n = 22) $\bar{x} \pm$ SD	MPDBEEG (n = 20) $\bar{x} \pm SD$	F ratio	P value
Age (yr)	50.6 ± 7.57	51.2 ± 7.50	53.8 ± 6.83	1.106	0.339
Height (m)	1.67 ± 0.04	1.66 ± 0.04	1.68 ± 0.04	2.185	0.331
Weight (Kg)	76.3 ± 9.95	75.2 ± 13.2	77.2 ± 10.8	0.156	0.856
BMI (Kg/m^2)	27.5 ± 4.20	27.3 ± 5.25	26.9 ± 3.89	0.093	0.912
VAS	6.56 ± 1.83	6.50 ± 1.71	6.60 ± 1.79	0.017	0.983
SE	36.7 ± 11.8	37.3 ± 13.4	39.2 ± 18.6	0.162	0.851
DE	11.7 ± 2.63	11.3 ± 2.10	11.3 ± 4.27	0.129	0.879
SRPE	13.5 ± 2.12	12.5 ± 2.01	12.2 ± 1.73	2.870	0.064
DRPE	14.1 ± 2.55	14.1 ± 2.16	13.4 ± 1.05	0.986	0.380

Alpha level was set at $P < 0.05$.
Key:
MPG: McKenzie Protocol Group.
MPSBEEG: McKenzie Protocol plus Static Back Endurance Exercise Group.
MPDBEEG: McKenzie Protocol plus Dynamic Back Endurance Exercise Group.
$\bar{x}$: Mean.
SD: Standard deviation.
VAS: Visual Analogue Scale.
SE: Static Endurance.
DE: Dynamic Endurance.
SRPE: Rate of perceived exertion to Biering-Sørensen test of Static Muscular Endurance.
DRPE: Rate of perceived exertion to Repetitive Arch-Up Test.

TABLE 2: Repeated measures ANOVA and post hoc multiple comparisons of the clinical variables across the 3 timepoints of the study.

Outcome	Baseline $\bar{x} \pm$ SD	4th week $\bar{x} \pm$ SD	8th week $\bar{x} \pm$ SD	F ratio	P value
MPG (n = 25)					
SE	36.7 ± 11.8^a	51.4 ± 10.2^b	66.4 ± 10.2^c	47.402	0.001
DE	11.2 ± 2.63^a	14.6 ± 2.52^b	20.0 ± 2.92^c	62.126	0.001
SRPE	13.4 ± 2.12^a	12.6 ± 2.16^a	9.06 ± 2.16^b	22.419	0.025
DRPE	14.1 ± 2.55^a	13.7 ± 2.11^a	10.7 ± 2.11^b	16.767	0.001
MPSBEEG (n = 22)					
SE	37.3 ± 13.4^a	83.1 ± 10.9^b	98.1 ± 10.1^c	159.362	0.001
DE	11.3 ± 2.10^a	24.2 ± 10.0^b	29.4 ± 8.93^c	13.981	0.001
SRPE	12.5 ± 2.02^a	10.5 ± 2.08^b	7.05 ± 2.08^c	38.069	0.001
DRPE	14.2 ± 2.16^a	12.7 ± 1.91^b	9.68 ± 1.91^c	29.448	0.001
MPDBEEG (n = 20)					
SE	39.2 ± 18.6^a	56.2 ± 18.5^b	75.2 ± 18.5^c	15.011	0.001
DE	11.3 ± 4.27^a	22.0 ± 8.45^b	27.9 ± 8.27^c	26.890	0.001
SRPE	12.2 ± 1.73^a	10.8 ± 2.19^b	7.80 ± 2.19^c	23.652	0.001
DRPE	13.4 ± 1.05^a	9.35 ± 1.35^b	6.35 ± 1.35^c	158.731	0.001

Alpha level was set at $P < 0.05$.
Superscripts ($^{a, b, c}$).
For a particular variable, mean values with different superscript are significantly ($P < 0.05$) different. Mean values with same superscripts are not significantly ($P > 0.05$) different. The pair of cell means that is significant has different superscripts.
Key:
$\bar{x}$: Mean.
SD: standard deviation.
VAS: Visual Analogue Scale.
SE: Static Endurance.
DE: Dynamic Endurance.
SRPE: rate of perceived exertion to Biering-Sørensen test of Static Muscular Endurance.
DRPE: rate of perceived exertion to Repetitive Arch-Up Test.

TABLE 3: One-way ANOVA and least significant difference post hoc multiple comparison of the participants' treatment outcomes (mean change) at weeks four and eight of the study.

Outcome	MPG (n = 25) $\overline{x} \pm$ SD	MPSBEEG (n = 22) $\overline{x} \pm$ SD	MPDBEEG (n = 20) $\overline{x} \pm$ SD	F ratio	P value
Week four					
SE	14.6 ± 8.44^{a}	45.7 ± 17.0^{b}	17.1 ± 10.2^{a}	43.703	0.001
DE	2.88 ± 1.88^{a}	12.9 ± 11.1^{b}	10.7 ± 6.51^{b}	12.088	0.001
SRPE	12.6 ± 2.16^{a}	10.1 ± 2.08^{b}	10.8 ± 2.19^{b}	3.916	0.025
DRPE	13.7 ± 2.11^{a}	12.7 ± 1.91^{a}	9.35 ± 1.35^{b}	60.250	0.001
Week eight					
SE	29.6 ± 8.44^{a}	60.7 ± 17.1^{b}	32.1 ± 10.2^{a}	41.620	0.001
DE	8.36 ± 2.22^{a}	18.1 ± 10.1^{b}	16.6 ± 6.24^{b}	13.981	0.001
SRPE	3.88 ± 1.67^{a}	5.41 ± 2.32^{b}	4.35 ± 1.63^{b}	5.616	0.012
DRPE	3.40 ± 1.00^{a}	4.55 ± 1.30^{a}	7.05 ± 1.05^{b}	60.210	0.001

Alpha level was set at $P < 0.05$.
Superscripts (^{a,b,c}).
For a particular variable, mean values with different superscript are significantly ($P < 0.05$) different. Mean values with same superscripts are not significantly ($P > 0.05$) different. The pair of cell means that is significant has different superscripts.
Key:
$\overline{x}$: Mean.
SD: standard deviation.
SE: Static Endurance.
DE: Dynamic Endurance.
SRPE: rate of perceived exertion to Biering-Sørensen Test of Static Muscular Endurance.
DRPE: rate of perceived exertion to Repetitive Arch-Up Test.

a shift in trunk mass [54]. Also, it is adduced that the increased mechanical loading resulting from the change in spinal posture during a static hold or posturing in prone-extension may put a stress on the musculature of the back extensors. The previously stated assertion is corroborated by studies that indicated that changes in spinal posture may lead to alterations in length-tension relationships and function of paraspinal musculature [55], moment arm lengths, and force vector orientations [56]. In addition, increased mechanical loading may have a reactivating effect on the paraspinal musculature [57–59] and this may account for one of the ways static back endurance exercise achieves it therapeutic effect. Conversely, mechanical loading that exceeds the fatigue threshold of the back muscles is deleterious [60–63]. However, change in muscles properties in response to static contraction is proposed to be dependent on the relationship between motor unit activity and conduction velocity of the muscle fiber membrane [64, 65]. Nonetheless, it is difficult to compare the result of this study directly with other previous findings without caution; this is because of the variability that exists in mode, load, frequency, and volume of exercise training. Also, some of the previous studies did not clearly delineate resistance training of the lumbar extensor as either strength or endurance, static or dynamic.

Within-group comparison across the 3 timepoints (weeks 0–4, 4–8, and 0–8) of the study revealed that MP plus Dynamic Back Endurance Exercise (MPDBEE) had significant effects on muscle fatigue and static and dynamic endurance, respectively. Over the past decades, different types of dynamic exercises have been employed in the management of patients with LBP with varying reported successes [66–69]. Johannsen et al. [70] found that dynamic endurance training improved isokinetic back muscle strength and endurance, while Arokoski et al. [71] reported that they are effective in activating the paraspinal muscles. The basis for dynamic exercises in low-back rehabilitation in most of the previous studies was due to the fact that, in reality, some daily tasks involve dynamic movement and may require dynamic endurance more than static endurance [33, 72, 73]. During dynamic tasks, it has been shown that the force generation and muscle recruitment activities associated with twisting change significantly as a function of the trunk posture [74] and the activity of the trunk muscles can be used to speculate the stress on the lumbar intervertebral joints [57–59, 75]. Consequently, the dynamic tasks could possibly lead to LBP [76]. Therefore, the concept of dynamic training for the trunk muscles to act in a synchronous manner to maintain stability [72] is supported by reported link between mechanical instability of the lumbar spine and LBP disorders [77] and the association of LBP with muscle dysfunction [78]. However, to the knowledge of the researchers, there seems to be an apparent dearth of studies that have examined the effects of combining the MP and dynamic endurance training of the back extensors.

The efficacy of each of the MP, MPSBEE, and MPDBEE as observed in this study could be as a result of the fact that each of the regimen-contained active exercise was carried out in extension positions. Some studies submitted that exercises and postures in extension improve and resolve symptoms in patients with specific and nonspecific LBP [79–82]. Active exercise is described as functional exercise performed by the patient or client. Previous studies have shown that active exercise, irrespective of the type, is more effective in the management of patients with long-term LBP than passive therapy [83–85]. Active exercises in their different forms in long-term LBP are aimed at restoring back function by improving movement, strength, endurance, and general fitness [86]. The MP utilizes a system of patient self-generated force to mobilize or manipulate the spine through a series of active repeated movements or static positioning and it is based on the patient's pain response to certain movements and postures during assessment [35]. Similarly, endurance exercises are active exercises that require static posturing or repeated movements in order to initiate overload stimuli on the musculature.

Mbada et al. [40] summarized that pain is the major impairment of long-term LBP and it results in deconditioning of the musculoskeletal system leading to loss of motion, stiffness, cartilage degeneration, fear-avoidance behaviour, iatrogenic muscular inhibition, and muscle atrophy [28, 29]. Like a vicious cycle, the deconditioning syndrome may also precipitate and perpetuate pain which consequents in recurrent or acute-on-chronic LBP. Pain leads to muscle guarding or splinting of all movements in the affected region, splinting or disuse leads to muscular atrophy, which in turn results in weakness [28]. The weakness, therefore, may be secondary to inhibition caused by the noxious stimuli caused by pain [28]. The movement component of treatment regimens as used in this study may have resulted in reconditioning of the patients by making them expand the limits to their physical functioning, retard muscle atrophy, enhance their pain control ability, and improve the psychosocial factors affected by LBP. This is in order to counteract the effect of long-term LBP which precipitates inhibition of movements and thus results in physical inactivity and consequent neurological and physiological changes of the paraspinal musculature resulting in back muscles' inhibition, selective loss of Type 2 muscle fibers, weakness, and shortening [85, 87–89].

Apart from the observed significant effects of each of the treatment regimens on back static and dynamic back extensors endurance and muscular fatiguability in this study, comparatively, MP plus Static Back Endurance Exercise (MPSBEE) led to higher significant improvement on static and dynamic endurance and reduction in muscle fatiguability at weeks four and eight, respectively. From the post-hoc results across the 3 time points of the study, it was observed that the different treatment regimens had significant effect at week four on static and dynamic endurance except on muscular fatiguability of the MP group that was only significant at the week eight. Previous studies indicated that static training programme was effective for increasing isometric (static) endurance of the trunk extensor muscles in healthy [25, 90] and patient populations [27, 91–93], respectively. Another study among healthy male adults found that static training can increase both isometric and dynamic endurance while dynamic training can increase dynamic endurance only [76]. The treatment methodology for the participants in this group involved both movement and mechanical loading components. The treatment regimen may have possible stimulating and reactivating effect on the inhibited muscles of the back extensors caused by long-term LBP. This is because skeletal muscle tissues adapt to higher level of stimulus. An overload stimulus is believed to improve neural control, muscle contractile protein size, and muscular hypertrophy [28]. Addition of load to movement is reported to enhance predominantly fast motor unit recruitment [94]. The physiological principle on which static endurance training depends is the overload principle. This principle states simply that the strength, endurance, and hypertrophy of a muscle will increase only when the muscle performs for a given period of time at its maximum strength and endurance capacity, that is, against workloads that are above those normally encountered [76].

5. Conclusion

From the finding of this study, it was concluded that the McKenzie protocol alone, or in combination with static or dynamic back extensor muscles endurance exercise, was effective in the rehabilitation of back extensor muscles endurance and fatiguability in patients with long-term LBP. However, the addition of static endurance exercise to the McKenzie protocol led to significantly higher positive effect.

References

[1] T. Sihvonen, J. Partanen, O. Hanninen, and S. Soimakallio, "Electric behavior of low back muscles during lumbar pelvic rhythm in low back pain patients and healthy controls," *Archives of Physical Medicine and Rehabilitation*, vol. 72, no. 13, pp. 1080–1087, 1991.

[2] J. E. Cassisi, M. E. Robinson, P. O'Conner, and M. MacMillan, "Trunk strength and lumbar paraspinal muscle activity during isometric exercise in chronic low-back pain patients and controls," *Spine*, vol. 18, no. 2, pp. 245–251, 1993.

[3] T. Sihvonen, M. Huttunen, M. Makkonen, and O. Airaksinen, "Functional changes in back muscle activity correlate with pain intensity and prediction of low back pain during pregnancy," *Archives of Physical Medicine and Rehabilitation*, vol. 79, no. 10, pp. 1210–1212, 1998.

[4] C. Richardson, G. Jull, P. Hodges, and J. Hides, *Therapeutic Exercise for Spinal Segmental Stabilization in Low Back Pain*, Churchill Livingstone, London, UK, 1999.

[5] J. T. Cottingham and J. Maitland, "A three-paradigm treatment model using soft tissue mobilization and guided movement-awareness techniques for a patient with chronic low back pain: a case study," *Journal of Orthopaedic and Sports Physical Therapy*, vol. 26, no. 3, pp. 155–167, 1997.

[6] J. Hildebrandt, M. Pfingsten, P. Saur, and J. Jansen, "Prediction of success from a multidisciplinary treatment programme for chronic low-back pain," *Spine*, vol. 22, no. 1, pp. 990–1001, 1997.

[7] H. Frost, S. E. Lamb, and C. H. Shackleton, "A functional restoration programme for chronic low back pain," *Physiotherapy*, vol. 86, no. 6, pp. 285–293, 2000.

[8] Clinical Standards Advisory Group CSAG, *Report on Back Pain*, HMSO, London, UK, 1994.

[9] J. Rainville, J. Sobel, C. Hartigan, G. Monlux, and J. Bean, "Decreasing disability in chronic back pain through aggressive spine rehabilitation," *Journal of Rehabilitation Research and Development*, vol. 34, no. 4, pp. 383–393, 1997.

[10] D. M. Carpenter and B. W. Nelson, "Low back strengthening for the prevention and treatment of low back pain," *Medicine and Science in Sports and Exercise*, vol. 31, no. 1, pp. 18–24, 1999.

[11] C. Demoulin, M. Vanderthommen, C. Duysens, and J.-M. Crielaard, "Spinal muscle evaluation using the Sorensen test: a critical appraisal of the literature," *Joint Bone Spine*, vol. 73, no. 1, pp. 43–50, 2006.

[12] D. C. Cherkin, R. A. Deyo, M. Battié, J. Street, and W. Barlow, "A comparison of physical therapy, chiropractic manipulation, and provision of an educational booklet for the treatment of patients with low back pain," *The New England Journal of Medicine*, vol. 339, no. 15, pp. 1021–1029, 1998.

[13] R. McKenzie and S. May, *The Lumbar Spine. Mechanical Diagnosis & Therapy*, vol. 1, Spinal Publications, Waikanae, New Zealand, 2nd edition, 2003.

[14] L. A. Carneiro Machado, M. V. S. De Souza, P. H. Ferreira, and M. L. Ferreira, "The McKenzie method for low back pain: a systematic review of the literature with a meta-analysis approach," *Spine*, vol. 31, no. 9, pp. E254–E262, 2006.

[15] O. Ayanniyi, O. T. Lasisi, B. O. A. Adegoke, and M. O. Oni-Orisan, "Management of low back pain: attitudes and treatment preferences of physiotherapists in Nigeria," *African Journal of Biomedical Research*, vol. 101, pp. 41–49, 2007.

[16] R. Donelson, G. Silva, and K. Murphy, "Centralization phenomenon. It usefulness in evaluating and treating referred pain," *Spine*, vol. 15, no. 3, pp. 211–213, 1990.

[17] M. R. Bookhout, "Biomechanical assessment of low back pain," *Journal of Back Back Musculoskeletal Rehabilitation*, vol. 1, pp. 33–45, 1991.

[18] M. R. Underwood, "Patients' beliefs as to the cause of their low back pain," *Journal of Back and Musculoskeletal Rehabilitation*, vol. 9, no. 1, pp. 65–67, 1997.

[19] I. Fiebert and C. D. Keller, "Are "passive" extension exercises really passive?" *Journal of Orthopaedic and Sports Physical Therapy*, vol. 19, no. 2, pp. 111–116, 1994.

[20] F. Biering-Sorensen, "Physical measurements as risk indicators for low-back trouble over a one-year period," *Spine*, vol. 9, no. 2, pp. 106–119, 1984.

[21] S. V. Risch, N. K. Norvell, M. L. Pollock et al., "Lumbar strengthening in chronic low back pain patients: physiologic and psychological benefits," *Spine*, vol. 18, no. 2, pp. 232–238, 1993.

[22] S. Luoto, M. Heliövaara, H. Hurri, and H. Alaranta, "Static back endurance and the risk of low-back pain," *Clinical Biomechanics*, vol. 10, no. 6, pp. 323–324, 1995.

[23] J. Mayer, V. Mooney, and S. Dagenais, "Evidence-informed management of chronic low back pain with lumbar extensor strengthening exercises," *Spine Journal*, vol. 8, no. 1, pp. 96–113, 2008.

[24] P. Plum and J. F. Rehfeld, "Muscular training for acute and chronic back pain," *The Lancet*, vol. 1, no. 8426, pp. 453–454, 1985.

[25] M. T. Moffroid, L. D. Haugh, A. J. Haig, S. M. Henry, and M. H. Pope, "Endurance training of trunk extensor muscles," *Physical Therapy*, vol. 73, no. 1, pp. 10–17, 1993.

[26] S. M. LeFort and T. E. Hannah, "Return to work following an aquafitness and muscle strengthening program for the low back injured," *Archives of Physical Medicine and Rehabilitation*, vol. 75, no. 11, pp. 1247–1255, 1994.

[27] B. Chok, R. Lee, J. Latimer, and S. B. Tan, "Endurance training of the trunk extensor muscles in people with subacute low back pain," *Physical Therapy*, vol. 79, no. 11, pp. 1032–1042, 1999.

[28] B. Holmes, S. Leggett, V. Mooney, J. Nichols, S. Negri, and A. Hoeyberghs, "Comparison of female geriatric lumbar-extension strength: asymptotic versus chronic low back pain patients and their response to active rehabilitation," *Journal of Spinal Disorders*, vol. 9, no. 1, pp. 17–22, 1996.

[29] B. W. Nelson, D. M. Carpenter, T. E. Dreisinger, M. Mitchell, C. E. Kelly, and J. A. Wegner, "Can spinal surgery be prevented by aggressive strengthening exercises? A prospective study of cervical and lumbar patients," *Archives of Physical Medicine and Rehabilitation*, vol. 80, no. 1, pp. 20–25, 1999.

[30] M. L. Pollock, S. H. Leggett, J. E. Graves, A. Jones, M. Fulton, and J. Cirulli, "Effect of resistance training on lumbar extension strength," *American Journal of Sports Medicine*, vol. 17, no. 5, pp. 624–629, 1989.

[31] B. E. Udermann, J. M. Mayer, J. E. Graves, and S. R. Murray, "Quantitative assessment of lumbar paraspinal muscle endurance," *Journal of Athletic Training*, vol. 38, no. 3, pp. 259–262, 2003.

[32] D. A. Thompson, *Sensitivity of paraspinal EMG spectral analysis to training. Two preliminary studies [Doctoral thesis]*, Queens University, Kingston, Canada, 1992.

[33] J. P. Leigh and R. M. Sheetz, "Prevalence of back pain among fulltime United States workers," *British Journal of Industrial Medicine*, vol. 46, no. 9, pp. 651–657, 1989.

[34] C. N. Burnett, T. M. Glenn, C. Kisner, and L. A. Colby, "Principles of aerobic exercise," in *Therapeutic Exercise: Foundations and Techniques*, pp. 111–142, Jaypee Brothers, New Delhi, India, 3rd edition, 1996.

[35] R. A. McKenzie, *The Lumbar Spine: Mechanical Diagnosis and Therapy Spinal Publication*, Spinal Publication, Waikanae, New Zealand, 1981.

[36] V. Mora, "Chronic mechanical back pain strategies for intervention when conservative treatment fails," *Journal of the American Academy of Physician Assistants*, vol. 17, no. 7, pp. 12–16, 2004.

[37] G. Waddell, "Low back pain: a twentieth century health care enigma," *Spine*, vol. 21, no. 24, pp. 2820–2825, 1996.

[38] G. A. V. Borg, "Psychophysical bases of perceived exertion," *Medicine and Science in Sports and Exercise*, vol. 14, no. 5, pp. 377–381, 1982.

[39] H. Alaranta, "Strength and endurance testing," in *The Clinical Application of Outcomes Assessment*, S. G. Yeomans, Ed., pp. 158–162, Appleton & Lange, Stamford, Calif, USA, 2000.

[40] C. E. Mbada, O. Ayanniyi, and S. O. Ogunlade, "Effect of static and dynamic back extensor muscles endurance exercise on pain intensity, activity limitation and participation restriction in patients with Long-Term Mechanical Low-Back Pain," *Rehabilitacja Medyczna*, vol. 15, no. 3, pp. 11–20, 2011.

[41] J. D. Childs, J. M. Fritz, T. W. Flynn et al., "A clinical prediction rule to identify patients with low back pain most likely to benefit from spinal manipulation: a validation study," *Annals of Internal Medicine*, vol. 141, no. 12, pp. 1032–1042, 2004.

[42] E. M. Hagen, E. Svensen, and H. R. Eriksen, "Predictors and modifiers of treatment effect influencing sick leave in subacute low back pain patients," *Spine*, vol. 30, no. 24, pp. 2717–2723, 2005.

[43] M. R. Underwood, V. Morton, and A. Farrin, "Do baseline characteristics predict response to treatment for low back pain? Secondary analysis of the UK BEAM dataset [ISRCTN32683578]," *Rheumatology*, vol. 46, no. 8, pp. 1297–1302, 2007.

[44] R. Stankovic and O. Johnell, "Conservative treatment of acute low-back pain. A prospective randomized trial: McKenzie

method of treatment versus patient education in "mini back school"," *Spine*, vol. 15, no. 2, pp. 120–123, 1990.

[45] T. Reddeck, "An evaluation of the McKenzie regimen-validity of the disc model," in *Proceedings of the 10th Biennial Conference of Manipulative Physiotherapists Association of Australia*, Melbourne, Autralia, November 1997.

[46] University of Iowa UoI, "Biological Link Between Pain and Fatigue Discovered," 2008, http://www.sciencedaily.com/.

[47] R. B. Armstrong, "Mechanism of exercise-induced delayed onset muscular soreness: a brief review," *Medicine and Science in Sports and Exercise*, vol. 16, no. 6, pp. 529–538, 1984.

[48] S. H. Roy and L. I. E. Oddsson, "Classification of paraspinal muscle impairments by surface electromyography," *Physical Therapy*, vol. 78, no. 8, pp. 838–851, 1998.

[49] C. Manniche, L. Bentzen, G. Hesselsoe, I. Christensen, and E. Lundberg, "Clinical trial for intensive muscle training for chronic low back pain," *The Lancet*, vol. 2, no. 8626-8627, pp. 1473–1476, 1988.

[50] I. Lindström, C. Ohlund, C. Eek, L. Wallin, L.-E. Peterson, and A. Nachemson, "Mobility, strength, and fitness after a graded activity program for patients with subacute low back pain: a randomized prospective clinical study with a behavioral therapy approach," *Spine*, vol. 17, no. 6, pp. 641–652, 1992.

[51] B. Gundewall, M. Liljeqvist, and T. Hansson, "Primary prevention of back symptoms and absence from work: a prospective randomized study among hospital employees," *Spine*, vol. 18, no. 5, pp. 587–594, 1993.

[52] M. T. Moffroid, "Endurance of trunk muscles in persons with chronic low back pain: assessment, performance, training," *Journal of Rehabilitation Research and Development*, vol. 34, no. 4, pp. 440–447, 1997.

[53] M. Kjær, "Role of extracellular matrix in adaptation of tendon and skeletal muscle to mechanical loading," *Physiological Reviews*, vol. 84, no. 2, pp. 649–698, 2004.

[54] D. J. Pearsall and J. G. Reid, "Line of gravity relative to upright vertebral posture," *Clinical Biomechanics*, vol. 7, no. 2, pp. 80–86, 1992.

[55] P. B. O'Sullivan, K. M. Grahamslaw, M. Kendell, S. C. Lapenskie, N. E. Möller, and K. V. Richards, "The effect of different standing and sitting postures on trunk muscle activity in a pain-free population," *Spine*, vol. 27, no. 11, pp. 1238–1244, 2002.

[56] S. M. McGill, R. L. Hughson, and K. Parks, "Changes in lumbar lordosis modify the role of the extensor muscles," *Clinical Biomechanics*, vol. 15, no. 10, pp. 777–780, 2000.

[57] T. M. Cook, S. Mann, and G. E. Lovested, "Dynamic comparison of the two-hand stoop and assisted one-hand lift methods," *Journal of Safety Research*, vol. 21, no. 2, pp. 53–59, 1990.

[58] S. M. McGill, "Electromyographic activity of the abdominal and low back musculature during the generation of isometric and dynamic axial trunk torque: implications for lumbar mechanics," *Journal of Orthopaedic Research*, vol. 9, no. 1, pp. 91–103, 1991.

[59] R. S. Delitto and S. J. Rose, "An electromyographic analysis of two techniques for squat lifting and lowering," *Physical Therapy*, vol. 72, no. 6, pp. 438–448, 1992.

[60] J. L. Kelsey, P. B. Githens, and T. O'Conner, "Acute prolapsed lumbar intervertebral disc. An epidemiologic study with special reference to driving automobiles and cigarette smoking," *Spine*, vol. 9, no. 6, pp. 608–613, 1984.

[61] M. A. Adams and W. C. Hutton, "The effect of posture on the role of the apophysial joints in resisting intervertebral compressive forces," *Journal of Bone and Joint Surgery. British*, vol. 62, no. 3, pp. 358–362, 1980.

[62] M. A. Adams, D. W. McMillan, T. P. Green, and P. Dolan, "Sustained loading generates stress concentrations in lumbar intervertebral discs," *Spine*, vol. 21, no. 4, pp. 434–438, 1996.

[63] M. Kankaanpää, S. Taimela, C. L. Webber Jr., O. Airaksinen, and O. Hänninen, "Lumbar paraspinal muscle fatigability in repetitive isoinertial loading: EMG spectral indices, Borg scale and endurance time," *European Journal of Applied Physiology and Occupational Physiology*, vol. 76, no. 3, pp. 236–242, 1997.

[64] C. Krogh-Lund and K. Jorgensen, "Modification of myo-electric power spectrum in fatigue from 15% maximal voluntary contraction of human elbow flexor muscles, to limit of endurance: reflection of conduction velocity variation and/or centrally mediated mechanisms?" *European Journal of Applied Physiology and Occupational Physiology*, vol. 64, no. 4, pp. 359–370, 1992.

[65] A. G. Crenshaw, S. Karlsson, B. Gerdle, and J. Friden, "Differential responses in intramuscular pressure and EMG fatigue indicators during low- vs. high-level isometric contractions to fatigue," *Acta Physiologica Scandinavica*, vol. 160, no. 4, pp. 353–361, 1997.

[66] C. Manniche, E. Lundberg, I. Christensen, L. Bentzen, and G. Hesselsøe, "Intensive dynamic back exercises for chronic low back pain: a clinical trial," *Pain*, vol. 47, no. 1, pp. 53–63, 1991.

[67] H. W. Lee, "Progressive muscle synergy and synchronization in movement patterns: an approach to the treatment of dynamic lumbar instability," *Journal of Manual and Manipulative Therapy*, vol. 2, pp. 133–142, 1994.

[68] D. S. Elia, R. W. Bohannon, D. Cameron, and R. C. Albro, "Dynamic pelvic stabilization during hip flexion: a comparison study," *Journal of Orthopaedic and Sports Physical Therapy*, vol. 24, no. 1, pp. 30–36, 1996.

[69] H. Bentsen, F. Lindgärde, and R. Manthorpe, "The effect of dynamic strength back exercise and/or a home training program in 57-year-old women with chronic law back pain. Results of a prospective randomized study with a 3-year follow-up period," *Spine*, vol. 22, no. 13, pp. 1494–1500, 1997.

[70] F. Johannsen, L. Remvig, P. Kryger et al., "Exercises for chronic low back pain: a clinical trial," *Journal of Orthopaedic and Sports Physical Therapy*, vol. 22, no. 2, pp. 52–59, 1995.

[71] J. P. A. Arokoski, M. Kankaanpää, T. Valta et al., "Back and hip extensor muscle function during therapeutic exercises," *Archives of Physical Medicine and Rehabilitation*, vol. 80, no. 7, pp. 842–850, 1999.

[72] S. M. McGill, A. Childs, and C. Liebenson, "Endurance times for low back stabilization exercises: clinical targets for testing and training from a normal database," *Archives of Physical Medicine and Rehabilitation*, vol. 80, no. 8, pp. 941–944, 1999.

[73] E. Zinzen, D. Caboor, M. Verlinden et al., "Will the use of different prevalence rates influence the development of a primary prevention programme for low-back problems?" *Ergonomics*, vol. 43, no. 10, pp. 1789–1803, 2000.

[74] W. S. Marras, K. G. Davis, and K. P. Granata, "Trunk muscle activities during asymmetric twisting motions," *Journal of Electromyography and Kinesiology*, vol. 8, no. 4, pp. 247–256, 1998.

[75] R. E. Seroussi and M. H. Pope, "The relationship between trunk muscle electromyography and lifting moments in the sagittal and frontal planes," *Journal of Biomechanics*, vol. 20, no. 2, pp. 135–146, 1987.

[76] C. Pinupong, *Effects of isometric and dynamic endurance training on fatigability of back extensor muscle in male [Ph.D. thesis]*,

2005, submitted in a partial fulfilment of the requirements for the degree of master of science physiotherapy of the faculty of graduate studies Mahidol university.

[77] J. Cholewicki and S. M. McGill, "Mechanical stability of the in vivo lumbar spine: implications for injury and chronic low back pain," *Clinical Biomechanics*, vol. 11, no. 1, pp. 1–15, 1996.

[78] P. B. O'Sullivan, L. Twomey, and C. T. Allison, "Dysfunction of the neuro-muscular system in the presence of low back pain-implications for physical therapy management," *Journal of Manual and Manipulative Therapy*, vol. 5, no. 1, pp. 20–26, 1997.

[79] D. J. Ponte, G. J. Jensen, and B. E. Kent, "A preliminary report on the use of the McKenzie protocol versus Williams protocol in the treatment of low back pain," *Journal of Orthopaedic and Sports Physical Therapy*, vol. 6, no. 2, pp. 130–139, 1984.

[80] J. R. Kopp, A. H. Alexander, and R. H. Turocy, "The use of lumbar extension in the evaluation and treatment of patients with acute herniated nucleus pulposus. A preliminary report," *Clinical Orthopaedics and Related Research*, vol. 202, pp. 211–218, 1986.

[81] A. H. Alexander, A. M. Jones, and D. H. Rosenbaum Jr., "Nonoperative management of herniated nucleus pulposus: patient selection by the extension sign: long-term follow-up," *Orthopaedic Review*, vol. 21, no. 2, pp. 181–188, 1992.

[82] G. Nwuga and V. C. B. Nwuga, "Relative therapeutic efficacy of the Williams and McKenzie protocols in back pain management," *Physiotherapy Practice*, vol. 1, no. 2, pp. 99–105, 1985.

[83] H. Frost, J. A. Klaber Moffett, J. S. Moser, and J. C. T. Fairbank, "Randomised controlled trial for evaluation of fitness programme for patients with chronic low back pain," *British Medical Journal*, vol. 310, no. 6973, pp. 151–154, 1995.

[84] M. Kankaanpää, S. Taimela, O. Airaksinen, and O. Hänninen, "The efficacy of active rehabilitation in chronic low back pain: effect on pain intensity, self-experienced disability, and lumbar fatigability," *Spine*, vol. 24, no. 10, pp. 1034–1042, 1999.

[85] J. Rainville, C. A. Jouve, C. Hartigan, E. Martinez, and M. Hipona, "Comparison of short- and long-term outcomes for aggressive spine rehabilitation delivered two versus three times per week," *Spine Journal*, vol. 2, no. 6, pp. 402–407, 2002.

[86] J. Rainville, C. Hartigan, E. Martinez, J. Limke, C. Jouve, and M. Finno, "Exercise as a treatment for chronic low back pain," *Spine Journal*, vol. 4, no. 1, pp. 106–115, 2004.

[87] D. K. Ahern, D. J. Hannon, A. J. Goreczny, M. J. Follick, and J. R. Parziale, "Correlation of chronic low-back pain behavior and muscle function examination of the flexion-relaxation response," *Spine*, vol. 15, no. 2, pp. 92–95, 1990.

[88] J. Rainville, D. K. Ahern, and L. Phalen, "Altering beliefs about pain and impairment in a functionally oriented treatment program for chronic low back pain," *Clinical Journal of Pain*, vol. 9, no. 3, pp. 196–201, 1993.

[89] A. Rissanen, H. Kalimo, H. Alaranta, and R. G. Hazard, "Effect of intensive training on the isokinetic strength and structure of lumbar muscles in patients with chronic low back pain," *Spine*, vol. 20, no. 3, pp. 333–340, 1995.

[90] B. O. A. Adegoke and F. O. Babatunde, "Effect of an exercise protocol on the endurance of trunk extensor muscles—a randomized control trial," *Hong Kong Physiotherapy Journal*, vol. 25, pp. 2–9, 2007.

[91] A. F. Mannion, S. Taimela, M. Müntener, and J. Dvorak, "Active therapy for chronic low back pain part 1. Effects on back muscle activation, fatigability, and strength," *Spine*, vol. 26, no. 8, pp. 897–908, 2001.

[92] T. Petersen, P. Kryger, C. Ekdahl, S. Olsen, and S. Jacobsen, "The effect of McKenzie therapy as compared with that of intensive strengthening training for the treatment of patients with subacute or chronic low back pain: a randomized controlled trial," *Spine*, vol. 27, no. 16, pp. 1702–1708, 2002.

[93] B. E. Udermann, J. M. Mayer, R. G. Donelson, J. E. Graves, and S. R. Murray, "Combining lumbar extension training with McKenzie therapy: effects on pain; disability; and psychosocial functioning in chronic low back pain patients," *Gundersen Lutheran Medical Journal*, vol. 32, pp. 7–12, 2004.

[94] W. D. McArdle, F. I. Katch, and V. L. Katch, *Exercise Physiology*, Williams & Wilkins, Baltimore, Md, USA, 4th edition, 1996.

Gait Performance and Lower-Limb Muscle Strength Improved in Both Upper-Limb and Lower-Limb Isokinetic Training Programs in Individuals with Chronic Stroke

Marie-Hélène Milot,[1,2] Sylvie Nadeau,[2] Denis Gravel,[2] and Daniel Bourbonnais[2]

[1] *Centre de Recherche sur le Vieillissement, École de Réadaptation, Faculté de Médecine et des Sciences de la Santé, Université de Sherbrooke, 1036 Belvédère sud, Sherbrooke, QC, Canada J1H 4C4*
[2] *Institut de Réadaptation Gingras-Lindsay-de-Montréal, Centre de Recherche Interdisciplinaire en Réadaptation (CRIR), Université de Montréal, C.P. 6128 Succ. Centre-Ville, Montréal, QC, Canada H3S 1M9*

Correspondence should be addressed to Marie-Hélène Milot; marie-helene.milot@usherbrooke.ca

Academic Editors: A. Danielsson, B. Dugue, K. Hashimoto, A. Ozcan Edeer, and C. I. Renner

Background. Limited improvement in gait performance has been noted after training despite a significant increase in strength of the affected lower-limb muscles after stroke. A mismatch between the training program and the requirements of gait could explain this finding. *Objective.* To compare the impact of a training program, matching the requirements of the muscle groups involved in the energy generation of gait, to a control intervention, on gait performance and strength. *Methods.* 30 individuals with chronic stroke were randomly assigned into two groups ($n = 15$), each training three times/week for six weeks. The experimental group trained the affected plantarflexors, hip flexors, and extensors, while the control group trained the upper-limb muscles. Baseline and posttraining values of gait speed, positive power (muscles' concentric action during gait), and strength were retained and compared between groups. *Results.* After training, both groups showed a similar and significant increase in gait speed, positive power of the hip muscles, and plantarflexors strength. *Conclusion.* A training program targeting the lower-limb muscles involved in the energy generation of gait did not lead to a greater improvement in gait performance and strength than a training program of the upper-limb muscles. Attending the training sessions might have been a sufficient stimulus to generate gains in the control group.

1. Introduction

It is well recognized that residual muscle strength on the affected side secondary to a stroke has a great impact on activities of daily living, especially on gait performance. The self-selected and maximal gait speeds of individuals with stroke have been positively related to the residual strength of the affected plantarflexors [1–3], hip flexors [1–3], knee extensors, and flexors [1, 2]. Gait asymmetry has also been negatively related to the residual strength of various muscle groups including the plantarflexors and the knee extensors [1]. Knowing that muscle weakness can jeopardize the fulfillment of a functional gait in individuals with stroke, muscle strengthening of the affected lower-limb has become a recognized therapy in the field of rehabilitation.

Many studies have verified the impact of resistance-strengthening programs on the muscle strength of the affected lower extremity of chronic individuals who have had a stroke (>3 months after stroke). Static, dynamic or isokinetic training protocols applied for less than three months resulted in a mean strength increase ranging from 7% to 155% and, generally speaking, this increase was clinically significant, with an effect size greater than one [4–9]. The large discrepancy in the relative increase could be related to differences in the form and intensity of the training protocols as well as in the evaluation procedures, namely, body positioning, stabilization [10], or torque measurements (peak torque versus strength taken at a common angle), for example.

The impact of resistance-strengthening programs on functional performance has been reported in most of the previous studies. The mean change in the self-selected gait speed ranges from 0 to 0.22 m/s [7–9, 11] and, expressed as a relative gain, it represents 0% to 25% of the pretraining values. Thus, resistance-strengthening programs have had a lower impact on self-selected gait speed than on strength among individuals with stroke.

The discrepancy between strength gain and gait changes may be related to the fact that the strengthening protocols did not match the requirements of the functional task in terms of range of motion, velocity, position, and trained muscles [12]. As opposed to strength training, functional training, defined as the practice of a context-specific task, has the advantage of directly practicing a problematic functional activity (e.g., gait), rather than focusing on the impairments (e.g., strength) negatively influencing its performance [13]. Significant gains in several activities of daily living have been reported following various functional trainings (see [14]). However, functional training alone not only allows less control of the intensity of effort produced [15], but its impact on gait is as limited as the one of strengthening programs [16]. One practical way to promote a match between strength-training parameters and a functional task, as well as allow a better control for the intensity of effort, is to use isokinetic devices. In addition, these dynamometers can accommodate the individual's strength throughout the range of motion and allow weakened muscles to be trained using various speeds and types of contraction [10]. It seems that no studies have yet explored the impact of an isokinetic-strengthening program specifically designed to match muscle requirements during gait on the biomechanical gait parameters. Only one study, by Teixeira-Salmela et al. [17], has assessed the impact of a conditioning program on gait speed and related biomechanical parameters. However, their conditioning program was general (strength and aerobic exercises) and not intended to correspond to the specific prerequisites of gait. Furthermore, the biomechanical gait parameters were analyzed only descriptively, thus restraining interpretation of the data.

Considering that transfer of strength gain into an improvement in functional performance could be related to the training program itself, the aim of the current randomized controlled trial was to compare the effect of a task-specific isokinetic training program, corresponding to the requirements of the concentric action in gait of the affected plantarflexors, hip flexors, and extensors, on gait performance and muscle strength, to an isokinetic training program targeting the affected upper-limb muscles. Selection of the lower-limb muscles was based on their significant involvement in energy generation during gait [18] and on the fact that their reduced moment and power production following a stroke have a great impact on gait speed after stroke [3]. Based on these findings, the main hypothesis of the present study was that the task-specific training of the affected lower-limb muscles would produce greater changes in gait performance and strength than a control intervention not aiming at training these muscle groups.

2. Materials and Methods

2.1. Participants. To take part in the study, individuals with a stroke had to meet the following criteria: (1) have a chronic (six months or more) unilateral stroke, (2) be able to walk 10 meters independently with or without a cane, (3) present residual weakness at the affected lower-limb (strength deficit > 10% compared to the unaffected side), and (4) have an activity tolerance of at least two hours with a rest period. The exclusion criteria were as follows: (1) receptive aphasia, (2) incontinence, (3) unstable medical condition, (4) history of injury, and (5) anesthesia at the lower limbs. Authorization by the primary-care physician was obtained if needed. All potential participants signed an informed consent form prior to the assessment session and the study was in accord with the ethical standards of the institutional ethics committee concerned.

2.2. Evaluation Sessions. In the week prior to each training program, participants attended a clinical, strength and gait evaluations that were split into three half-day evaluation sessions. The strength, and gait evaluations were repeated at the end of each training program.

2.2.1. Clinical Evaluation. In order to complete the characterization of all the participants, a trained physical therapist, blinded to the group assignment, collected demographic data and various outcome measures. For the outcome measures, the lower-limb physical impairment at the leg and foot, the perception threshold of touch-pressure of the affected foot and the function and dexterity of the affected upper extremity were evaluated by means of the Chedoke-McMaster Stroke Assessment [19], the calibrated Semmes-Weinstein filaments, and the Action Research Arm Test (ARAT) [20], respectively. Spasticity at the ankle was measured by the Composite Spasticity Index [21]. This scale evaluated three components of spasticity: resistance to full-range passive ankle dorsiflexion (0 = normal and 8 = maximal opposition), Achilles tendon jerks (0 = normal and 4 = hyperreflexia), and the amount and duration of ankle clonus (1 = none and 4 = tireless). Summed scores ranging from 0 to 5, 6 to 9, 10 to 12, and 13 to 16 corresponded to normal muscle tone, mild spasticity, moderate spasticity, and severe spasticity at the ankle, respectively. Also, balance was assessed with the Berg Balance Scale [22] and self-selected and maximal clinical gait speeds were quantified by means of the 5-meter walk test [23]. Finally, to measure a participant's activity level and his/her perceived health status, the Human Activity Profile (HAP) questionnaire (adjusted score) [24] and the Short Form 36 Health Survey were used, respectively [25].

2.2.2. Strength Evaluation. The maximal voluntary concentric strength in plantarflexion, hip flexion, and extension of the affected muscles was measured with a Biodex dynamometric system (Biodex Medical Systems, NY, USA).

The positioning and testing of each muscle groups are described elsewhere [26]. Briefly, the joint position was selected to closely represent that found during the muscles' maximal concentric effort in gait. Therefore, for the testing of plantarflexors, participants were seated with their affected knee strapped in nearly full extension, whereas for the hip muscles, participants were in an horizontal position with their evaluated lower-limb positioned in a leg-rest device that maintained the knee at 25° of flexion [18]. Because individuals with stroke have difficulty generating maximal exertion throughout the entire range of movement at high velocity [8, 26], especially at the hip joint [26], a 30°/s testing velocity was chosen to evaluate the effectiveness of each training program. A rest period of 30 seconds was given between contractions, and a 2-minute rest period was allowed between directions of movement for the hip joint. For each testing condition, two trials were done for each muscle group and the trial showing the highest torque value was retained. Passive torque was also recorded for gravity correction at each angle of the movements assessed.

From the torque-angle curves of each joint, strength values were extracted at the first common angle (external range of motion) reached by all participants, which was 7° of dorsiflexion for the plantarflexors, 0° (hip in neutral position) for the hip flexors, and 40° of hip flexion for the hip extensors.

2.2.3. Gait Evaluation. Kinematic and kinetic data were recorded with an Optotrak system (Northern Digital Inc.) and three AMTI force platforms during five gait cycles at self-selected and maximal speeds, respectively. The ankle and hip joint positions were combined with the ground reaction forces to estimate the net muscular moment using an inverse dynamic approach. Positive power phases, meaning that a concentric action was performed by a muscle group, were identified when the angular velocity multiplied by the local net muscular moment at the ankle and hip joints presented the same polarity [18]. At the ankle joint, the concentric phase of the plantarflexors, A2, begins at about 40% of the gait cycle and ends at toe off (~60%), which corresponds to the push-off phase. At the hip joint, two concentric phases are observed: H1, corresponding to hip extensor activity at the beginning of the gait cycle, and H3, representing the pull-off phase by the hip flexors to swing the limb forward and upward (~50–80% of the gait cycle) [18]. Within these concentric phases, the peak positive power was retained for each muscle group at both speeds and the values were normalized to body mass to remove the influence of individual mass.

The stride characteristics of each gait cycle were computed with footswitches located on the sole of the shoe at the heel, the metatarsal heads, and midfoot. These signals and those from the vertical ground reaction force were used by in-house developed software to determine the gait cycles, which were normalized to 100%. Three trials out of five, showing the most similar values of speed and cadence, were averaged.

2.3. Randomization. A 4 × 2 blocked randomization allowed the main author (MHM) to allocate participants to an experimental group (EXP), that is, task-specific isokinetic strengthening program of the affected lower-limb muscles, or to a control group (CTL), that is, isokinetic-strengthening program of the affected upper-limb muscles. Randomization was based on the baseline results of the 5-meter walk test at self-selected speed and the ARAT. A speed value higher or lower than 0.4 m/s was used as a delimiter because this can be considered the cutoff speed for community walking [27] whereas for the ARAT, a score higher or lower than 10/57 was retained because it could represent the lower limit for a functional upper arm [28] (see Figure 1). Because participants were not blinded to the group assignment, they were instructed not to reveal their training group status to the physical therapist in charge of the clinical evaluation to avoid any bias.

Table 1: Strengthening program for both training groups and each muscle group.

Training parameters	Weeks of training					
	1	2	3	4	5	6
Intensity (% MSC*)	65	70	70	80	80	80
Repetitions	6	6	8	6	8	10
Series	2	2	2	2	2	2

*MSC: maximal static contraction.

2.4. Strengthening Program. The strengthening program was conducted three times a week for six weeks for a total of 18 sessions. Each session lasted between 60 and 90 minutes and started with a 5-min warm-up period followed by a cool-down period of about 15 minutes. For each group, a trained physical therapist, blinded to the experimental and clinical evaluations, supervised the session and was in charge of the progression of the training based on the established protocol. The protocol started with a maximal static contraction in the external range of motion of the trained joint. This contraction allowed the physical therapist to determine the maximal torque that could be reached right at the beginning of the movement. Based on the maximal torque obtained, the intensity of the training session was determined and a target line, corresponding to the requested intensity, provided the participants with a retroaction of the force level to be reached. The dynamometer was put in an isokinetic passive mode and participants were asked to produce repeated submaximal dynamic contractions in the desired direction of movement, maintaining their effort throughout the movement. Progression of the training was based on intensity and repetitions in accordance with the recommendations of the American College of Sports Medicine for a strengthening program [29] (see Table 1), and all training sessions missed were noted in the participant's chart.

For the EXP group, the plantarflexors, hip flexors, and extensors were trained concentrically with a Biodex dynamometer. Submaximal contractions were preceded by a static preloading to closely correspond to the muscle conditions during their concentric action in gait and participants trained at slow and moderate velocities of 30°/s and 90°/s, respectively. These velocities were chosen to cover the joint angular velocity observed during the power generation

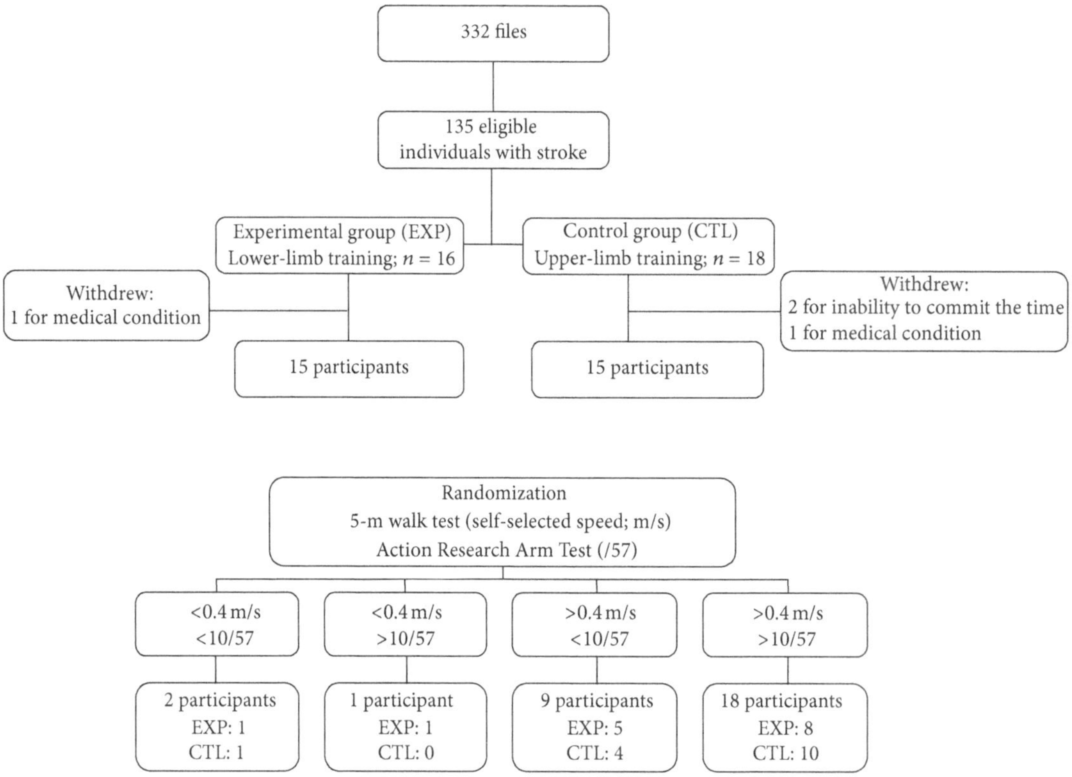

FIGURE 1: Chart of the recruitment and randomization procedures.

phase (concentric action) of gait when the maximal net moment is reached by the muscle group. Range of motion was individually adapted to each participant's gait kinematics. The positions of the adjacent joints were identical to those in the strengthening evaluation. For participants allocated to the CTL group, they took part in a training program targeting their upper-limb muscles. This was done to ensure that these participants had a training regimen as demanding and motivating as the EXP group, but without having any impact on the strength of the lower-limb muscles. Thus, participants trained concentrically their shoulder flexors, elbow flexors, and wrist extensors with a Cybex dynamometer (Cybex Medical, Ronkonkoma, USA) at slow and moderate velocities of 15°/s and 60°/s, respectively. The positioning and ranges of motion were in accordance with the Cybex manual. In addition, grip muscles were trained isotonically with a Martin vigorimeter (Chattanooga, United Kingdom). These muscles were chosen because they are related to the upper-limb function [30, 31]. The training programs of the EXP and CTL groups were conducted at the Institut de réadaptation Gingras-Lindsay-de Montréal pavilion Gingras and pavilion Lindsay, respectively. Therefore, both groups had to walk approximately the same distance to go to their training session.

2.5. Statistical Analysis. The main outcome measure was a change in gait speed and peak positive power following training. The secondary outcome measure was a change in strength at the plantarflexors, hip flexors, and extensors. Descriptive statistics (mean and SD) were calculated for the demographic and clinical data. The baseline comparison of the two training groups was assessed with the Wilcoxon's rank-sum test for the clinical evaluations and independent t-tests for the primary (gait speed and peak positive power) and secondary (strength values) outcomes. Also, two-way repeated measures ANOVA with a "group of subjects" between factors compared the main effect of time on gait performance and strength values for each gait speed and each muscle group, respectively. The P value was set at 0.05. All statistical analyses were performed using SPSS software Windows (version 18, Chicago, IL, USA).

3. Results

3.1. Participants. Out of 332 files scanned for potential candidates, 135 individuals with stroke met the study inclusion criteria and were sent a recruitment letter. Of these, 34 answered and agreed to participate. They were randomly divided into the EXP group ($n = 16$) and the CTL group ($n = 18$). After one week of training, one participant in the EXP group withdrew because of a medical condition and two others in the CTL group withdrew because they were unable to commit the time. Another participant in the CTL group dropped out after five weeks of training because of a medical condition. These participants were excluded from the analysis. Thus, a convenience sample of 30 chronic individuals with stroke, 15 in each training group, completed the study (see Figure 1). Overall, compared to healthy individuals evaluated from a previous study [32], participants showed a 34% decrease in their self-selected gait speed and presented strength deficits at the affected plantarflexors, hip flexors, and hip extensors of 64%, 40% and 34%, respectively. At baseline, both groups showed similar demographic characteristics, clinical, gait, and strength data ($P > 0.05$) (see Table 2).

3.2. Gait Changes. A significant increase in the self-selected ($F_{1,28} = 14.62$, $P = 0.001$) and maximal ($F_{1,28} = 5.6$, $P = 0.025$) gait speeds was noted after the 6-week strengthening program for both groups (between group $P > 0.1$). For the EXP group, this increase corresponded to a 9% (−13 to 42%) and 12% (−17 to 97%) mean change for the self-selected and maximal gait speeds, respectively. For the CTL group, the corresponding values were 19% (−11 to 48%) and 6% (−10 to 33%).

After training, a significant increase in the peak positive power bursts of the hip flexors at self-selected speed ($F_{1,28} = 5.34$, $P = 0.028$) and hip extensors at maximal speed ($F_{1,28} = 4.58$, $P = 0.042$) was noted for both groups (between group $P > 0.1$). For the hip flexors, the change in peak positive power corresponded to a mean increase of 31% (−33 to 122%) and 35% (−33 to 171%) for the EXP and CTL groups, respectively. For the hip extensors, the corresponding mean increase in the peak positive power was 43% (−78 to 151%) and 51% (−82 to 224%) (see Table 3). No change in the peak positive power of the plantarflexors was found for both groups and at both speeds. Note that for the plantarflexors, participants wearing an ankle support were excluded from the data analysis.

3.3. Strength Changes. No group difference was noted for the strength gains obtained at the plantarflexors, hip flexors, and extensors (between group $P > 0.2$). For both groups, a significant increase in the strength of the plantarflexors was found ($F_{1,28} = 11.21$, $P = 0.002$), representing a 51% (−31 to 180%) and 40% (−22 to 179%) mean strength gain for the EXP and CTL groups, respectively. A trend towards an increase in strength for the hip flexors ($F_{1,28} = 4.01$, $P = 0.055$) and hip extensors ($F_{1,28} = 3.82$, $P = 0.061$) was also noted (see Table 4).

4. Discussion

A 6-week task-specific isokinetic strengthening program, targeting the affected plantarflexors, hip flexors, and extensor muscles in the context of their concentric action during gait, did not produce greater gains in gait speed, peak positive power, and strength than a similar training targeting the affected upper-limb muscles. This finding suggests a generalized improvement in physical function rather than a training-specific effect of the isokinetic strengthening program. Therefore, it seems that the important point in rehabilitation of individuals in the chronic phase of their stroke is to promote physical activity regardless of the training they are provided with.

4.1. Effect of the Training Program on Gait Performance. The training of the EXP group was task-specific to the phase of gait substantially influencing walking speed, that is the energy generation phase of gait [18]. For that reason, the absence of a significant difference in the gains obtained in the gait parameters between the EXP and CTL groups is very surprising, especially since the CTL group did not train the lower-limb muscles. It is thought that attending the rehabilitation centres had a possible training effect for the CTL group. After stroke, very low levels of physical activity are reported [33] resulting in several negative health issues. In the current study, based on the baseline HAP score, most of the participants of the CTL group fell into the impaired to moderately active categories. Thus, attending a demanding training program 3 times a week for 6 weeks could be a sufficient stimulus to induce gains in gait performance in this subset of stroke survivors. Based on that, the intensity of training seems to be a key element in rehabilitation after stroke in order to enhance functional improvement.

Although our task-specific isokinetic training program matched the gait parameters found during the energy generation phase of gait, it could be thought that the training was not task-specific enough to the requirements of gait to translate into greater gains in gait and strength than the CTL group. Incorporating the practice of gait into the training program might have been more relevant to ensure a greater transfer between strength gain and gait speed [34]. However, it seems that functional training alone does not cause greater improvement in gait speed than resistance training, with a mean change as low as 0.04 m/s [16]. From the results of the current study and previous ones, it seems that the type of training (e.g., task-specific training or resistance training) does not seem to be the key element to generate improved gait performance since various training programs produced comparable gains in gait performance. This is in line with the review by Dickstein on rehabilitation of gait speed after stroke, where the author reported that other variables such as amount and intensity within a training program were common denominators of interventions that facilitated more improvement in function after stroke than the treatment mode [35].

For both groups, the improvement in self-selected and maximal gait speeds was modest and appeared to be mainly associated with an increase in hip power. This indicates that the hip compensatory strategy, typical of gait after stroke [3, 26, 36], is used even more after the training period. These results are in line with previous studies [17, 37] that assessed the impact of various training programs on gait speed and related biomechanical parameters. These studies reported marked changes in ankle and hip power after training, associated with significant improvement in gait speed.

4.2. Effects of the Training Program on Strength. No difference in strength gains was noted between both groups, for the plantarflexors, hip flexors, and extensors. This is not the first study to be plagued with a nonspecific effect of a training program as similar results were found by Flansbjer et al. [4], Ouellette et al. [7], and Kim et al. [8]. The lack of statistically

Table 2: Demographic and clinical characteristics of the experimental (lower-limb training) and control (upper-limb training) groups at pretraining.

Characteristics	Experimental group (n = 15)		Control group (n = 15)	
	Mean (SD)	n (%)	Mean (SD)	n (%)
Age (yr)	58.5 (14.9)		54.7 (14.6)	
Body mass (kg)	78.3 (11.3)		72.5 (13.4)	
Height (cm)	170.6 (7.3)		166.5 (9.5)	
Time since stroke (months)	56.9 (43.8)		85.5 (111.9)	
5-meter walk test: self-selected speed (m/s)	0.65 (0.24)		0.79 (0.29)	
5-meter walk test: maximal speed (m/s)	0.98 (0.38)		1.10 (0.50)	
Chedoke McMaster Stroke Assessment (/7)				
Leg	4.3 (1.2)		4.5 (1.4)	
Foot	3.5 (1.1)		3.9 (1.8)	
Action Research Arm Test (/57)	28.3 (25.2)		29.9 (24.9)	
Balance Scale (/56)	49.8 (5.3)		49.5 (5.8)	
Spasticity Index (/16)	7.4 (3.3)		6.7 (2.9)	
Human Activity Profile (adjusted score/94)	51.4 (14.3)		58.3 (16.5)	
SF-36 (%)				
Physical functioning	52.3 (24.9)		56.7 (23.2)	
Mental status	71.2 (16.4)		68.8 (23.4)	
Involved side				
Left		9 (60)		9 (60)
Right		6 (40)		6 (40)
Gender				
Female		6 (40)		6 (40)
Male		9 (60)		9 (60)
Ankle support		4 (26.6)		5 (33.3)
Hypoesthesia of the affected foot		2 (13.3)		2 (13.3)

significant difference between groups could be related to the variability of the response to the training programs. A phenomenon that is scarcely mentioned or explained in studies evaluating resistance training in individuals with chronic stroke is the fact that not all participants seem to benefit from the exercise protocol. Gains in strength are reported mainly as a mean for an entire group but the related standard deviation clearly indicates that strength gain is variable among participants. Variation in strength gain is not typical of individuals with stroke; earlier studies have acknowledged this phenomenon in the able-bodied [38, 39]. It is known that not all muscle groups have a similar rate of strength development and this, combined with the pretraining status of individuals [38, 39], could partly explain the variability in individual training responses.

In the current study, the plantarflexor strength showed the greatest change in both groups. This could be explained by the fact that because the plantarflexors showed a greater strength deficit at baseline than the hip flexors or extensors as compared to the unaffected side (data not presented), there was more possibility for an increase in strength than in the hip joint. This result concurs with the study of Kim et al. [8] who found that the plantarflexors showed a greater mean percentage change than the hip flexors and extensors. The fact that the plantarflexors of the CTL group presented a gain in strength allows the hypothesis that mechanisms other than the direct effect of the strengthening program itself are involved. One of these could be the presence of involuntary contractions of the lower-limb muscles associated with the training of the upper extremity. These contractions could be related to the necessity of the lower-limb muscles to stabilize the body to allow efficient maximal exertion of the tested upper-limb muscles. During training of the upper extremity, the feet of participants were positioned on a resting platform, possibly allowing them to use the platform as an anchor for the lower-limb muscles to provide stability for the body. As mentioned for the changes in gait performance, a more likely mechanism explaining the gain in strength of the plantarflexors of the CTL group could be the possible training effect caused by attending the rehabilitation centres for the training sessions. In fact, during gait, the affected plantarflexors are the most involved muscle group at self-selected speed, with a muscular level of effort (mean ± 1 SD) reaching 64% ± 19% of their maximal strength [26, 36]. This intensity of muscular effort during gait could act as an appropriate training stimulus especially for the plantarflexors, which were weaker than the hip muscles.

4.3. Discrepancy between Strength and Gait Changes. A disproportion between the increase (%) in the current muscle strength and the change in gait speeds was observed.

TABLE 3: Mean (SD), range, and 95% confidence interval (CI) for the laboratory self-selected and maximal gait speeds (m/s) and mean (SD) for the related peak positive power of the affected plantarflexors, hip flexors, and extensors for the experimental (lower-limb training—$n = 15$) and control (upper-limb training—$n = 15$) groups at pre- and posttraining.

Statistics	Self-selected speed (m/s)					Maximal speed (m/s)				
	Experimental		Control		P^b	Experimental		Control		P^b
	Pre	Post	Pre	Post		Pre	Post	Pre	Post	
Mean (SD)	0.56 (0.19)	0.59[a] (0.18)	0.68 (0.30)	0.78[a] (0.28)	0.1	0.92 (0.41)	0.98[a] (0.39)	1.08 (0.43)	1.13[a] (0.46)	0.3
Range:										
Min	0.29	0.35	0.30	0.38		0.29	0.35	0.30	0.40	
Max	0.93	0.95	1.39	1.24		1.65	1.74	1.71	1.89	
95% CI:										
Lower bound	0.45	0.49	0.51	0.63		0.69	0.77	0.84	0.88	
Upper bound	0.66	0.69	0.84	0.94		1.15	1.19	1.32	1.38	
Peak positive power (W/kg)										
Plantarflexors	0.63 (0.43)	0.74 (0.53)	1.19 (1.25)	1.32 (1.09)	0.2	1.14 (0.74)	1.39 (0.77)	1.86 (1.46)	1.62 (1.30)	0.3
Hip flexors	0.37 (0.17)	0.43[a] (0.14)	0.45 (0.37)	0.55[a] (0.41)	0.3	0.85 (0.67)	0.90 (0.47)	0.88 (0.64)	1.05 (0.61)	0.7
Hip extensors	0.12 (0.08)	0.14 (0.12)	0.19 (0.17)	0.29 (0.38)	0.1	0.43 (0.34)	0.48[a] (0.37)	0.61 (0.43)	0.91[a] (0.82)	0.1

[a] $P < 0.05$ (pretraining value versus posttraining value).
[b] P value is comparison between experimental and control groups.

This is not typical of this work and other studies evaluating the impact of various training programs for the affected lower-limb muscles have obtained similar results where greater effect size for muscle strength change was observed aftertraining in comparison to that for the self-selected gait speed [4, 5, 9, 34]. Unfortunately, there is a lack of explanation for this fact. One reason could be the specificity of the strength-training outcomes. For example, it was observed that static training at one specific angle produced mainly strength gains at this angle [40]. Specificity of training was also noted for velocity and type of contraction [41]. It seems that strength gains are not transferable to various testing conditions other than those used in the training protocol. Consequently, the transfer of strength gain to a functional task such as gait could be more problematic because the muscles have to function in conditions where velocity and type of contractions are constantly changing. In the current work, in addition to ensuring a correspondence between the trained muscle groups and those known to influence gait speed, careful attention was paid to the selection of the angle, velocity, and type of contraction to make them biomechanically comparable to the muscle conditions observed at their maximal concentric effort in gait. It was thought that creating predominantly a gain in strength during the above conditions would have benefited more gait speed. However, because the training program was performed in a sitting or horizontal position, the additional demand related to the role played by some muscle groups in maintaining balance during gait [18] was not required during training. It could be thought that dynamic balance control could also be an important determinant of the participants' capacity to increase gait speed rather than strength or power gains alone.

A second explanation for the divergence between strength and gait changes could come from the muscular levels of effort that need to be produced during gait. It was demonstrated that participants with stroke unconsciously used the gain in strength to reduce the muscular levels of effort during gait instead of substantially increasing their gait speed [42]. This concurrently helped them decrease the mechanical requirements of walking.

4.4. Limitations. It should be remembered that the present sample was small, consisting of chronic individuals with stroke. Considering the large failure in voluntary activation in the first months following a stroke, it could be thought that, in the subacute period of a stroke, intense overloading of the weakened muscles by resistance training would produce perhaps more significant results regarding strength and gait performance. Also, the rate of force development of the affected lower-limb muscles was not assessed and could have provided relevant explanations of the current results since it has a great impact on function after stroke [43]. Moreover, the activity that participants were doing outside the training was not monitored. Gathering of this information might have helped explain the absence of difference in the gains observed between groups. Overall, despite the low impact of strength gain on gait speed and power, the fact that the effort produced during gait could be decreased with an increase in strength [42] makes the necessity to increase strength following a stroke still highly relevant.

5. Conclusion

Although some individuals with stroke benefited from a task-specific isokinetic training program, the impact of the gains in strength on gait performance was limited, and no difference was observed between the EXP and CTL groups. Future research aiming at improving gait following a stroke should thoroughly determine the parameters of the strengthening program in order to maximize the transfer of strength gain to functional activities. The impact of a combination of upper- and lower-limb isokinetic training

TABLE 4: Mean (SD), range, and 95% confidence interval (CI) for the maximal torque (Nm) taken at a common angle of 7° of ankle dorsiflexion, 0° (hip in neutral position), and 40° of hip flexion for the plantarflexors, hip flexors, and extensors, respectively, for the experimental (lower-limb training—$n = 15$) and control (upper-limb training—$n = 15$) groups at pre- and posttraining.

Statistics	Plantarflexors					Hip flexors					Hip extensors				
	Experimental		Control		P^b	Experimental		Control		P^b	Experimental		Control		P^b
	Pre	Post	Pre	Post		Pre	Post	Pre	Post		Pre	Post	Pre	Post	
Mean (SD)	58.9 (42.0)	75.1[a] (37.1)	48.7 (36.3)	56.3[a] (35.1)	0.3	73.6 (29.7)	91.3 (36.9)	65.4 (33.9)	67.8 (31.3)	0.2	103.8 (40.7)	105.4 (34.4)	79.7 (47.7)	101.3 (60.5)	0.4
Range:															
Min	8.2	15.9	5.0	13.9		17.6	21.5	6.6	0		43.2	42.5	18.6	37.3	
Max	163.2	138.1	122.6	117.6		121.5	146.2	153.3	120.2		180.8	164.7	201.1	259.2	
95% CI:															
Lower bound	35.6	54.5	28.6	36.4		57.1	70.9	46.7	50.4		81.3	86.3	53.3	67.8	
Upper bound	82.2	95.6	68.8	75.7		90.0	111.8	84.2	85.1		126.3	124.4	106.1	134.8	

[a] $P < 0.05$ (pretraining value versus posttraining value).

[b] P value is comparison between experimental and control groups.

program on gait parameters should be further assessed since it might help maximize gait performance in stroke survivors. Because participants could have chosen to use the gain in strength to lower their lower-limb muscular levels of effort; as opposed to strongly increasing their gait speed, strengthening of the affected lower-limb muscles remains highly relevant following a stroke.

Conflict of Interests

The authors declare that there is no conflict of interests.

Acknowledgments

The project was supported by the Canadian Institutes of Health Research (Grant no. 44059). M. H. Milot held a scholarship from the CIHR and Fonds de la Recherche en Santé du Québec (FRSQ), S. Nadeau was a Senior Scientist Salary from FRSQ when the study was realized. The authors offer their heartfelt thanks to the physical therapists of the Institut de Réadaptation Gingras-Lindsay-de Montréal (Pauline Cross, Josianne Fecteau, Susan Crabb, Sonia Nguyen, Josiane De Serres, and Julie Lecours) and the research assistants of the Pathokinesiology and Functional Activities Laboratory (Fabiana Antunes, Alexandra Duranceau, and Nathaly Gaudreault) for their participation in the project. Pierre Desjardins, Michel Goyette, Daniel Marineau, and André Dumoulin are also acknowledged for their technical support.

References

[1] A. L. Hsu, P. F. Tang, and M. H. Jan, "Analysis of impairments influencing gait velocity and asymmetry of hemiplegic patients after mild to moderate stroke," *Archives of Physical Medicine and Rehabilitation*, vol. 84, no. 8, pp. 1185–1193, 2003.

[2] C. Maria Kim and J. J. Eng, "The relationship of lower-extremity muscle torque to locomotor performance in people with stroke," *Physical Therapy*, vol. 83, no. 1, pp. 49–57, 2003.

[3] S. Nadeau, D. Gravel, A. B. Arsenault, and D. Bourbonnais, "Plantarflexor weakness as a limiting factor of gait speed in stroke subjects and the compensating role of hip flexors," *Clinical Biomechanics*, vol. 14, no. 2, pp. 125–135, 1999.

[4] U. B. Flansbjer, M. Miller, D. Downham, and J. Lexell, "Progressive resistance training after stroke: effects on muscle strength, muscle tone, gait performance and perceived participation," *Journal of Rehabilitation Medicine*, vol. 40, no. 1, pp. 42–48, 2008.

[5] T. R. Hill, T. I. Gjellesvik, P. M. Moen et al., "Maximal strength training enhances strength and functional performance in chronic stroke survivors," *American Journal of Physical Medicine & Rehabilitation*, vol. 91, no. 5, pp. 393–400, 2012.

[6] M. J. Lee, S. L. Kilbreath, M. F. Singh, B. Zeman, and G. M. Davis, "Effect of progressive resistance training on muscle performance after chronic stroke," *Medicine and Science in Sports and Exercise*, vol. 42, no. 1, pp. 23–34, 2010.

[7] M. M. Ouellette, N. K. LeBrasseur, J. F. Bean et al., "High-intensity resistance training improves muscle strength, self-reported function, and disability in long-term stroke survivors," *Stroke*, vol. 35, no. 6, pp. 1404–1409, 2004.

[8] C. M. Kim, J. J. Eng, D. L. MacIntyre, and A. S. Dawson, "Effects of isokinetic strength training on walking in persons with stroke: a double-blind controlled pilot study," *Journal of Stroke and Cerebrovascular Diseases*, vol. 10, no. 6, pp. 265–273, 2001.

[9] S. L. Morris, K. J. Dodd, and M. E. Morris, "Outcomes of progressive resistance strenght training following stroke: a systematic review," *Clinical Rehabilitation*, vol. 18, no. 1, pp. 27–39, 2004.

[10] N. Hammami, F. O. Coroian, M. Julia et al., "Isokinetic muscle strengthening after acquired cerebral damage: a literature review," *Annals of Physical and Rehabilitation Medicine*, vol. 55, no. 4, pp. 279–291, 2012.

[11] S. A. Sharp and B. J. Brouwer, "Isokinetic strength training of the hemiparetic knee: effects on function and spasticity," *Archives of Physical Medicine and Rehabilitation*, vol. 78, no. 11, pp. 1231–1236, 1997.

[12] J. Eng, "Strength training in individuals with stroke," *Physiotherapy Canada*, vol. 56, pp. 189–201, 2004.

[13] I. J. Hubbard, M. W. Parsons, C. Neilson, and L. M. Carey, "Task-specific training: evidence for and translation to clinical practice," *Occupational Therapy International*, vol. 16, no. 3-4, pp. 175–189, 2009.

[14] B. French, L. Thomas, M. Leathley et al., "Does repetitive task training improve functional activity after stroke? A Cochrane systematic review and meta-analysis," *Journal of Rehabilitation Medicine*, vol. 42, no. 1, pp. 9–15, 2010.

[15] C. Mercier, D. Bourbonnais, S. Bilodeau, J. F. Lemay, and P. Cross, "Description of a new motor re-education programme for the paretic lower limb aimed at improving the mobility of stroke patients," *Clinical Rehabilitation*, vol. 13, no. 3, pp. 199–206, 1999.

[16] C. M. Dean, C. L. Richards, and F. Malouin, "Task-related circuit training improves performance of locomotor tasks in chronic stroke: a randomized, controlled pilot trial," *Archives of Physical Medicine and Rehabilitation*, vol. 81, no. 4, pp. 409–417, 2000.

[17] L. F. Teixeira-Salmela, S. Nadeau, I. Mcbride, and S. J. Olney, "Effects of muscle strengthening and physical conditioning training on temporal, kinematic and kinetic variables during gait in chronic stroke survivors," *Journal of Rehabilitation Medicine*, vol. 33, no. 2, pp. 53–60, 2001.

[18] D. A. Winter, *The Biomechanics and Motor Control of Human Gait: Normal, Elderly and Pathological*, University of Waterloo Press, Waterloo, Canada, 2nd edition, 1991.

[19] C. Gowland, P. Stratford, M. Ward et al., "Measuring physical impairment and disability with the Chedoke-McMaster Stroke Assessment," *Stroke*, vol. 24, no. 1, pp. 58–63, 1993.

[20] M. H. Rabadi and F. M. Rabadi, "Comparison of the action research arm test and the Fugl-Meyer assessment as measures of upper-extremity motor weakness after stroke," *Archives of Physical Medicine and Rehabilitation*, vol. 87, no. 7, pp. 962–966, 2006.

[21] M. F. Levin and C. Hui-Chan, "Are H and stretch reflexes in hemiparesis reproducible and correlated with spasticity?" *Journal of Neurology*, vol. 240, no. 2, pp. 63–71, 1993.

[22] K. Berg, S. Wood-Dauphinee, and J. I. Williams, "The balance scale: reliability assessment with elderly residents and patients with an acute stroke," *Scandinavian Journal of Rehabilitation Medicine*, vol. 27, no. 1, pp. 27–36, 1995.

[23] N. M. Salbach, N. E. Mayo, J. Higgins, S. Ahmed, L. E. Finch, and C. L. Richards, "Responsiveness and predictability of gait

speed and other disability measures in acute stroke," *Archives of Physical Medicine and Rehabilitation*, vol. 82, no. 9, pp. 1204–1212, 2001.

[24] J. Fix and D. Daughton, *Human Activity Profile: Professional Manual*, Psychological Assessment Resources, Odessa, Fla, USA, 1988.

[25] J. E. Ware Jr., K. K. Snow, M. Kosinski, and B. Gandek, *SF-36 Health Survey: Manual and Interpretation Guide*, The Health Institute, New England Medical Center, Boston, Mass, USA, 1993.

[26] M. H. Milot, S. Nadeau, and D. Gravel, "Muscular utilization of the plantarflexors, hip flexors and extensors in persons with hemiparesis walking at self-selected and maximal speeds," *Journal of Electromyography and Kinesiology*, vol. 17, no. 2, pp. 184–193, 2007.

[27] J. Perry, M. Garrett, J. K. Gronley, and S. J. Mulroy, "Classification of walking handicap in the stroke population," *Stroke*, vol. 26, no. 6, pp. 982–989, 1995.

[28] H. Van der Lee, *Forced Use of the Upper Extremity in Chronic Stroke Patients*, Vrije Universiteit, Amsterdam, The Netherlands, 2001.

[29] W. J. Kraemer, K. Adams, E. Cafarelli et al., "American College of Sports Medicine position stand; progression models in resistance training for healthy adults," *Medicine & Science in Sports & Exercise*, vol. 34, no. 2, pp. 364–380, 2002.

[30] M. C. Cirstea and M. F. Levin, "Compensatory strategies for reaching in stroke," *Brain*, vol. 123, no. 5, pp. 940–953, 2000.

[31] A. M. Bertrand, C. Mercier, P. L. W. Shun, D. Bourbonnais, and J. Desrosiers, "Effects of weakness on symmetrical bilateral grip force exertion in subjects with hemiparesis," *Journal of Neurophysiology*, vol. 91, no. 4, pp. 1579–1585, 2004.

[32] L. F. Requião, S. Nadeau, M. H. Milot, D. Gravel, D. Bourbonnais, and D. Gagnon, "Quantification of level of effort at the plantarflexors and hip extensors and flexor muscles in healthy subjects walking at different cadences," *Journal of Electromyography and Kinesiology*, vol. 15, no. 4, pp. 393–405, 2005.

[33] S. A. Moore, K. Hallsworth, T. Plotz et al., "Physical activity, sedentary behaviour and metabolic control following stroke: a cross-sectional and longitudinal study," *PloS One*, vol. 8, no. 1, Article ID e55263, 2013.

[34] I. G. L. Van de Port, S. Wood-Dauphinee, E. Lindeman, and G. Kwakkel, "Effects of exercise training programs on walking competency after stroke: a systematic review," *American Journal of Physical Medicine and Rehabilitation*, vol. 86, no. 11, pp. 935–951, 2007.

[35] R. Dickstein, "Rehabilitation of gait speed after stroke: a critical review of intervention approaches," *Neurorehabilitation and Neural Repair*, vol. 22, no. 6, pp. 649–660, 2008.

[36] M. H. Milot, S. Nadeau, D. Gravel, and L. F. Requião, "Bilateral level of effort of the plantar flexors, hip flexors, and extensors during gait in hemiparetic and healthy individuals," *Stroke*, vol. 37, no. 8, pp. 2070–2075, 2006.

[37] S. J. Mulroy, T. Klassen, J. K. Gronley, V. J. Eberly, D. A. Brown, and K. J. Sullivan, "Gait parameters associated with responsiveness to treadmill training with body-weight support after stroke: an exploratory study," *Physical Therapy*, vol. 90, no. 2, pp. 209–223, 2010.

[38] K. Hakkinen, "Factors influencing trainability of muscular strength during short term and prolonged training," *NSCA Journal*, vol. 7, no. 2, pp. 32–37, 1985.

[39] H. J. Hislop, "Quantitative changes in human muscular strength during isometric exercise," *Journal of the American Physical Therapy Association*, vol. 43, no. 1, pp. 21–38, 1963.

[40] M. Lindh, "Increase of muscle strength from isometric quadriceps exercises at different knee angles," *Scandinavian Journal of Rehabilitation Medicine*, vol. 11, no. 1, pp. 33–36, 1979.

[41] M. I. R. Pereira and P. S. C. Gomes, "Movement velocity in resistance training," *Sports Medicine*, vol. 33, no. 6, pp. 427–438, 2003.

[42] M. H. Milot, S. Nadeau, D. Gravel, and D. Bourbonnais, "Effect of increases in plantarflexor and hip flexor muscle strength on the levels of effort during gait in individuals with hemiparesis," *Clinical Biomechanics*, vol. 23, no. 4, pp. 415–423, 2008.

[43] S. J. Garland, V. L. Gray, and S. Knorr, "Muscle activation patterns and postural control following stroke," *Motor Control*, vol. 13, no. 4, pp. 387–411, 2009.

Risk Factors for Falls and Fragility Fractures in Community-Dwelling Seniors: A One-Year Prospective Study

Sacha Song,[1,2] Joy C. MacDermid,[3,4] and Ruby Grewal[3]

[1] *Schulich School of Medicine & Dentistry, University of Western Ontario, London, ON, Canada N6A 5C1*
[2] *University of Windsor, Medical Education Building Room 1100, 401 Sunset Avenue, Windsor, ON, Canada N9B 3P4*
[3] *Division of Orthopedic Surgery, University of Western Ontario, Hand and Upper Limb Center, St. Joseph's Health Care, 268 Grosvenor Street, London, ON, Canada N6A 4L6*
[4] *School of Rehabilitation Sciences, McMaster University, 1400 Main Street West, Hamilton, ON, Canada L8S 1C7*

Correspondence should be addressed to Ruby Grewal; rgrewa@uwo.ca

Academic Editors: P. Czarnecki, E. E. Hansson, and H. Unalan

Objective. To evaluate risk factors for falls and fragility fractures in healthy seniors. *Methods.* Assessing 50 ambulatory community-dwelling volunteers ≥65 for demographics, BMI, bone mineral density (BMD) (DEXA), fracture risk (FRAX), balance (Biodex), fear of falling (Modified Falls Efficacy Scale (MFES)), and activity level (RAPA). One-year followup was done through phone interviews. *Results.* Most participants (17 males, 33 females; mean age 72.0 ± 5.5 years) had normal BMD and were active with little to no fear of falling. Balance did not correlate with FRAX or fear of falling. Activity level did not correlate with FRAX, but the active group had less fear of falling. Most scored below age specific norms on balance testing. Fear of falling was not significantly different between genders but did correlate with FRAX, indicating that patients with higher fracture risk were also more afraid of falling. Individuals who fell after one year had increased fear of falling and decreased activity levels. *Conclusions.* Community-dwelling seniors with higher risk of future fractures were more afraid of falling. Although healthy and active, this cohort had poor balance compared to age matched norms. Further research on how to best assess fall risk and improve balance to prevent fractures is needed.

1. Introduction

Fractures resulting from a fall from standing height (fragility fractures) account for significant morbidity and health care expenses in older patients [1–3]. The 65-year and older age bracket is the fastest growing demographic around the world in both industrialized and developing countries [4, 5]. In industrialized countries, an estimated one-third of individuals ≥65 experience at least one fall each year [6, 7]. In 2008-2009, more than half of the cases of injurious falls were experienced by individuals ≥65, and within this age group, falls were responsible for 74% of major injuries suffered and approximately 10% to 15% resulted in fracture [8].

Regardless of whether a fracture occurs, falls can lead to a reduced quality of life and a functional decline for the individual [1, 7]. Falls in this age group are also more likely to result in longer and more expensive hospitalizations [1–3]. Annually, the cost to treat falls is 0.85% to 1.5% of the total health care expenditure [2, 3]. Fractures are the most costly result of falls; Stevens et al. found that although fractures accounted for only 35% of injuries sustained from falls, they were responsible for 61% of related health care costs [2].

Since a fracture event is determined both by risk of falling and bone susceptibility, factors that adversely affect either predispose individuals for fracture. Balance impairments are a common cause of falls in the elderly population. Bone mineral density (BMD) has also been established as a risk factor for fall-related fractures. Fear of falling relates to an individual's perception of risk, past experiences, and attitudes about future falls. There is little research investigating the interrelationships between fear of falling, balance deficits, BMD, and estimated risk of fracture. Thus, it is unclear whether patients' stated views about their fear of future falls provide sufficient guidance for clinicians to take action or whether more detailed investigations are necessary.

One factor that has been shown in studies to be related to fall risk is activity level in older adults [2, 9, 10]. Decreased activity levels are believed to lead to functional decline, predisposing to falls [2, 9, 10]. In order to implement appropriate interventions to keep older adults active and to prevent functional decline, we need to understand what the current activity level of the community-dwelling population is so that we can assess their current risk of falls and fractures.

In order to prevent falls and their consequences, individuals who are at risk of falling need to be identified so that appropriate interventions and preventative measures can be put in place.

A better understanding of the role of balance, fear of falling, activity level, and BMD in fracture risk may lead to the development of more effective preventive measures that encompass multiple risk factors. As well, the incorporation of FRAX scores as a clinical tool in evaluating fracture risk will be considered. The purpose of this study was to assess risk factors for fragility fractures and correlations between these risk factors in a population of healthy volunteers aged ≥65 living independently in the community. Risk factors assessed include fear of falling, activity level, balance, BMD, and FRAX scores. These individuals were then reassessed at the one-year mark to gain a better understanding of how these risk factors actually influenced whether individuals suffered a fall or fragility fracture. As well, gender differences of these risk factors were also assessed.

2. Methods

2.1. Study Design. All study procedures were reviewed and approved by the Health Sciences Research Ethics Board at the University of Western Ontario for this prospective cohort study.

Fifty ambulatory subjects aged ≥65 were recruited from the community (via poster advertisements). Individuals who were living in an institution, required the use of walking aids, had sustained a fragility fracture within the past year, or had a known balance disorder were excluded.

Participants completed a data collection form to determine their general health. Additional data collected included weight and height, which was used to calculate body mass index (BMI) as well as age and gender. The participant's fall and fracture history, family history of hip fracture, medical comorbidities, medications, and smoking and alcohol use were also collected in this survey. This information, along with BMD, was then used to determine the participant's ten-year probability of osteoporotic and hip fracture using the Fracture Risk Assessment Tool (FRAX) [11–13].

FRAX is a tool that can help assess fracture risk. Launched by the World Health Organization (WHO) in 2008, FRAX is a web-based algorithm that calculates an individual's ten-year probability of both osteoporotic and hip fracture based on clinical information and BMD [11–13]. The information obtained from FRAX is meant to help guide clinicians in their treatment decisions but should be used in conjunction with clinical presentation and judgment [11–13]. In addition, FRAX has been calibrated for use in specific countries based on epidemiological data, making it a valid fracture model for specific populations [12, 13].

The Modified Falls Efficacy Scale (MFES) was administered at this time. The MFES is a reliable valid means of evaluating an individual's fear of falling by asking them to rate their confidence level in performing 14 different daily activities without falling (zero indicates no confidence, ten indicates complete confidence) [14]. The overall fear of falling score is determined by averaging the scores for each activity.

Participants also completed the Rapid Assessment of Physical Activity (RAPA) questionnaire. The RAPA is a highly sensitive self-reported questionnaire that has been validated to measure the physical activity levels of individuals over age 50 [15]. It categorizes individuals as sedentary, underactive, underactive regular—light activities, underactive regular, and active as well as assesses strength and flexibility [15].

A balance assessment was performed using the Biodex Balance System SD [16, 17]. The Biodex Balance System SD consists of a movable platform that objectively measures an individual's dynamic balance abilities. The fall risk test categorized participants as normal or above/below normal when compared to the age specified norms predetermined by the Biodex Balance SD program.

BMD of the femoral neck and spine was measured with a DEXA GE-Lunar scanner. The BMD values (in g/cm^2) for the femoral neck and L2-L4 were collected, along with Z-scores and T-scores. We also noted whether an individual was osteoporotic or osteopenic or had normal bone density. One participant recently had a BMD scan independent of this study. Because only T-scores were available, this patient was excluded from most analyses, but we were able to calculate a FRAX score.

Participants were followed prospectively at the one-year mark through phone calls where information was collected on their fall history over the past year. A followup MFES was administered at this time to assess the participant's current stance on fear of falling. A modified version of the RAPA, the Telephone Assessment of Physical Activity (TAPA), was also given to evaluate current activity levels and to observe any changes in activity [18].

2.2. Statistical Analysis. Data analysis was performed using IBM SPSS Statistics for Windows, Version 21.0, Armonk, NY: IBM Corp. Data were checked for normality by examining skewness and kurtosis. Data analysis was performed for the group; the relationship between age, gender, BMI, activity level, fear of falling, and FRAX was examined. Data analyses were also disaggregated to examine gender differences. Bivariate relationships between continuous variables were determined using Pearson's correlation. Differences between categorical groups (male/female) were determined using Student's t-test and ANOVA and categorical variables with chi-square tests.

3. Results

3.1. Demographics. Of the 50 participants in this study, 17 were males and 33 were females with a mean age of 72.0 ± 5.5 years (range, 65–84 years) (Table 1). The average BMI was 29.3 ± 5.8 (range, normal—obese class III) (Table 1) [19]. The majority of participants (55%) had a normal BMD at the

TABLE 1: Demographic information.

	Males	Females	Both
Mean age	73.9 ± 5.8	71.1 ± 5.2	72.0 ± 5.5
Mean BMI	27.8 ± 3.0	30.1 ± 6.7	29.3 ± 5.8
BMI category			
Underweight (BMI < 18.5)	0	0	0
Normal (BMI 18.5–24.9)	2 (12%)	6 (18%)	8 (16%)
Overweight (BMI 25.0–29.9)	12 (71%)	12 (36%)	24 (48%)
Obese class I (BMI 30.0–34.9)	2 (12%)	9 (27%)	11 (22%)
Obese class II (BMI 35.0–39.9)	1 (6%)	3 (9%)	4 (8%)
Obese class III (BMI ≥ 40.0)	0	3 (9%)	3 (6%)
BMD			
Osteoporosis	0	1 (3%)	1 (2%)
Osteopenia	3 (18%)	18 (56%)	21 (43%)
Normal	14 (82%)	13 (41%)	27 (55%)
Balance			
Better than normal	0	4 (12%)	4 (8%)
Normal	3 (18%)	11 (33%)	14 (28%)
Poor	14 (82%)	18 (55%)	32 (64%)
RAPA			
Sedentary	0	0	0
Underactive	0	0	0
Under-active regular—light activities	1 (6%)	8 (24%)	9 (18%)
Under-active regular	3 (18%)	11 (33%)	14 (28%)
Active	13 (76%)	14 (42%)	27 (54%)
FRAX			
FRAX osteoporotic fracture (%)	6.12 ± 2.83*	10.79 ± 5.12*	9.20 ± 4.97
FRAX hip fracture (%)	1.88 ± 2.11	2.10 ± 2.07	2.02 ± 2.06

*$P < 0.05$.

TABLE 2: Correlation between age, BMI, MFES scores, and FRAX osteoporotic and hip fracture scores for both genders.

	Age	BMI	MFES score	FRAX osteoporotic fracture score	FRAX hip fracture score
Age	—	—	—	—	—
BMI	−0.32*	—	—	—	—
MFES score	−0.15	0.02	—	—	—
FRAX osteoporotic fracture score	0.31*	−0.30*	−0.34*	—	—
FRAX hip fracture score	0.55**	−0.39**	−0.24	0.83**	—

*$P < 0.05$, **$P < 0.01$.

femoral neck, while 43% of the sample had osteopenia (one female with osteoporosis) (Table 1).

3.2. Fear of Falling. The average MFES score was 9.47 ± 0.97 (best possible score 10), indicating that this cohort had little to no fear of falling. There were no significant differences in MFES scores between males (9.69 ± 0.59) and females (9.35 ± 1.11) ($P = 0.26$). There was no significant relationship between the fear of falling and age, BMI, or FRAX ten-year probability of hip fracture scores (Table 2). There was also no significant difference in fear of falling among balance fall risk categories ($P = 0.32$) or BMD categories ($P = 0.71$) (Table 3). Males differ from the combined gender analysis and the female analysis in that there was a significant difference in fear of falling and balance fall risk categories (Table 3). The average MFES score for males with normal balance was 9.02 ± 1.15, and the average score for males with poor balance was 9.83 ± 0.32. This difference was significant ($P = 0.03$).

Males had less fear of falling with poorer balance. This was the opposite trend when compared to females, who had greater fear of falling with poorer balance. A significant correlation was found between fear of falling and FRAX ten-year probability of major osteoporotic fracture scores ($r = -0.34$, $P = 0.02$). When analysis of fear of falling was done within gender groups, there were a few notable differences. Fear of falling for females still had a significant and negative

TABLE 3: MFES scores* among balance fall risk, BMD, and RAPA categories.

	Males	Females	Both
Balance			
Better than normal	0	9.80 ± 0.40	9.80 ± 0.40
Normal	9.02 ± 1.15**	9.15 ± 1.51	9.12 ± 1.40
Poor	9.83 ± 0.32**	9.38 ± 0.94	9.58 ± 0.76
BMD			
Osteoporotic	0	8.86 ± 0	8.86 ± 0
Osteopenic	10.00 ± 0	9.27 ± 1.17	9.38 ± 1.11
Normal	9.62 ± 0.64	9.46 ± 1.12	9.54 ± 0.89
RAPA			
Under-active regular—light activities	9.00 ± 0	9.32 ± 0.81	9.28 ± 0.77
Under-active regular	9.02 ± 1.15**	8.97 ± 1.72	8.98 ± 1.58**
Active	9.90 ± 0.22**	9.68 ± 0.38	9.78 ± 0.33**

*Higher scores indicate less fear of falling.
**$P < 0.05$.

correlation with FRAX osteoporotic fracture scores ($r = -0.36$, $P = 0.04$); however, this same correlation for males was nonsignificant and positive ($r = 0.07$, $P = 0.79$).

The relationship between fear of falling and RAPA categories approached statistical significance ($P = 0.07$). In particular, the difference in fear of falling between the active and underactive regular RAPA categories was significant ($P = 0.03$), with the active group having a mean MFES score of 9.78 ± 0.33 and the underactive regular group having a mean MFES score of 8.98 ± 1.58 (Table 3). A significant difference was found between fear of falling and RAPA categories for males ($P = 0.02$), but this difference was not significant for females ($P = 0.31$) (Table 3).

3.3. Fall Risk Balance Testing. Baseline results of the fall risk balance testing showed that a majority of the sample (64%) had poor balance (Table 1). The difference in balance between males and females was not significant ($P = 0.11$) (Table 1). There was no significant relationship between balance and age, BMI, the FRAX risk of major osteoporotic fracture, or FRAX risk of hip fracture. The relationship between age and balance approached statistical significance ($P = 0.06$), with the mean ages of the better than normal, normal, and poor balance groups being 66.5±1.0, 72.4±6.0, and 72.5±5.4 years, respectively. The relationship between BMI and balance for females also approached statistical significance ($P = 0.06$). The mean BMI of the better than normal balance group was 25.65 ± 5.45, the normal balance group was 26.89 ± 2.53, and the poor balance group was 33.12 ± 7.45. Activity level was not significantly impacted by balance for both genders ($P = 0.69$).

3.4. Rapid Assessment of Physical Activity. No participants were categorized as sedentary or underactive. Based on the RAPA questionnaire, the majority of the participants were categorized as active, with males more active than females (Table 1). This difference approached statistical significance ($P = 0.06$). Activity level did not have a significant relationship with age, BMI, FRAX osteoporotic fracture score, or FRAX hip fracture score for males, females, and both genders combined.

3.5. Bone Mineral Density. Gender had a significant impact on BMD ($P = 0.02$) (Table 1). There was no significant relationship between BMD when compared to age and BMI. BMD had a significant relationship with both the FRAX osteoporotic fracture score ($P < 0.01$) and the FRAX hip fracture score ($P < 0.01$) for both genders combined and females. While there was a significant relationship between BMD and the FRAX osteoporotic fracture score ($P = 0.03$) for males, the relationship of BMD with the FRAX hip fracture score was not significant ($P = 0.20$).

3.6. FRAX Scores. The average ten-year probability of major osteoporotic fracture as determined by FRAX was 9.20% ± 4.97% (range, 3.30%–23.00%). Females had a significantly higher ten-year probability of major osteoporotic fracture than males ($P < 0.01$) (Table 1). The ten-year probability of hip fracture based on the FRAX score was 2.02% ± 2.06% (range, 0.00%–8.40%). No significant difference was found in the ten-year probability of hip fracture between males and females ($P = 0.72$) (Table 1). Age was found to have a significant and positive correlation with both FRAX scores for both genders combined and females; however, this correlation was not significant for males (Tables 2, 4, and 5). BMI, on the other hand, had a significant and negative correlation with both FRAX scores for both genders, males, and females (Tables 2, 4, and 5). The two FRAX scores had a significant and strong correlation with each other (Tables 2, 4, and 5).

3.7. One-Year Followup. Out of the original 50 participants in this study, 42 took part in the one-year followup (84%). Among the eight lost to followup, we were unable to contact two participants and the other six withdrew from the study. The remaining 14 males and 28 females had a mean age of 72.4±5.7 years (range, 66–85 years) and a mean BMI of 29.0± 5.7 (range, normal—obese class III) (Table 6) [19].

Table 4: Correlation between age, BMI, MFES scores, and FRAX osteoporotic and hip fracture scores for males.

	Age	BMI	MFES score	FRAX osteoporotic fracture score	FRAX hip fracture score
Age	—	—	—	—	—
BMI	−0.44	—	—	—	—
MFES score	−0.10	−0.07	—	—	—
FRAX osteoporotic fracture score	0.42	−0.61*	0.07	—	—
FRAX hip fracture score	0.47	−0.61*	−0.02	0.93*	—

*$P < 0.01$.

Table 5: Correlation between age, BMI, MFES scores, and FRAX osteoporotic and hip fracture scores for females.

	Age	BMI	MFES score	FRAX osteoporotic fracture score	FRAX hip fracture score
Age	—	—	—	—	—
BMI	−0.27	—	—	—	—
MFES score	−0.24	0.07	—	—	—
FRAX osteoporotic fracture score	0.54**	−0.43*	−0.36*	—	—
FRAX hip fracture score	0.64**	−0.38*	−0.31	0.93**	—

*$P < 0.05$, **$P < 0.01$.

The average MFES score at one-year followup was 9.35 ± 0.94. Consistent with our initial results, no significant difference was found between fear of falling for males (9.47 ± 1.09) and females (9.29 ± 0.86) ($P = 0.56$). The trend that older males are more active than older females was found to be significant at one-year followup ($P < 0.01$) (Table 6). However, the activity level was not found to have a significant association with age ($P = 0.61$), BMI ($P = 0.13$), or fear of falling ($P = 0.86$).

Eight individuals (two males, six females) experienced a fall in the previous year, with one female participant experiencing multiple falls. On initial testing, five of these participants had poor balance when compared to the norms for their age group. Two female participants had normal balance, and one female participant had better than normal balance. Average FRAX score for major osteoporotic fracture was 11.51% ± 5.58% and the average FRAX score for hip fracture was 2.88% ± 2.38%. Three participants had a normal BMD (one male, two females), four were osteopenic (one male, three females), and one female was osteoporotic. These individuals also became more afraid of falling, with an initial average MFES score of 9.23 ± 1.44 decreasing to 9.11 ± 1.12 one-year later, though this was not a significant change ($P = 0.83$). They also became less active, though again the change from baseline to the one-year point was not significant ($P = 0.48$). Initially seven individuals were considered active with one female participant being underactive regular. After one-year, only three individuals were still active (one male, two females), with four being underactive regular (one male, three females) and one female being underactive.

Seven participants did not sustain any injuries due to their falls, except for one female participant who suffered a fractured foot and subsequently required the use of a walker to ambulate. The female participant who suffered a fracture was one of the oldest participants in the study at 84 years old. Prior to her fragility fracture she had been active. She was osteopenic with poor balance and FRAX scores of 15.00% and 4.10% for osteoporotic and hip fractures, respectively. After her fragility fracture she became much more afraid of falling, with her MFES score decreasing from 9.54 to 7.64.

4. Discussion

The participants in this study consisted of ambulatory community-dwelling volunteers. They were generally healthy and physical active, with no sedentary individuals. Nearly half were overweight and one had osteoporosis, and they had little to no fear of falling and were fairly healthy and active; however, their balance scores were generally poor. In addition, the difference in balance between males and females approached statistical significance ($P = 0.11$), which may suggest a trend that older males have poorer balance than older females. The overall poor balance is an unexpected finding because physically activity is believed to improve balance and reduce the risk of falls [9, 20, 21]. We did not find a significant relationship between balance and activity level and fall and fracture risk; however, this may be due to our small sample size. This finding is of concern because it suggests that many older adults are unaware of their capability with respect to balance. Therefore, balance screening and training is important even in active healthy nonosteoporotic individuals to decrease future fall and fracture risk.

Our finding of no difference in fear of falling between males and females contradicts the literature. Several studies examining fear of falling in community-dwelling seniors have shown that women are significantly more afraid of falling than men [22–24]; however, our findings may have been influenced by a small sample size and selection bias. Although we did not find a gender difference, fear of falling can have serious implications. Our cohort overall had very little fear of falling; even the lower MFES scores that were recorded for this sample are considered to have little fear of falling. However, even between the small range of scores significant differences were found.

Table 6: One-year followup data on demographics and TAPA* categories.

	Males	Females	Both
Mean age	74.8 ± 6.0	71.1 ± 5.3	72.4 ± 5.7
Mean BMI	27.6 ± 2.9	29.7 ± 6.7	29.0 ± 5.7
BMI category			
Underweight (BMI < 18.5)	0	0	0
Normal (BMI 18.5–24.9)	2 (14%)	8 (29%)	10 (24%)
Overweight (BMI 25.0–29.9)	10 (72%)	7 (25%)	17 (40%)
Obese class I (BMI 30.0–34.9)	1 (7%)	8 (29%)	9 (21%)
Obese class II (BMI 35.0–39.9)	1 (7%)	3 (10%)	4 (10%)
Obese class III (BMI ≥ 40.0)	0	2 (7%)	2 (5%)
TAPA*			
Under-active	0	11 (39%)	11 (26%)
Under-active regular	4 (29%)	9 (32%)	13 (31%)
Active	10 (71%)**	8 (29%)**	18 (43%)

*Telephone assessment of physical activity [18].
**$P < 0.01$.

It has been well documented in the literature that osteoporosis is more prevalent in women than in men [25–27]. Therefore, our finding that gender significantly impacts BMD was expected. This also likely contributed to our finding that females had a significantly greater risk of osteoporotic fracture, as determined by FRAX scores. As well, considering that BMD is one of the components used to calculate FRAX scores, it was no surprising that BMD had a strong relationship with both the FRAX osteoporotic fracture score and the FRAX hip fracture score.

BMI is another risk factor that has been shown to have some influence on fragility fractures [7, 28]. A low BMI is believed to increase fracture risk because there is less soft tissue protecting the bones [7, 28]. Therefore, our finding of a negative relationship between BMI and FRAX is expected as a higher BMI would be expected to reduce fracture risk as the individual would have more soft tissue.

Individuals who have a greater fear of falling have a significantly greater risk of sustaining a major osteoporotic fracture based on the FRAX score. There are a number of potential reasons that may explain this. It may be that individuals with a poor BMD have some awareness of their bone health issues either because these have been previously addressed by health professionals or because they have health problems or symptoms that initiate concern and as a result have a greater fear of falling. Since BMD has a strong association with osteoporotic fracture risk [26, 27, 29, 30], this appears like a plausible explanation. However, fall and fracture risk is multifactorial and does not rely solely on BMD [5, 8, 11, 12, 30]. The relationship between fear of falling and BMD was not significant, suggesting that the increased fracture risk in the more fearful individuals was influenced by risk factors other than BMD (i.e., other factors used to calculate FRAX scores such as previous fracture, parent with a fractured hip, smoking and excessive alcohol consumption, long-term glucocorticoid use, rheumatoid arthritis, and causes of secondary osteoporosis) [11–13].

Another factor influencing fall and fracture risk is activity level. It is believed that decreasing activity levels leads to a functional decline, predisposing individuals to fall [2, 9, 10]. Fear of falling is a common reason for older individuals to decrease their activity level [2, 10, 22, 31–33], which supports our finding that more active individuals have less fear of falling. Individuals who suffered a fall at the one-year followup had experienced some increased fear of falling and decreased activity level compared to those who did not fall. In addition, our findings suggest that fear of falling affects activity levels of males more than females. Balance is also believed to be closely related to activity level and fall and fracture risk [20], but we did not find a significant relationship between these factors. Even though we found an association between fear of falling and activity level, with fear of falling known to influence osteoporotic fracture risk, we did not find a relationship between activity level and fracture risk.

The individuals who experienced a fall at one-year followup had higher FRAX scores for major osteoporotic fracture and hip fracture than those who did not fall. As well, many of the individuals who fell experienced a decrease in their activity level and became more afraid of falling, whereas individuals who did not fall did not experience much change in their activity or fear of falling. This supports the notion that falls, even if they do not cause injury, increase fear of falling, and can lead to decreased activity and potentially a functional decline in older adults [7, 14, 22, 23]. Although specific measures to improve or maintain activity level were not evaluated in this study, encouraging older adults to stay active should help minimize their fear of falling and falls. Future studies are needed to assess specific activities that will help maintain balance and prevent falls.

The results of this study may be influenced by selection bias since the cohort consisted of healthy volunteers. Another limitation is that the number of males who participated was small; therefore, conclusions based around the male gender are not as robust as the conclusions for females. As well, the one-year followup relied upon accurate reporting by the participants. Considering that there was no contact between the researchers and the study participants over a period of 12 months, it is possible that recall bias influenced fall reporting. We might have been able to obtain a more precise picture of fall risk with more regular followup with the participants. In spite of these limitations, this study was able to successfully follow a cohort longitudinally over one-year. In doing this, we were able to identify the differences in risk factors between individuals who did and did not suffer a fall.

5. Conclusions

Our baseline data showed that individuals with greater fear of falling had an increased fracture risk. The finding that overall balance was poor in this healthy, active population was unexpected. More attention should be dedicated towards balance interventions in this population to minimize fall risk. Individuals who fell after one-year experienced an increase in their fear of falling as well as decreased activity levels. This emphasizes the need for methods to reduce fear of falling in active healthy seniors in order to prevent future falls, fractures, and functional decline.

Abbreviations

BMI: Body mass index
BMD: Bone mineral density
DEXA: Dual-energy X-ray absorptiometry
FRAX: Fracture Risk Assessment Tool
MFES: Modified Falls Efficacy Scale
RAPA: Rapid Assessment of Physical Activity
TAPA: Telephone Assessment of Physical Activity
WHO: World Health Organization.

Acknowledgment

This work was supported by an operating grant received from the Canadian Institute of Health Research (CIHR) under project titled Identification of Risk of Adverse Activity Transtition following a Distal Radius Fracture. PIs are MacDermid JC and Grewal R and Coinvestigators are McIntyre N and Richardson J. Award no. MOP-93372.

References

[1] V. Scott, M. Pearce, and C. Pengelly, "Technical report: hospitalizations due to falls among Canadians age 65 and over," Tech. Rep. HP25-1/20005E, Public Health Agency of Canada, Ottawa, Canada, 2005.

[2] J. A. Stevens, P. S. Corso, E. A. Finkelstein, and T. R. Miller, "The costs of fatal and non-fatal falls among older adults," *Injury Prevention*, vol. 12, no. 5, pp. 290–295, 2006.

[3] S. Heinrich, K. Rapp, U. Rissmann, C. Becker, and H.-H. König, "Cost of falls in old age: a systematic review," *Osteoporosis International*, vol. 21, no. 6, pp. 891–902, 2010.

[4] K. Malik, "Development Report 2013," Tech. Rep., United Nations Development Programme, New York, NY, USA, 2013.

[5] Canadian Demographics at a Glance, Catalogue 91-003-X, Statistics Canada, Ottawa, Canada, 2008.

[6] M. E. Tinetti, M. Speechley, and S. F. Ginter, "Risk factors for falls among elderly persons living in the community," *The New England Journal of Medicine*, vol. 319, no. 26, pp. 1701–1707, 1988.

[7] S. D. Berry and R. R. Miller, "Falls: epidemiology, pathophysiology, and relationship to fracture," *Current Osteoporosis Reports*, vol. 6, no. 4, pp. 149–154, 2008.

[8] National Trauma Registry 2011 Report: Hospitalizations for Major Injury in Canada, 2008-2009 Data, Toronto, Canada, Canadian Institute for Health Information, 2011.

[9] C. M. Arnold, M. M. Sran, and E. L. Harrison, "Exercise for fall risk reduction in community-dwelling older adults: a systematic review," *Physiotherapy Canada*, vol. 60, pp. 358–372, 2008.

[10] D. G. Bruce, A. Devine, and R. L. Prince, "Recreational physical activity levels in healthy older women: the importance of fear of falling," *Journal of the American Geriatrics Society*, vol. 50, no. 1, pp. 84–89, 2002.

[11] J. A. Kanis, E. V. McCloskey, H. Johansson, A. Oden, O. Ström, and F. Borgström, "Development and use of FRAX in osteoporosis," *Osteoporosis International*, vol. 21, supplement 2, pp. S407–S413, 2010.

[12] N. B. Watts, "The fracture risk assessment tool (FRAX): applications in clinical practice," *Journal of Women's Health*, vol. 20, no. 4, pp. 525–531, 2011.

[13] A. Papaioannou, S. Morin, A. M. Cheung et al., "2010 clinical practice guidelines for the diagnosis and management of osteoporosis in Canada: summary," *Canadian Medical Association Journal*, vol. 182, no. 17, pp. 1864–1873, 2010.

[14] K. D. Hill, J. A. Schwarz, A. J. Kalogeropoulos, and S. J. Gibson, "Fear of falling revisited," *Archives of Physical Medicine and Rehabilitation*, vol. 77, no. 10, pp. 1025–1029, 1996.

[15] T. D. Topolski, J. LoGerfo, D. L. Patrick, B. Williams, J. Walwick, and M. B. Patrick, "The Rapid Assessment of Physical Activity (RAPA) among older adults," *Preventing Chronic Disease*, vol. 3, no. 4, p. A118, 2006.

[16] K. Y. Oh, S. A. Kim, S. Y. Lee et al., "Comparison of manual balance and balance board tests in healthy adults," *Annals of Physical and Rehabilitation Medicine*, vol. 35, pp. 873–879, 2011.

[17] M. L. Pickerill and R. A. Harter, "Validity and reliability of limits-of-stability testing: a comparison of 2 postural stability evaluation devices," *Journal of Athletic Training*, vol. 46, no. 6, pp. 600–606, 2011.

[18] C. J. Mayer, L. Steinman, B. Williams, T. D. Topolski, and J. LoGerfo, "Developing a Telephone Assessment of Physical Activity (TAPA) questionnaire for older adults," *Preventing Chronic Disease*, vol. 5, no. 1, p. A24, 2008.

[19] Health Canada, "Description of the Canadian Guidelines for Body Weight Classification in Adults," 2003, http://www.hc-sc.gc.ca/fn-an/nutrition/weights-poids/guide-ld-adult/weight_book-livres_des_poids-03-table1-eng.php.

[20] A. Barnett, B. Smith, S. R. Lord, M. Williams, and A. Baumand, "Community-based group exercise improves balance and reduces falls in at-risk older people: a randomised controlled trial," *Age and Ageing*, vol. 32, no. 4, pp. 407–414, 2003.

[21] L. Clemson, M. A. Fiatarone Singh, A. Bundy et al., "Integration of balance and strength training into daily life activity to reduce rate of falls in older people (the LiFE study): randomised parallel trial," *British Medical Journal*, vol. 345, Article ID e4547, 2012.

[22] R. Boyd and J. A. Stevens, "Falls and fear of falling: burden, beliefs and behaviours," *Age and Ageing*, vol. 38, no. 4, pp. 423–428, 2009.

[23] H. W. Lach, "Incidence and risk factors for developing fear of falling in older adults," *Public Health Nursing*, vol. 22, no. 1, pp. 45–52, 2005.

[24] G. A. R. Zijlstra, J. C. M. van Haastregt, J. T. M. van Eijk, E. van Rossum, P. A. Stalenhoef, and G. I. J. M. Kempen, "Prevalence and correlates of fear of falling, and associated avoidance of activity in the general population of community-living older people," *Age and Ageing*, vol. 36, no. 3, pp. 304–309, 2007.

[25] P. M. Cawthon, "Gender differences in osteoporosis and fractures," *Clinical Orthopaedics and Related Research*, vol. 469, no. 7, pp. 1900–1905, 2011.

[26] N. E. Lane, "Epidemiology, etiology, and diagnosis of osteoporosis," *American Journal of Obstetrics and Gynecology*, vol. 194, no. 2, supplement, pp. S3–S11, 2006.

[27] NIH Consensus Development Panel on Osteoporosis Prevention, Diagnosis, "Osteoporosis prevention, diagnosis, and therapy," *Journal of the American Medical Association*, vol. 285, pp. 785–795, 2001.

[28] C. De Laet, J. A. Kanis, A. Odén et al., "Body mass index as a predictor of fracture risk: a meta-analysis," *Osteoporosis International*, vol. 16, no. 11, pp. 1330–1338, 2005.

[29] O. Johnell, J. A. Kanis, A. Oden et al., "Predictive value of BMD for hip and other fractures," *Journal of Bone and Mineral Research*, vol. 20, pp. 1185–1194, 2005.

[30] J. A. Kanis, "Osteoporosis III: diagnosis of osteoporosis and assessment of fracture risk," *The Lancet*, vol. 359, no. 9321, pp. 1929–1936, 2002.

[31] D. Rand, W. C. Miller, J. Yiu, and J. J. Eng, "Interventions for addressing low balance confidence in older adults: a systematic review and meta-analysis," *Age and Ageing*, vol. 40, no. 3, pp. 297–306, 2011.

[32] G. I. J. M. Kempen, J. C. Van Haastregt, K. J. McKee, K. Delbaere, and G. R. Zijlstra, "Socio-demographic, health-related and psychosocial correlates of fear of falling and avoidance of activity in community-living older persons who avoid activity due to fear of falling," *BMC Public Health*, vol. 9, article 170, 2009.

[33] H. Shimada, S. R. Lord, H. Yoshida, H. Kim, and T. Suzuki, "Predictors of cessation of regular leisure-time physical activity in community-dwelling elderly people," *Gerontology*, vol. 53, no. 5, pp. 293–297, 2007.

22

An Overview of Cognitive Remediation Therapy for People with Severe Mental Illness

Cherrie Galletly[1,2,3] **and Ashlee Rigby**[2,3]

[1] *Adelaide Health Service, Northern Mental Health Directorate, Department of Health and Ageing, Adelaide, SA 5000, Australia*
[2] *Mental Health Services (SA), Ramsay Health Care, The Adelaide Clinic, Adelaide, SA 5082, Australia*
[3] *Discipline of Psychiatry, School of Medicine, The University of Adelaide, Adelaide, SA 5000, Australia*

Correspondence should be addressed to Cherrie Galletly; cherrie.galletly@adelaide.edu.au

Academic Editors: K. Hashimoto, K.-H. Lin, and M. Schmitter-Edgecombe

Cognitive remediation refers to nonpharmacological methods of improving cognitive function in people with severe mental disorders. Cognitive remediation therapy (CRT) can be delivered via computerised programs, of varying length and complexity, or can be undertaken one-on-one by a trained clinician. There has been a considerable interest in cognitive remediation, driven by recognition that cognitive deficits are a major determinant of outcome in people with severe, chronic mental illnesses. CRT has been shown to be effective, especially if combined with vocational rehabilitation.

1. Cognitive Impairment in Severe Mental Illness

The term "severe mental illness" (SMI) is generally taken to encompass chronic psychotic disorders. Whilst many people in this category suffer from schizophrenia, disorders such as schizoaffective disorder, delusional disorder and bipolar disorder are also commonly associated with persistent symptoms, cognitive impairment and long-term disability [1]. Data collected from 1875 people with SMI demonstrated that their current cognitive ability was markedly impaired, compared to the general population. On average, people with psychosis scored 1.6 standard deviations below the general population on a test of information processing speed [1].

There are some differences between diagnostic groups. Children who later develop schizophrenia are more likely to be slow to learn to speak [2] and to have impaired language and arithmetic ability during childhood [3], reflecting neurodevelopmental processes underlying adult schizophrenia [4]. In contrast, people with bipolar disorder tend to have average or superior educational achievement as children, suggesting a different illness trajectory [5]. Nevertheless, despite premorbid differences, cognitive impairment is evident in both affective psychoses (bipolar disorder and psychotic depression) and nonaffective psychoses (schizophrenia) [6] even in the early stages of the disorder. Cognitive impairment is generally most profound and pervasive in schizophrenia [7].

Vocational outcomes are poor in people with SMI, with many experiencing long-term unemployment and welfare dependence, despite evidence that they could gain considerable benefit from engagement in paid employment [8]. Numerous studies have demonstrated an association between the severity of cognitive impairment and functional, social, and occupational outcomes in schizophrenia [9, 10]. Similarly, in bipolar disorder, cognitive deficits have been shown to be associated with reduced psychosocial function [11, 12]. Cognitive impairment is an important determinant of poor engagement with vocational rehabilitation services [13] and failure to maintain job tenure [14]. Research into measures to improve cognition is therefore driven by the hope that such improvements might lead to better long-term economic as well as functional outcomes, along with greater opportunities for social inclusion.

A number of medications have been trialled, specifically targeting cognitive function [15]. Treatment with clozapine is associated with improvements in working memory although normal levels of performance are not achieved [16]. Whilst other atypical antipsychotic drugs have been shown to be associated with improved cognition, it appears that much of this improvement is an artefact of study design with failure to properly address practice effects [17].

Very high levels of tobacco use are found amongst people with schizophrenia [18, 19], and interestingly nicotine improves their ability to filter out irrelevant information and to manage complex environments [20]. Drugs acting on nicotinic receptors may therefore have a role in enhancing cognition in schizophrenia. A number of other targets for drug development have been identified, but so far none of the drugs available have shown substantial benefit in clinical trials [15]. This lack of progress in psychopharmacology has highlighted the need for effective nonpharmacological methods of cognitive remediation.

2. Cognitive Remediation: Study Populations

Virtually all of the research regarding cognitive remediation in SMI has been undertaken in people with schizophrenia, perhaps because, as described above, schizophrenia has been shown to be associated with the most severe cognitive deficits. There has been one study comparing cognitive remediation in schizophrenia and schizoaffective disorder [21] which found that cognitive enhancement therapy, a two-year intervention including both computer training and social cognitive group sessions, was equally effective in both groups. Harvey et al. (2010) suggest that people with bipolar disorder might also benefit from the treatments used to address cognitive deficits in schizophrenia [22]. Deckersbach et al. (2010) have reported that a 14-session cognitive remediation program designed to treat both residual depressive symptoms and cognitive impairment in people with bipolar disorder, and delivered to each participant individually, was effective in reducing depression and improving occupational and psychosocial functioning. This was a small study ($N = 18$) with no control group, but it does provide an indication that further research into cognitive remediation in bipolar disorder is warranted [23].

3. Methods of Cognitive Remediation

An expert consensus group has defined cognitive remediation Therapy (CRT) as "a behavioural-training based intervention that aims to improve cognitive processes (attention, memory, executive function, social cognition, or metacognition) with the goal of durability and generalization" [24]. A variety of different methods of cognitive remediation have been described in the research literature. The starting point for this research was to establish whether it is possible to achieve any improvement in cognitive function in schizophrenia using non-pharmacological methods. Some of the earliest studies demonstrated that people with schizophrenia could be taught to improve their performance on the Wisconsin Card Sorting Test [25, 26]. Simple strategies such as vocalisation (speaking aloud whilst performing the task) have been shown to improve performance on complex tasks [27]. In other early studies, computer programs developed to retrain attentional deficits due to closed-head injury were used with people with schizophrenia. Results were mixed, with some studies reporting improvement [28, 29] while others found no change [24, 30].

Next, programs were developed to target the cognitive deficits characteristic of schizophrenia. These programs differ considerably in their theoretical underpinnings, methods, duration, and target outcomes. CRT programs generally take one of two approaches, either rehearsal learning, also termed drill and practice, or strategy coaching, where participants are helped to develop effective strategies to undertake cognitive tasks. Combinations of these two approaches can be utilised [31].

Whilst earlier studies often used clinician-administered CRT, recent studies most commonly utilise computerised CRT. Computerised methods have the advantages of being standardised and more efficient. Less staff time is needed as one staff member can supervise several participants, and staff do not require specialised skills. The larger and more successful studies have used programs such as Cogpack [32] and CogRehab [31]. Cogpack and Cogrehab consist of a series of computer-based programs which address a range of cognitive functions. Cognitive domains including memory, attention, visual information processing, language, and motor function are targeted using interactive training programs. Genevsky et al. (2010) randomly assigned participants to either 50 hours of playing computer games, or to 50 hours of computerised training of auditory perception and aural speech reception for 10 weeks. These exercises were used as it is thought that early auditory processing deficits are associated with impaired verbal memory, reading ability and emotional recognition. Subjects who undertook this training showed improvements in working memory, verbal learning and memory, and global cognition compared to the comparison group [33]. These programs allow therapy to be extended through independent exercise on a home computer. Computer-delivered programs are generally acceptable to participants, especially younger people for whom these programs resemble recreational computer games. Some studies use a combination of the two methods; for example, Royer et al. (2012) describe a combination of psychologist-assisted pencil and paper exercises and a computerised training program [34].

4. Outcome Measures

There is a considerable variation in outcome measures, and this makes comparison between studies difficult. The National Institute of Mental Health (NIMH) MATRICS (Measurement and Treatment Research to Improve Cognition in Schizophrenia) initiative attempted to address the lack of standardization of instruments used to measure cognition in schizophrenia. A consensus neuropsychological battery of 10 tests [35, 36] was developed to evaluate performance across seven domains previously shown to be impaired in schizophrenia. These domains are speed of processing, attention/vigilance, working memory, verbal learning, visual learning; reasoning and problem solving; and social cognition. Normative data for the MATRICS test battery has been obtained on 300 adults [35]. However, despite the availability of the MATRICS battery, a wide range of outcome measures continue to be used in research evaluating CRT [36].

5. Efficacy of CRT

Wykes et al. (2007) described a study using a clinician-delivered CRT program in young people with schizophrenia. The program required 40 hours of individual work with each patient [37]. Tasks were designed to improve information processing strategies and included memory, complex planning, and problem solving. Three cognitive outcome measures were selected, and comparisons between the CRT group and the control group found statistically significant improvement in only one of these measures, with no significant effect of CRT on symptom severity or social functioning. There was some controversy about whether such modest gains are worth the investment of time and expertise [38].

However, in a meta-analysis of 40 studies of cognitive remediation in schizophrenia, Wykes et al. (2011) found that CRT resulted in significant improvements in global cognition with a mean effect size of 0.45. Nearly all cognitive domains, including attention and vigilance, speed of processing, working memory, reasoning, problem solving, and social cognition demonstrated significant effect sizes ranging from 0.25 to 0.65. Importantly, the effects on global cognition were sustained 3–12 months after CRT was completed (effect size = 0.43). The average length of treatment was 32.3 hours provided across 16.7 weeks; however the sample size in most studies was small, ranging from 10 to 145 people. Wykes et al. (2011) concluded that CRT can provide benefits to patients with cognitive difficulties independent of therapy characteristics such as individual versus group therapy, patient characteristics or sample size [39].

Wykes et al. (2011) also proposed that nearly all cognitive domains respond to remediation in the treatment of schizophrenia. As cognitive remediation is not domain specific they propose that the outcome measure of any cognitive remediation therapy should be the effect it has on community functioning [39].

6. Real-World Applications of CRT

Improving performance on cognitive tests is not in itself of benefit; the goals of CRT are to improve real-world outcomes such as work, socialisation, and independent living skills. One of the shortcomings in CRT research has been that this therapy has often been provided without concurrent rehabilitation programs, and the more successful studies do combine CRT and psychosocial and/or vocational rehabilitation. For example, McGurk and Meltzer (2000) found that a combination of computer-aided CRT and vocational rehabilitation was more successful in returning people to work than vocational rehabilitation alone [32]. A meta-analysis by McGurk et al. (2007) reported that studies that included adjunctive psychiatric rehabilitation had significantly better outcomes, compared with cognitive remediation alone [40]. This makes sense as participants have the opportunity to apply their improved cognitive skills directly to the challenges of the workplace, resulting in iterative learning opportunities.

This is supported by a meta-analysis that concluded that CRT was more effective when it was provided with other adjunctive psychiatric rehabilitation [39]. In the short term, the CRT programs which focussed solely on cognitive skills had a small to medium effect size but demonstrated no significant difference at followup assessment [39]. These results indicate that in order to maximise the benefits of CRT, participants should be working or be involved in employment-focused rehabilitation. This important finding, reported more than a decade ago, has nevertheless not been widely translated into services for people with SMI.

CRT has also been shown to improve symptoms in schizophrenia. Participants in a study by Lecardeur et al. (2009) received 2 novel CRTs, one targeting mental state attribution, and the other, mental flexibility, and compared both groups with a control group given treatment as usual. Symptoms decreased after therapy, but not in the control group. The mental flexibility group showed the most improvement [41]. Additionally, this study reported that participants described a subjective reduction of their cognitive deficits.

On the whole, CRT has been shown to have moderate improvements on global cognition and to a lesser extent functioning. However, greater improvement in functional outcomes can be achieved by combining psychosocial rehabilitation and CRT [40].

7. Remediation of Social Cognitive Deficits

Social cognition is a domain of cognitive function that includes the ability to understand and manage social interactions. Social cognition refers to aspects of cognition that are critical for social functioning and interpersonal relationships, such as accurate perception of the emotions of others, the ability to recognize important social cues, theory of mind (TOM), and the management of emotions in social situations [42]. Various components of social cognition have been found to be impaired in people with schizophrenia [43, 44]. Lindenmayer et al. (2012) concluded that CRT combined with emotion perception remediation produced greater improvements in emotion recognition, emotion discrimination, social functioning, and neurocognition compared with CRT alone in chronic schizophrenia [45]. Furthermore, as has been shown previously in cognitive remediation research, training in one area of cognition can generalise to other social cognition domains which were not the primary focus of treatment [46]. Penadés et al. (2010) reported that improvement in executive functioning predicted improved daily functioning and social cognition among people with schizophrenia who had negative symptoms and neuropsychological impairment [47]. This provides further support for the generalizability of CRT training to a variety of cognitive domains. A meta-analysis of computerised CRT found a significant medium effect size of 0.64 (CI 0.29–0.99) for Social Cognition [48].

8. Remediation of Cognitive Biases

Cognitive illusions or biases are perceptions or judgements that deviate from reality in a systematic way and reflect inherent thinking errors made in processing information. Metacognitive training (MCT) has been developed as a treatment for people with schizophrenia to address cognitive biases thought to contribute to delusions [49]. MCT is a combination of psychoeducation, cognitive remediation, and cognitive-behavioural therapy (CBT). CBT is a focussed approach to therapy that helps individuals to identify unhelpful thoughts or behaviours and to learn healthy thought patterns and habits. By contrast, CRT is conceptualised as a behavioural-based training program for various areas of neurocognition and executive functioning which has generalizable effects on functioning. By combining these two therapeutic approaches MCT educates people about their cognitive biases and teaches them strategies to deal with biases which may impact on functioning [49].

MCT has been shown to be effective in retraining the "jumping to conclusions" bias and in theory of mind [50]. Balzan et al. (in press) enrolled 24 participants with schizophrenia and a history of delusions to a metacognitive training program. In one-hour individual sessions, participants were encouraged to think about the cognitive underpinnings of delusional ideation and to consider that their delusions may be maintained by a hypersalience of evidence-hypothesis matches [51]. Hypersalience of evidence-hypothesis matches is one type of "jumping to conclusions" bias, where people make strong connections between existing beliefs and weak evidence [51, 52]. After two weeks of MCT, the severity of the delusions, and the extent of delusional preoccupation and conviction, had decreased compared to a treatment as usual comparison group [51].

9. The Future of CRT

As yet, CRT has not been commonly adopted in clinical practice. Wykes, writing in Nature (2010), proposes that the future of CRT lies in a more personalised approach. She suggests that research participants should be stratified, perhaps according to age or learning style, to identify the methods that are most effective according to these individual factors [38]. The goal would be to tailor an optimal remediation program for each individual. Ultimately, biological research methods utilising biomarkers or brain imaging might have a role in investigating the effects of CRT on brain function, and eventually in matching the treatment approach to the individual patient.

Clinically the future of CRT most likely lies in developing effective programs that combine CRT and psychosocial and vocational rehabilitation. Although the outcome measures differ, comparison between the results of clinician-delivered programs [37] and computerised CRT programs suggest that the computerised programs are generally equally effective [48]. Computerised programs are more likely to be adopted in clinical practice, with clinician-delivered programs used primarily for research. CRT programs would need to be standardised with built in measures of efficacy, so that they easily set up in community mental health services, require minimal staff supervision, and demonstrate sufficient improvement to justify the ongoing commitment of resources. Future research in this area should continue to look at the optimal modality for CRT and the effects on particular domains of cognition as well as evaluating the impact on general functional outcome.

References

[1] V. A. Morgan, A. Waterreus, and A. Jablensky, "People living with psychotic illness 2010," Report on the Second Australian National Survey, Australian Government Department of Health and Ageing, Canberra, Australia, 2011.

[2] P. Jones, B. Rodgers, R. Murray, and M. Marmot, "Child developmental risk factors for adult schizophrenia in the British 1946 birth cohort," *The Lancet*, vol. 344, no. 8934, pp. 1398–1402, 1994.

[3] D. J. Done, T. J. Crow, E. C. Johnstone, and A. Sacker, "Childhood antecedents of schizophrenia and affective illness: social adjustment at ages 7 and 11," *British Medical Journal*, vol. 309, no. 6956, pp. 699–703, 1994.

[4] R. M. Murray, P. Sham, J. Van Os, J. Zanelli, M. Cannon, and C. McDonald, "A developmental model for similarities and dissimilarities between schizophrenia and bipolar disorder," *Schizophrenia Research*, vol. 71, no. 2-3, pp. 405–416, 2004.

[5] T. Toulopoulou, S. Quraishi, C. McDonald, and R. M. Murray, "The Maudsley Family study: premorbid and current general intellectual function levels in familial bipolar I disorder and schizophrenia," *Journal of Clinical and Experimental Neuropsychology*, vol. 28, no. 2, pp. 243–259, 2006.

[6] S. K. Hill, J. L. Reilly, M. S. H. Harris et al., "A comparison of neuropsychological dysfunction in first-episode psychosis patients with unipolar depression, bipolar disorder, and schizophrenia," *Schizophrenia Research*, vol. 113, no. 2-3, pp. 167–175, 2009.

[7] J. Zanelli, A. Reichenberg, K. Morgan et al., "Specific and generalized neuropsychological deficits: a comparison of patients with various first-episode psychosis presentations," *American Journal of Psychiatry*, vol. 167, no. 1, pp. 78–85, 2010.

[8] D. J. Martino, E. Marengo, A. Igoa et al., "Neurocognitive and symptomatic predictors of functional outcome in bipolar disorders: a prospective 1 year follow-up study," *Journal of Affective Disorders*, vol. 116, no. 1-2, pp. 37–42, 2009.

[9] M. Kukla, G. R. Bond, and H. Xie, "A prospective investigation of work and nonvocational outcomes in adults with severe mental illness," *Journal of Nervous and Mental Disease*, vol. 200, no. 3, pp. 214–222, 2012.

[10] M. F. Green, R. S. Kern, D. L. Braff, and J. Mintz, "Neurocognitive deficits and functional outcome in schizophrenia: are we measuring the "right stuff"?" *Schizophrenia Bulletin*, vol. 26, no. 1, pp. 119–136, 2000.

[11] R. S. E. Keefe, M. Poe, T. M. Walker, J. W. Kang, and P. D. Harvey, "The schizophrenia cognition rating scale: an interview-based assessment and its relationship to cognition, real-world functioning, and functional capacity," *American Journal of Psychiatry*, vol. 163, no. 3, pp. 426–432, 2006.

[12] B. Solé, C. M. Bonnin, C. Torrent et al., "Neurocognitive impairment and psychosocial functioning in bipolar II disorder," *Acta Psychiatrica Scandinavica*, vol. 125, no. 4, pp. 309–317, 2012.

[13] M. K. O'Connor, L. Mueller, A. van Ormer et al., "Cognitive impairment as barrier to engagement in vocational services

among veterans with severe mental illness," *Journal of Rehabilitation Research and Development*, vol. 48, no. 5, pp. 597–607, 2011.

[14] J. M. Gold, R. W. Goldberg, S. W. McNary, L. B. Dixon, and A. F. Lehman, "Cognitive correlates of job tenure among patients with severe mental illness," *American Journal of Psychiatry*, vol. 159, no. 8, pp. 1395–1402, 2002.

[15] C. Galletly, "Recent advances in treating cognitive impairment in schizophrenia," *Psychopharmacology*, vol. 202, no. 1–3, pp. 259–273, 2009.

[16] C. A. Galletly, C. R. Clark, A. C. McFarlane, and D. L. Weber, "The effect of clozapine on the speed and accuracy of information processing in schizophrenia," *Progress in Neuro-Psychopharmacology and Biological Psychiatry*, vol. 24, no. 8, pp. 1329–1338, 2000.

[17] A. Szöke, A. Trandafir, M.-E. Dupont, A. Méary, F. Schürhoff, and M. Leboyer, "Longitudinal studies of cognition in schizophrenia: meta-analysis," *British Journal of Psychiatry*, vol. 192, no. 4, pp. 248–257, 2008.

[18] J. De Leon and F. J. Diaz, "A meta-analysis of worldwide studies demonstrates an association between schizophrenia and tobacco smoking behaviors," *Schizophrenia Research*, vol. 76, no. 2-3, pp. 135–157, 2005.

[19] J. Cooper, S. G. Mancuso, R. Borland, T. Slade, C. Galletly, and D. Castle, "Tobacco smoking among people living with a psychotic illness: the second Australian survey of psychosis," *Australian and New Zealand Journal of Psychiatry*, vol. 46, no. 9, pp. 851–863, 2012.

[20] R. S. Barr, M. A. Culhane, L. E. Jubelt et al., "The effects of transdermal nicotine on cognition in nonsmokers with schizophrenia and nonpsychiatric controls," *Neuropsychopharmacology*, vol. 33, no. 3, pp. 480–490, 2008.

[21] K. E. Lewandowski, S. M. Eack, S. S. Hogarty, D. P. Greenwald, and M. S. Keshavan, "Is cognitive enhancement therapy equally effective for patients with schizophrenia and schizoaffective disorder?" *Schizophrenia Research*, vol. 125, no. 2-3, pp. 291–294, 2011.

[22] P. D. Harvey, A. P. Wingo, K. E. Burdick, and R. J. Baldessarini, "Cognition and disability in bipolar disorder: lessons from schizophrenia research," *Bipolar Disorders*, vol. 12, no. 4, pp. 364–375, 2010.

[23] T. Deckersbach, A. A. Nierenberg, R. Kessler et al., "Cognitive rehabilitation for bipolar disorder: an open trial for employed patients with residual depressive symptoms," *CNS Neuroscience and Therapeutics*, vol. 16, no. 5, pp. 298–307, 2010.

[24] R. H. B. Benedict, A. E. Harris, T. Markow, J. A. McCormick, K. H. Nuechterlein, and R. F. Asarnow, "Effects of attention training on information processing in schizophrenia," *Schizophrenia Bulletin*, vol. 20, no. 3, pp. 537–546, 1994.

[25] S. L. Rossell and A. S. David, "Improving performance on the WCST: variations on the original procedure. Wisconsin Card Sorting Test," *Schizophrenia Research*, vol. 28, no. 1, pp. 63–76, 1997.

[26] P. Stratta, F. Mancini, P. Mattei et al., "Remediation of Wisconsin Card Sorting Test performance in schizophrenia. A controlled study," *Psychopathology*, vol. 30, no. 2, pp. 59–66, 1997.

[27] K. E. Harvey, C. A. Galletly, C. Field, and M. Proeve, "The effects of verbalisation on cognitive performance in schizophrenia: a pilot study using tasks from the Delis Kaplan Executive Function System," *Neuropsychological Rehabilitation*, vol. 19, no. 5, pp. 733–741, 2009.

[28] M. Hermanutz and J. Gestrich, "Computer-assisted attention training in schizophrenics. A comparative study," *European Archives of Psychiatry and Clinical Neuroscience*, vol. 240, no. 4-5, pp. 282–287, 1991.

[29] A. Medalia, M. Aluma, W. Tryon, and A. E. Merriam, "Effectiveness of attention training in schizophrenia," *Schizophrenia Bulletin*, vol. 24, no. 1, pp. 147–152, 1998.

[30] C. D. Field, C. Galletly, D. Anderson, and P. Walker, "Computer-aided cognitive rehabilitation: possible application to the attentional deficit of schizophrenia, a report of negative results," *Perceptual and Motor Skills*, vol. 85, no. 3, pp. 995–1002, 1997.

[31] G. E. Hogarty, S. Flesher, R. Ulrich et al., "Cognitive enhancement therapy for schizophrenia: effects of a 2-year randomized trial on cognition and behavior," *Archives of General Psychiatry*, vol. 61, no. 9, pp. 866–876, 2004.

[32] S. R. McGurk and H. Y. Meltzer, "The role of cognition in vocational functioning in schizophrenia," *Schizophrenia Research*, vol. 45, no. 3, pp. 175–184, 2000.

[33] A. Genevsky, C. T. Garrett, P. P. Alexander, and S. Vinogradov, "Cognitive training in schizophrenia: a neuroscience-based approach," *Dialogues in Clinical Neuroscience*, vol. 12, no. 3, pp. 416–421, 2010.

[34] A. Royer, A. Grosselin, C. Bellot et al., "Is there any impact of cognitive remediation on an ecological test in schizophrenia?" *Cognitive Neuropsychiatry*, vol. 17, no. 1, pp. 19–35, 2012.

[35] P. D. Harvey and B. A. Cornblatt, "Pharmacological treatment of cognition in schizophrenia: an idea whose method has come," *American Journal of Psychiatry*, vol. 165, no. 2, pp. 163–165, 2008.

[36] K. H. Nuechterlein, M. F. Green, R. S. Kern et al., "The MATRICS consensus cognitive battery, part 1: test selection, reliability, and validity," *American Journal of Psychiatry*, vol. 165, no. 2, pp. 203–213, 2008.

[37] T. Wykes, C. Reeder, S. Landau et al., "Cognitive remediation therapy in schizophrenia: randomised controlled trial," *British Journal of Psychiatry*, vol. 190, pp. 421–427, 2007.

[38] T. Wykes, "Cognitive remediation therapy needs funding," *Nature*, vol. 468, no. 7321, pp. 165–166, 2010.

[39] T. Wykes, V. Huddy, C. Cellard, S. R. McGurk, and P. Czobor, "A meta-analysis of cognitive remediation for schizophrenia: methodology and effect sizes," *American Journal of Psychiatry*, vol. 168, no. 5, pp. 472–485, 2011.

[40] S. R. McGurk, E. W. Twamley, D. I. Sitzer, G. J. McHugo, and K. T. Mueser, "A meta-analysis of cognitive remediation in schizophrenia," *American Journal of Psychiatry*, vol. 164, no. 12, pp. 1791–1802, 2007.

[41] L. Lecardeur, E. Stip, M. Giguere, G. Blouin, J. P. Rodriguez, and M. Champagne-Lavau, "Effects of cognitive remediation therapies on psychotic symptoms and cognitive complaints in patients with schizophrenia and related disorders: a randomized study," *Schizophrenia Research*, vol. 111, no. 1–3, pp. 153–158, 2009.

[42] M. F. Green, B. Olivier, J. N. Crawley, D. L. Penn, and S. Silverstein, "Social cognition in schizophrenia: recommendations from the MATRICS New Approaches Conference," *Schizophrenia Bulletin*, vol. 31, no. 4, pp. 882–887, 2005.

[43] E. Bora, M. Yucel, and C. Pantelis, "Theory of mind impairment in schizophrenia: meta-analysis," *Schizophrenia Research*, vol. 109, no. 1–3, pp. 1–9, 2009.

[44] P. Stratta, M. Bustini, E. Daneluzzo, I. Riccardi, M. D'Arcangelo, and A. Rossi, "Deconstructing theory of mind in schizophrenia," *Psychiatry Research*, vol. 190, no. 1, pp. 32–36, 2011.

[45] J-P. Lindenmayer, S. R. McGurk, and A. Khan, "Improving social cognition in schizophrenia: a pilot intervention combining computerized social cognition training with cognitive remediation," *Schizophrenia Bulletin*. In press.

[46] W. Wölwer and N. Frommann, "Social-cognitive remediation in schizophrenia: generalization of effects of the training of affect recognition (TAR)," *Schizophrenia Bulletin*, vol. 37, supplement 2, pp. S63–S70, 2011.

[47] R. Penadés, R. Catalán, O. Puig et al., "Executive function needs to be targeted to improve social functioning with Cognitive Remediation Therapy (CRT) in schizophrenia," *Psychiatry Research*, vol. 177, no. 1-2, pp. 41–45, 2010.

[48] O. Grynszpan, S. Perbal, A. Pelissolo et al., "Efficacy and specificity of computer-assisted cognitive remediation in schizophrenia: a meta-analytical study," *Psychological Medicine*, vol. 41, no. 1, pp. 163–173, 2011.

[49] S. Moritz, F. Vitzthum, S. Randjbar, R. Veckenstedt, and T. S. Woodward, "Detecting and defusing cognitive traps: metacognitive intervention in schizophrenia," *Current Opinion in Psychiatry*, vol. 23, no. 6, pp. 561–569, 2010.

[50] T. S. Woodward, R. Mizrahi, M. Menon, and B. K. Christensen, "Correspondences between theory of mind, jumping to conclusions, neuropsychological measures and the symptoms of schizophrenia," *Psychiatry Research*, vol. 170, no. 2-3, pp. 119–123, 2009.

[51] R. Balzan, P. Delfabbro, C. Galletly, and T. Woodward, "Metacognitive training for patients with schizophrenia: preliminary evidence for a targeted single-module program," In Submission.

[52] R. Balzan, P. Delfabbro, C. Galletly, and T. Woodward, "Reasoning heuristics across the psychosis continuum: the contribution of hypersalient evidence-hypothesis matches," *Cognitive Neuropsychiatry*, vol. 17, no. 5, pp. 431–450, 2012.

Permissions

The contributors of this book come from diverse backgrounds, making this book a truly international effort. This book will bring forth new frontiers with its revolutionizing research information and detailed analysis of the nascent developments around the world.

We would like to thank all the contributing authors for lending their expertise to make the book truly unique. They have played a crucial role in the development of this book. Without their invaluable contributions this book wouldn't have been possible. They have made vital efforts to compile up to date information on the varied aspects of this subject to make this book a valuable addition to the collection of many professionals and students.

This book was conceptualized with the vision of imparting up-to-date information and advanced data in this field. To ensure the same, a matchless editorial board was set up. Every individual on the board went through rigorous rounds of assessment to prove their worth. After which they invested a large part of their time researching and compiling the most relevant data for our readers. Conferences and sessions were held from time to time between the editorial board and the contributing authors to present the data in the most comprehensible form. The editorial team has worked tirelessly to provide valuable and valid information to help people across the globe.

Every chapter published in this book has been scrutinized by our experts. Their significance has been extensively debated. The topics covered herein carry significant findings which will fuel the growth of the discipline. They may even be implemented as practical applications or may be referred to as a beginning point for another development. Chapters in this book were first published by Hindawi Publishing Corporation; hereby published with permission under the Creative Commons Attribution License or equivalent.

The editorial board has been involved in producing this book since its inception. They have spent rigorous hours researching and exploring the diverse topics which have resulted in the successful publishing of this book. They have passed on their knowledge of decades through this book. To expedite this challenging task, the publisher supported the team at every step. A small team of assistant editors was also appointed to further simplify the editing procedure and attain best results for the readers.

Our editorial team has been hand-picked from every corner of the world. Their multi-ethnicity adds dynamic inputs to the discussions which result in innovative outcomes. These outcomes are then further discussed with the researchers and contributors who give their valuable feedback and opinion regarding the same. The feedback is then collaborated with the researches and they are edited in a comprehensive manner to aid the understanding of the subject.

Apart from the editorial board, the designing team has also invested a significant amount of their time in understanding the subject and creating the most relevant covers. They scrutinized every image to scout for the most suitable representation of the subject and create an appropriate cover for the book.

The publishing team has been involved in this book since its early stages. They were actively engaged in every process, be it collecting the data, connecting with the contributors or procuring relevant information. The team has been an ardent support to the editorial, designing and production team. Their endless efforts to recruit the best for this project, has resulted in the accomplishment of this book. They are a veteran in the field of academics and their pool of knowledge is as vast as their experience in printing. Their expertise and guidance has proved useful at every step. Their uncompromising quality standards have made this book an exceptional effort. Their encouragement from time to time has been an inspiration for everyone.

The publisher and the editorial board hope that this book will prove to be a valuable piece of knowledge for researchers, students, practitioners and scholars across the globe.

List of Contributors

Fiona J. Clay, Swati Shourie and Emily Kerr
Injury Outcomes Research Unit, Monash Injury Research Institute, Monash University, Building 70, Level 1, Clayton Campus, Melbourne, VIC 3800, Australia

Priscilla Robinson
School of Public Health, Faculty of Health Sciences, La Trobe University, Bundoora, Melbourne, VIC 3086, Australia

Donna McKenzie
Institute for Safety Compensation and Recovery Research, Monash University, Melbourne, VIC 3004, Australia

Norma J. MacIntyre
School of Rehabilitation Science, McMaster University, IAHS 403, 1400 Main Street West, Hamilton, ON, Canada L8S 1C7

Chris P. Recknor and Julie C. Recknor
United Osteoporosis Centres, 2350 Limestone Parkway, N.E., Gainesville, GA 30501, USA

Neha Dewan
School of Rehabilitation Sciences, McMaster University 1400, Main Street West, Hamilton, ON, Canada

Kavitha Raja
JSS College of Physiotherapy, JSS Hospital Campus, Mysore, Karnataka 570004, India

Ganesh Balthillaya Miyaru
Department of Physiotherapy, Manipal College of Allied Health Sciences, Manipal University, Manipal, Karnataka 576104, India

Joy C. Mac Dermid
School of Rehabilitation Sciences, McMaster University 1400, Main Street West, Hamilton, ON, Canada
Hand and Upper Limb Centre, St. Joseph's Health Centre, London, ON, Canada

Lisa Farrell
Adjunct Clinical Faculty, Nova Southeastern University, 3200 South University Drive, Fort Lauderdale, FL 33328, USA
OrthoSport, Inc., 5200 South University Drive, Suite 105, Fort Lauderdale, FL 33328, USA

Rose Marie Rine
Specialty Therapy Source LLC, 12948 Palmetto Glade Drive, Jacksonville, FL 32246, USA

Bhasker Amatya
Department of Rehabilitation Medicine, Royal Melbourne Hospital, 34-54 Poplar Road, Parkville, Melbourne, Victoria 3052, Australia
Louisa Ng and Mary Galea
Department of Rehabilitation Medicine, Royal Melbourne Hospital, 34-54 Poplar Road, Parkville, Melbourne, Victoria 3052, Australia
Department of Medicine (Royal Melbourne Hospital), The University of Melbourne, Parkville, Victoria 3052, Australia

Fary Khan
Department of Rehabilitation Medicine, Royal Melbourne Hospital, 34-54 Poplar Road, Parkville, Melbourne, Victoria 3052, Australia
Department of Medicine (Royal Melbourne Hospital), The University of Melbourne, Parkville, Victoria 3052, Australia
School of Public Health and Preventive Medicine, Monash University, Clayton, Victoria 3800, Australia

Rachel L. Wright, Afia Masood, Elinor S. MacCormac and Alan M. Wing
School of Psychology, University of Birmingham, Edgbaston, Birmingham B15 2TT, UK

David Pratt
West Midlands Rehabilitation Centre, Birmingham Community Healthcare Trust, Birmingham B29 6HZ, UK

Catherine M. Sackley
School of Allied Health Professions, University of East Anglia, Norwich NR4 7TJ, UK

Valdeci Carlos Dionisio
Physical Therapy Course, Federal University of Uberlandia, Benjamin Constant Street No. 1286, 38400-678 Uberlandia, MG, Brazil

Bruna Maria Silva Azevedo and Daniela Abrahão Siqueira
Physical Therapy Course of the University Center of Triangulo, Nicomedes Alves dos Santos Avenue No. 4545, 38411-106 Uberlandia, MG, Brazil

Shirley S. M. Fong
Institute of Human Performance, The University of Hong Kong, Pokfulam, Hong Kong

X. Guo, Alice P. M. Cheung, Alex T. L. Jo, Gary K. W. Lui, Dennis K. C. Mo, Shamay S. M. Ng and William W. N. Tsang
Department of Rehabilitation Sciences, The Hong Kong Polytechnic University, Hung Hom, Hong Kong

Yvonne Tran
Rehabilitation Studies Unit, Sydney Medical School-Northern, The University of Sydney, P.O. Box 6, Ryde, Sydney, NSW 1680, Australia
Key University Centre for Health Technologies, University of Technology, Broadway, Sydney, NSW2007, Australia

Ashley Craig and Nirupama Wijesuriya
Rehabilitation Studies Unit, Sydney Medical School-Northern, The University of Sydney, P.O. Box 6, Ryde, Sydney, NSW 1680, Australia

Margaret K. Glenn
West Virginia University, P.O. Box 6122, 502 Allen Hall, Morgantown, WV 26506, USA

Duygu Cubukcu and Ferda Metinkisi
Department of Physical Medicine and Rehabilitation, Dr. Behcet Uz Children's Diseases Training and Research Hospital, Sezer Dogan Street No. 11, Konak, 35210 Izmir, Turkey

Unsal Yilmaz
Department of Pediatric Neurology, Dr. Behcet Uz Children's Diseases Training and Research Hospital, Sezer Dogan Street No. 11, Konak, 35210 Izmir, Turkey

Hakan Alkan
Department of Physical Medicine and Rehabilitation, Pamukkale University Faculty of Medicine, Kınıklı 20070, Denizli, Turkey

Muazzez Ozcan
Department of Otorhinolaryngology, Dr. Behcet Uz Children's Diseases Training and Research Hospital, Sezer Dogan Street No. 11, Konak, 35210 Izmir, Turkey

Vilai Kuptniratsaikul and Piyapat Dajpratham
Rehabilitation Medicine Department, Faculty of Medicine Siriraj Hospital, Mahidol University, 2 Prannok, Bangkok 10700, Thailand

Apichana Kovindha
Rehabilitation Medicine Department, Faculty of Medicine, Chiang Mai University, Chiang Mai 50200, Thailand

Krisna Piravej
Rehabilitation Medicine Department, Faculty of Medicine, Chulalongkorn University, Bangkok 10330, Thailand

Sandra H. Arnold and Thubi H. A. Kolobe
Department of Rehabilitation Sciences, College of Allied Health, University of Oklahoma Health Sciences Center, 1200 N Stonewall Avenue, P.O. Box 26901, Oklahoma City, OK 73126-0901, USA

David M. Thompson and Lindsay Boeckman
Department of Biostatistics and Epidemiology, University of Oklahoma Health Sciences Center, 801 N.E. 13th Street, P.O. Box 26901, Oklahoma City, OK 73126-0901, USA

Salene M. Wu
Group Health Research Institute, 1730 Minor Avenue, Seattle, WA 98101, USA

Dagmar Amtmann
Department of Rehabilitation Medicine, University of Washington, P.O. Box 354237, Seattle, WA 98195-4237, USA

Mitsuhiro Hayashibe, David Guiraud and Philippe Poignet
DEMAR Project, INRIA Sophia-Antipolis and LIRMM, CNRS, University of Montpellier, 34095 Montpellier, France

Elaine Duncan
Department of Psychology and Allied Health Sciences, Glasgow Caledonian University, Glasgow G4 0BA, UK

Yori Gidron
Faculty of Medicine & Pharmacy, Free University of Brussels (VUB), 1050 Brussels, Belgium

David Lavallee
School of Sport Stirling, University of Stirling, Stirling FK9 4LA, UK

Francesco Giallauria and Carlo Vigorito
Department of Translational Medical Sciences, Cardiac Rehabilitation Unit, University of Naples "Federico II," Via S. Pansini 5, 80131 Naples, Italy

Francesco Fattirolli
Department of Critical Care Medicine and Surgery, Cardiac Rehabilitation Unit, University of Florence and Azienda Ospedaliero-Universitaria Careggi, Via delle Oblate 4, 50141 Florence, Italy

Roberto Tramarin
Division of Cardiac Rehabilitation, Fondazione Europea di Ricerca Biomedica, Via Uboldo 56, 20063 Cernusco S/N, Italy

Marco Ambrosetti
Clinica "Le Terrazze," Via Foscolo 6/B, 21035 Cunardo, Italy

Raffaele Griffo
Cardiac Rehabilitation Unit, Department of Cardiology, La Colletta Hospital, Via del Giappone, 16011 Arenzano, Italy

Carmine Riccio
Azienda Ospedaliera S. Anna e S. Sebastiano di Caserta, Via Gennaro Tescione 1, 81100 Caserta, Italy

Halim Yilmaz, Gulten Erkin and Alparslan Ali İZKİ
The Department of Physical Medicine and Rehabilitation, Konya Education and Research Hospital, 42090 Konya, Turkey

Chidozie Emmanuel Mbada
Department of Medical Rehabilitation, College of Health Sciences, Obafemi Awolowo University, Ile-Ife, Nigeria

Olusola Ayanniyi
Department of Physiotherapy, College of Medicine, University of Ibadan, Ibadan, Nigeria

Samuel Olusegun Ogunlade
Department of Orthopaedic and Trauma, College of Medicine, University of Ibadan, Ibadan, Nigeria

Elkanah Ayodele Orimolade and Ajibola Babatunde Oladiran
Department of Orthopaedic Surgery and Traumatology, Obafemi Awolowo University Teaching Hospitals Complex, Ile-Ife, Nigeria

Abiola Oladele Ogundele
Department of Physiotherapy, Obafemi Awolowo University Teaching Hospitals Complex, Ile-Ife, Nigeria

Marie-Hélène Milot
Centre de Recherche sur le Vieillissement, Ecole de Readaptation, Faculte de Medecine et des Sciences de la Sante, Universite de Sherbrooke, 1036 Belvedere sud, Sherbrooke, QC, Canada
Institut de Readaptation Gingras-Lindsay-de-Montreal, Centre de Recherche Interdisciplinaire en Readaptation (CRIR), Universite de Montreal, C.P. 6128 Succ. Centre-Ville, Montreal, QC, Canada

Sylvie Nadeau, Denis Gravel and Daniel Bourbonnais
Institut de Readaptation Gingras-Lindsay-de-Montreal, Centre de Recherche Interdisciplinaire en Readaptation (CRIR), Universite de Montreal, C.P. 6128 Succ. Centre-Ville, Montreal, QC, Canada

Sacha Song
Schulich School of Medicine & Dentistry, University of Western Ontario, London, ON, Canada
University of Windsor, Medical Education Building Room 1100, 401 Sunset Avenue, Windsor, ON, Canada

Ruby Grewal
Division of Orthopedic Surgery, University of Western Ontario, Hand and Upper Limb Center, St. Joseph's Health Care, 268 Grosvenor Street, London, ON, Canada

Joy C. MacDermid
Division of Orthopedic Surgery, University of Western Ontario, Hand and Upper Limb Center, St. Joseph's Health Care, 268 Grosvenor Street, London, ON, Canada
School of Rehabilitation Sciences, McMaster University, 1400 Main Street West, Hamilton, ON, Canada

Cherrie Galletly
Adelaide Health Service, Northern Mental Health Directorate, Department of Health and Ageing, Adelaide, SA 5000, Australia
Mental Health Services (SA), Ramsay Health Care, The Adelaide Clinic, Adelaide, SA 5082, Australia
Discipline of Psychiatry, School of Medicine, The University of Adelaide, Adelaide, SA 5000, Australia

Ashlee Rigby
Mental Health Services (SA), Ramsay Health Care, The Adelaide Clinic, Adelaide, SA 5082, Australia
Discipline of Psychiatry, School of Medicine, The University of Adelaide, Adelaide, SA 5000, Australia